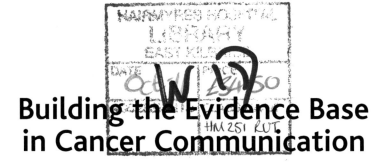

Building the Evidence Base
in Cancer Communication

HEALTH COMMUNICATION
Gary L. Kreps, Series Editor

Building the Evidence Base in Cancer Communication

edited by

Lila J. Finney Rutten
SAIC, Inc.,
National Cancer Institute

Bradford W. Hesse
National Institute of Health

Richard P. Moser
National Cancer Institute

Gary L. Kreps
George Mason University

HAMPTON PRESS, INC.
CRESSKILL, NEW JERSEY

Printed in the United States of America

Library of Congress Cataloging-in-Publication Data

Building the evidence base in cancer communication / edited by Lila J. Finney Rutten ... [et al.].
    p. ; cm. -- (Hampton Press communication series. Health communication)
    Includes bibliographical references and indexes.
    ISBN 978-1-57273-943-7 (hardbound) -- ISBN 978-1-57273-944-4 (paperbound)
    1. Communication in medicine. 2. Cancer--Information services. 3.
Cancer--Prevention. 4. Evidence-based medicine. I. Rutten, Lila J. Finney. II.
Series: Health communication (Cresskill, N.J.)
    [DNLM: 1. Neoplasms--prevention & control. 2. Communication. 3. Data
Collection. 4. Evidence-Based Medicine. 5. Health Care Surveys. QZ 200]
    RC262.B83 2010
    616.99'406--dc22
                                    2010036879

Hampton Press, Inc.
23 Broadway
Cresskill, NJ 07626

CONTENTS

II Extending Reach in Health Communication

III The Future of Health Communication and Informatics

Conclusion

1

HEALTH COMMUNICATION IN A WORLD GONE FLAT

Programmatic Overview of HINTS

Bradford W. Hesse
National Institutes of Health

> Give me 26 soldiers of lead and I shall conquer the world.
>
> —*Johannes Gutenberg*

There is little doubt that great (and small) revolutions in communication technology can be credited with bringing about momentous changes in the ways in which individuals work and live together. Introduction of movable type in 1493 set into motion a revolution in mass communication that has been credited with giving rise to massive reformations in religious and political governance, to scientific enlightenment, and to economic empowerment (Man, 2002). The telephone, once thought to be of little interest to anyone except factory workers, has altered the very fabric of social exchange by enabling conversations to occur in real time over great and small distances. Now it can be used to bring families together, to order goods and services, and to seek help in emergencies (Fischer, 1992). Wireless communications, such as radio and television, have created a global consciousness of images and norms that seemed to change the ways in which whole cultures evolved, leading social commentators such as Marshall McLuhan to proclaim that in the new world of mediated communication, the media had their own independent effect on living; that the "medium was the message" (McLuhan, 1967).

In his book *America Calling: A Social History of the Telephone to 1940*, Claude Fischer (Fischer, 1992) recounted a 1926 meeting of the Knights of Columbus Adult Education Committee focused on answering the question "Do modern inventions help or mar character and health?" (pp. 1-6). The answer, the group decided, was neither. Modern inventions allow people to do things (sometimes old things, sometimes new things) in new ways. It was up to each individual's character and creativity to decide how the new inventions could be used to improve—or detract from—the human condition. The Gutenberg revolution of the 16th century allowed for the dissemination of ideas and technical processes; but it was the creativity of William Shakespeare and the scientific prowess of Sir Isaac Newton that helped change the world. Technology was the accelerator, but it was the new ideas of visionary thinkers that created the future. This is where we are with health communication at the beginning of the 21st century.

THE COMMUNICATION REVOLUTION
AND POPULATION HEALTH

Arguably, population health is one of those areas that can be influenced— for better or worse—by twists and turns in the communication environment. Consider the state of the tobacco industry at the beginning of the 20th century. Tobacco as a cash crop had a budding, but very limited appeal to a small group of consumers in 1900. Confronted with a stagnant market, tobacco industry executives hired cutting-edge advertising firms to recreate the image associated with smoking using the innovations in communication technology becoming widespread at the time. The problem with the public's perception of tobacco use, the advertising executives clandestinely acknowledged, was that it was considered by many people to be a dirty, bothersome habit that seemed to lead to occasional health problems such as coughing and wheezing. To overturn that image, the tobacco-paid ad executives seized on images that were pervasive within the nascent movie industry to recreate the image of smoking as a masculine indulgence; something that "real men" did to show they were tough, and not bothered by petulant social norms. Images of cowboys and soldiers with cigarettes in their mouths helped reinforce a sense of rugged individualism. Tobacco consumption skyrocketed. So, too, did rates of lung and bronchus cancer, chronic obstructive pulmonary disease, emphysema, and stroke (Davis, Gilpin, Loken, Viswanath, & Wakefield, 2008).

By the early 1960s health scientists had accumulated enough evidence to know that a devastatingly strong causal link existed between cigarette smoking and lung disease. The surgeon general's report of 1964 warned the nation that cigarette smoking was harmful to the public's health (U.S. Department of Health, 1964), and kicked off a decade-long series of countermeasures to curtail the influence of the tobacco industry's propaganda. Regulations were placed on advertising, warning labels were placed on products, and over time restrictions were put in place to limit exposure to second-hand smoke. Public health professionals used the same media that spawned a national addiction to acquaint the American public with the facts: "Smoking kills" and with help anyone can quit smoking and begin pursuing a longer, healthier life.

Figure 1.1 illustrates what the battleground for public health concerning lung cancer looked like during much of the 20th century. The effects of mass marketing, powered by innovations from the industrial revolution (broad-circulation magazines, radio, and television), can be seen with a steady increase in per-capita consumption of cigarettes up until the time that the surgeon general's report was released. Following the increase in cigarette purchasing was the inevitable, delayed affect of an increase in per capita

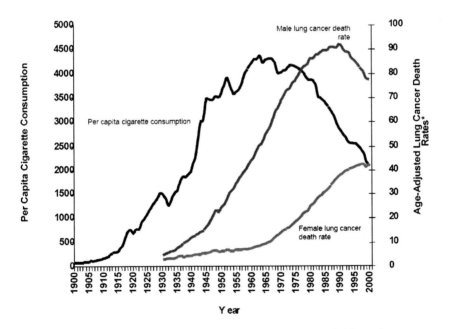

FIGURE 1.1. Per-capita cigarette consumption overlaid against age-adjusted lung cancer death rates for males and females.

(*Age-adjusted to 2000 U.S. standard population. Source: Death rates: US Mortality Public Use Tapes, 1960-2000. US Mortality Volumes, 1930-1959, National Center for health Statistics, Centers for Disease Control and Prevention, 2002. Cigarette consumption: US Department of Agriculture, 1900-2000.)

mortality due to lung and bronchus cancer. Figure 1.1 also illustrates how the public health impact of tobacco smoking mirrored the advertising strategy of the tobacco industry to specific demographics. Initially, advertising was aimed at men, with the greatest pick-up in smoking and later death from lung cancer showing up primarily among men. In the 1960s, confronted with decreasing markets caused by public health pressures, the cigarette advertising companies began exploiting a wave of feminism to market cigarette smoking to women. From Fig. 1.1 it can be seen that increases in smoking and subsequent mortality in women follow a similar, albeit delayed, pattern to that of men.

Something else Fig. 1.1 portrays is the cumulative effect of exposure to communication messages over time. Generally, the immediate effect in the population from exposure to messages in the media through communication campaigns is relatively small (Hornik, 2002). Industry wins at the advertising game by committing a steady flow of dollars to maintain exposure—total advertising for the tobacco industry in 2003 alone amounted to $15 billion (Federal Trade Commission, 2005). Needless to say, resources in public health are often much more limited than the generous advertising budgets of multinational companies. Nevertheless, public health planners can have access to other resources not afforded to commercial entities. Community activism, legislative regulation, support from the medical community, journalistic coverage, and access to scientifically based data and information can all serve as tools in the public health armamentarium. Over time, these combined approaches can exert their own positive influence on population health, as seen by the decrease in cancer mortality rates during the last two decades of the century in Fig. 1.1, one of the most pronounced public health victories of the latter part of the 20th century.

The U.S. National Institutes of Health (NIH) and the Centers for Disease Control and Prevention (CDC) have recognized that by using the tools of the communications revolution, public health planners can put into place evidence-based programs to counter the effects of unhealthy lifestyles and to warn the public in cases of emergency or acute need. Public service announcements, coordinated through radio, television, newspapers, and magazines, can increase exposure to positive health messages, exerting a slow but steady influence on population attitudes and awareness. Brochures and other types of "small media" can counter negative advertising through strategic placements in community centers, retail facilities, and physicians' offices. All of these strategies comprise a type of coordinated "push" of information into public consciousness. Telephone hotlines, smoking cessation "quitlines," clinics, government service offices, and a well-prepared cadre of advice nurses, social workers, and office staff can also be readied to deal with the "pull" of a public ready to seek information for healthier living. The U.S. National Cancer Institute's (NCI) Cancer Information Service, mandated by the National Cancer Act of 1971 to communicate accurate information about the disease directly to the public, stands as an exemplary resource of credible, evidence-based health communication for patients and their loved ones (Morra et al., 1993).

The accomplishments of active public health campaigns have contributed substantively to the nation's goals in creating a country of healthier and safer people. Nevertheless, the wheels of the communication revolution—now moving faster than ever before—have continued to roll on. As presaged by industry experts on the PBS *Lehrer News Hour* on October 19, 2006: "The pace of change [in communication options] over the next 5 years will dwarf the pace of change for the last 50 years." The change has been precipitated by a convergence of innovations in the area of digital technology that will alter the playing field for health communication.

THE INFORMATION REVOLUTION AND POPULATION HEALTH

"While we were sleeping," quipped author Thomas Friedman (2007), "we entered a new era of globalization . . . and it is flattening the global economic playing field in ways that we have never seen before." Unlike periods of globalization in previous centuries when countries colonized and companies internationalized, Friedman explained, the new globalization will be open to all individuals of every stripe and color as they learn to "plug and play" in a global communication network. What is this revolution Friedman is speaking about, and how is it changing the world we live in? Friedman talks about several "flattening forces" in his book including the fall of the Berlin Wall in 1989, but what really took center stage was another evolution of communication technology: the rise of the Internet.

The origins of the Internet can be traced back to the launch of Sputnik in 1957, which catalyzed a flurry of cold war funding activities in the United States designed to keep the country competitive in science and engineering. One of the most prescient thought pieces of the time was a white paper commissioned by the Advanced Research Projects Agency (ARPA) titled "Augmenting Human Intellect: A Conceptual Framework" (Engelbart, 1962). The paper borrowed heavily from the writings of Benjamin Lee Whorf, a communication scientist/linguist who theorized that the sophistication of language influences the sophistication of thought for those who understand and speak that language. Engineered correctly, the group reasoned, an information technology environment could serve in a capacity analogous to language; that is, it could serve as a vehicle for augmenting human thought by supporting highly sophisticated ways of communicating and thinking. The conceptual framework called for developing the technologies that would link people, data, and resources together in an electronic network of interconnected and distributed resources. Serving as the catalyst for four decades of technology development, the paper essentially functioned as the blueprint for development of windowed computer systems; the computer mouse and other digital pointing systems; the ARPAnet, predecessor to the Internet; the concept and technical application of hypertext; and eventually the World Wide Web (WWW) as we know it today (Bardini & Friedwald, 2002; Hesse, 2008).

The progression of technology advancement to the ubiquitous change in communication environment that surrounds health information seekers today proceeded in fits and starts. Several engineering powerhouses joined in making the enabling technology to support the vision of an augmentative, distributed computing system, but the revolutionary spirit of personal access to online information as a form of individual empowerment remained rooted in the counter-culture atmosphere of Silicon Valley in the 1960s and the 1970s (Markoff, 2005). This was quite literally the birthplace of the personal computer, and it would be the rallying point for such paradigm-shifting Internet giants as Yahoo!™ and Google™. It was the nexus for some of the first online social communities, such as the WELL (Rheingold, 2000), and the intellectual birthplace of "user-friendly" computing as embodied by the spirit and mission of Apple Computer (Hertzfeld & Capps, 2005). In many respects, it was this spirit of enabling individual, personal access to the world's connected information resources that gave form to the vision of a world "gone flat" as articulated decades later by Friedman. The vision boldly articulated by a pioneering set of engineers at the cusp of the cold war in 1961 had finally begun to materialize.

In the mid-1990s, the U.S. Congress voted to open up the benefits of the Internet and the WWW to the general public. Up to that point, these national information resources had been the exclusive domain of researchers, academics, and defense contractors. The rationale for opening this resource was to create an information infrastructure, or "information superhighway" as it was called at the time, that would change the ways in which individuals worked and thrived in a world of freely accessible information. If the adage is true that "information is power," Congress was electing to share that power with the masses in a collective experiment of electronic democratization. The stage was set to hand the reigns of personal health empowerment over to individual students, teachers, professionals, and nonprofessionals who would learn how to marshal the power of the new environment for critical life challenges (Gore, 1991).

One of the first indications that the revolutionary spirit of the Internet had begun influencing the ways in which people made decisions about their health came from the observation that members of the general public who had gone online were not shy in searching online for health information. In an early Harris Poll, survey administrators reported that nearly 70% of online users reported having looked online for information about a disease or health condition. Of the conditions searched, the top three included depression (19%), allergies (15%), and cancer (15%) (Rice, 2001). A study of WWW traffic at the CDC in 2000–2001 revealed that, contrary to expectations, the majority (66%) of unique visitors to the CDC Web site was not made up of public health professionals but of one-time, public visitors looking for health information (Hesse, Shaikh, Toward, & Edgar, 2002; Robinson, Hesse, Shaikh, Coss, & Crawford, 2003). The NCI, the Bureau of Labor Statistics, the Department of Education, the Internal Revenue Service, and other agencies reported similar phenomena: Individuals were bypassing traditional intermediaries to come straight to the source for credible information (Marchionini, Hert, Liddy, & Schneiderman, 2000).

A cautionary study conducted by researchers at RAND suggested that health scientists and government administrators were not necessarily ready for the influx of public health information seekers to their sites (Berland et al., 2001). Much of the accurate health content found on academic and government Web sites was written for a technical, professional audience and was not easily accessible to lay readers. In contrast, the content on nongovernment, nonacademic sites varied more dramatically in terms of accuracy and quality with ulterior profit motives coloring the presentation of facts and figures. In a twist on a Hollywood-inspired adage, when it came to health information on the Internet: we built it, they came, but we were not ready.

AN EXTRAORDINARY OPPORTUNITY

If advances in communication technology can influence personal and public health, then the era marked by the passing of the millennium in 1999–2000 heralded a period of extraordinary opportunity for research on the use of communication technology to improve population health. During that period of time, discussions of the latest "dot com" business venture dominated space on financial pages in newspapers and magazines; speculations abounded over how the Internet was going to change the world, with new terms from the digital age such as e-commerce, e-government, and e-health joining the national lexicon. Physicians found themselves going over printouts from the WWW as patients took advantage of time between appointments to research alternatives for treatment, a phenomenon that would lead the American Medical Association to issue a press release encouraging the American public to set a New Year's resolution not to bother going online to look for health information. The dawning of the 21st century was a time when policymakers found themselves entertaining speculations of both hope and doubt, of optimism and cynicism, in understanding the role that new information technologies would play in promulgating an era of improved public health.

In the area of disease control, especially cancer control, the implications of how the new assets of the information revolution could be marshaled for population health were tremendous. For the first time in the 20th century the public was exhibiting a generational shift in its attitudes toward health and health care. People were going online, actively looking for credible medical information to guide their decision making both before and after their visits to their doctors (Hesse et al., 2005). This level of patient activation has been considered vital by experts in health care redesign (Institute of Medicine, 2001; Wagner, 2004). Personal interest and motivation is a first, and vitally necessary, step toward making more efficient and proactive use of an economically distraught health care system (Cayton, 2006), and it is a crucial public health step in giving people the tools they need to live longer, more productive lives (President's Cancer Panel, 2007). The question facing policymakers, health-system engineers, physicians, and public health scientists is how to engineer the information environment so that it is patient-centric and supportive of positive life goals (Gustafson, Brennan, & Hawkins, 2007; Hesse, 2005; Kemper & Mettler, 2002; McLuhan, 1967; U.S. Department of Health and Human Services, 2008; Wagner, 2004).

The communication and information revolutions have particular relevance in the case of cancer (Viswanath, 2005). In the 1990s, hospital registry data tracked by the NCI and the CDC showed a decrease for the first time in a century in age-adjusted deaths from cancer (Hiatt & Rimer, 1999). Marked victories in the decades-old war were being won in the areas of lung and bronchus cancer, colorectal cancer, cervical cancer, breast cancer, stomach cancer, and prostate cancer. Each of these particular cancers can be influenced by behavioral factors (smoking cessation, diet, exercise, and early detection) despite the role of genetic predisposition. It was becoming obvious that after a long and arduous battle there were some things that the public could do now to reduce their cancer risks. Estimates are that behavioral changes alone would reduce more than 50% of cancer mortalities (Hiatt & Rimer, 1999; President's Cancer Panel, 2007; Viswanath, 2005).

It was questionable, however, whether the prevention messages were getting through to the public (The Royal Institution of Great Britain, 2001). Journalistic exposure was still focused on sensationalistic stories rather than on the activities people could engage in now to improve their health. In fact, there has been some indication, through content analysis, that an inverse correlation exists between the prevalence of a disease and its coverage in the press: Quite simply, rare diseases and deaths get all the press, whereas the steadfast threats are ignored (Frost, Frank, & Maibach, 1997). There was also concern that the people who needed health communication messages the most—those with low socioeconomic status, minorities, or the underserved—were precisely the ones being left out of the digital revolution (Kreps et al., 2007; Viswanath et al., 2006; Viswanath & Kreuter, 2007). Although death rates from cancer were dropping, these benefits have not been distributed equally across all segments of the population (Edwards et al., 2005). Knowledge gaps have been emerging between groups that are preventing them from participating actively in their own care or in the care of their families (Donohue, Tichenor, & Olien, 1975; Freimuth, 1993; Viswanath & Kreuter, 2007).

Confronted with this extraordinary situation at the national science level (Kreps & Viswanath, 2001), program directors at the U.S.-based NCI (one of the NIH) convened a working meeting of experts in the areas of risk communication and behavior to determine areas for focused research in the decades ahead (NCI, 1999). As the group contemplated the profound impact that a change in the cancer communication environment might have on public behavior, the experts advocated for a nationally representative survey to help researchers and policymakers monitor the changes that would surely be occurring in the health information environment. The survey, they reasoned, could be used to monitor the public's use of new communication technologies while investigating relationships between the health information environment and its subsequent influence on the public's knowledge, attitudes, and behaviors related to cancer control.

Following the experts' recommendations, the NCI launched the Health Information National Trends Survey (HINTS) in Spring 2001. The HINTS program was funded explicitly to serve as a unique source of data relating theoretical constructs in behavior change to the public's use of a changing communication environment over time. It was designed with the rigor of a scientifically sound surveillance sample, using carefully considered sampling techniques and meticulously derived weighting strategies, to produce national estimates on self-reported health behaviors. It was scoped as a biennial survey—not to be nimble in picking up transient fluctuations in the communication environment (something that a marketing-type survey can accomplish more effectively), but to provide a more carefully derived national anchor for unfolding structural changes within the health information environment (Nelson et al., 2004).

BUILDING THE EVIDENCE BASE: HINTS 2003 AND 2005

As program designers considered a sense of place for the newly minted survey, they drew on the recognition that cancer—like many of the most challenging health problems in the 21st century—must be solved with a transdisciplinary, team science approach (Abrams, 2006; Nass, Stillman, National Cancer Policy Board [U.S.]. Committee on Large-scale Science and Cancer Research, & National Research Council [U.S.]. Division on Earth and Life Studies, 2003). Thus, program designers argued that the HINTS program should be built on values of "data sharing" and "collective intelligence," hallmarks of the type of collaborative science that will be needed to solve some of the more perplexing and complicated problems emerging in the new century (Nass, Stillman, National Cancer Policy Board [U.S.]. Committee on Large-scale Science and Cancer Research, & National Research Council [U.S.]. Division on Earth and Life Studies, 2003). The survey's methodology itself, which inherently depends on assumptions about communication channels, should be open to change as the communication environment shifts and morphs in response to societal trends. The items within the survey should be linked to other national surveillance efforts, such as the CDC's Behavioral Risk Factor Surveillance System (BRFSS) and National Health Interview Survey (NHIS), in order to enable data linkages. It should also serve as a complement to efforts outside of the government, such as those by the Pew Foundation's Internet and American Life series, aimed at understanding some of the same changes in American life affected by changes in communications technology. Finally, the survey should work hand-in-glove with the efforts of individual researchers looking to tie their findings across levels of analysis (Smith & Suls, 2004) to expand generalizability and enhance translation of evidence-based practices into real-world settings (Kerner et al., 2005).

The inaugural administration of the HINTS data-collection effort was implemented as a random-digit dial (RDD) telephone survey in Fall 2002 and ended in Spring 2003. Data were collected from 6,369 Americans age 18 years and older throughout the general, noninstitutionalized population. The data were cleaned, appropriately weighted, and delivered to the NCI later in 2003, and then mounted for public use on the NCI Web site in February 2004. To encourage community participation, the NCI hosted a community symposium on HINTS findings in January 2005. Health communication scientists from around the country participated in the 2-day symposium, sharing the results of analyses conducted on the baseline data and offering their own suggestions for how these types of data could be used to improve the science and practice of health communication. A "call for papers" was issued after the conference to provide participants with an opportunity to publish their work in a specially positioned supplement to the *Journal of Health Communication*. The supplement, oriented around the theme of conducting research at the baseline, was released in Spring 2006.

A set of embedded experiments was also included in the administration of the 2003 HINTS, both to serve as a mechanism for investigating hypothesized relationships among subpopulations and to evaluate the comparative effectiveness of different administration techniques. The inclusion of these embedded experiments distinguished HINTS from many other federally funded or privately funded communication surveys. They allowed the research community to evaluate hypothesized relationships between variables within and among different subpopulations. It also allowed the

HINTS community to explore differences in various methodological techniques designed to improve total survey quality by reducing sampling error, exploring issues or coverage, bolstering (ever diminishing) response rates, and reduce measurement error (Dillman, 2007).

The second administration of the HINTS data collection effort was funded in Fall 2003, with data collection completed in calendar year 2005. Program directors preserved common items for purposes of exploring trends between the 2 years of the survey. Approximately 50% of the items in the survey remained constant. The remaining portion of the instrument was populated with new items to learn more about respondents' mental conceptualizations of cancer as a disease (or, more accurately, a series of diseases), to explore the nuances of patient–provider communication, to observe the proliferation of new tobacco-related products, and to document the diffusion of new cancer control prevention therapies, such as human papillomavirus immunization. Also, as with HINTS 2003, a methodological study was included; this one to investigate the contributions of a Web-based survey as a complement to the diminishing telephone-only audience of a RDD technique.

The HINTS 2005 data were released to the public in March 2006. Release of the new data gave researchers an opportunity to begin working with some of the same variables at two points in time and to begin experimenting with the statistical techniques needed to evaluate trends across the cross-sectional surveys. Several new studies were published on the new data release, both to begin reporting on what appeared to be the initial stages of usage trends and to provide population estimates on the new variables under investigation from the later survey. In 2007, the NCI published a compilation of frequencies in book form, juxtaposing data from the 2 years of the program and separating the data by key demographic characteristics for support in strategic communication planning (Rutten, Moser, Beckjord, Hesse, & Croyle, 2007). The program also updated its online Web site to portray sample and population estimates as separate tabs within the site's dynamically generated user interface.

On the methodological side, survey response rates were lower in 2005 than in 2003, reflecting a general decrease in RDD telephone response rates throughout the nation. Overall, screening rates dipped down to 34% of all those contacted (calculated according to criteria from the American Association for Public Opinion Research [AAPOR]) while extended interview completion rates fell down to 61%. The Web-based arm of the data collection, although explored as a hope for improving response rates in an era of "do not call lists" and caller ID, did not appear to improve response rates for the general population survey. To the contrary, there was some evidence to suggest that the methodology for completing the Web-based survey may have reduced likelihood that a sampled person would move from the screening/identification phase to completion of an extended interview.

In May 2007, the NCI hosted the second of its biennial meetings designed to bring together the HINTS research community to discuss results, issues, and future directions. The timing was propitious in that it allowed methodological experts to discuss proposed remedies for addressing issues of declining response rates (a problem compounded by changes in the information environment) at the same time that content experts were working to evaluate the stability of trends hinted at in the first two administrations of the survey. The meeting occurred at a time when the NCI had begun experimenting with methods for catalyzing change in the cancer research and practice communities. The NCI's own Division of Cancer Control and Population Sciences, soon to reach its 10-year anniversary, stood as a sentinel for a new type of health science research: one based on assumptions for data sharing, commonality of purpose, transdisciplinarity, and translational effectiveness.

To understand what it means to collect an evidence base in health communication at a time of extraordinary change, the NCI invited experts from multiple disciplines to discuss their insights across a number of different content areas. Experts in survey methodology were invited to discuss the implications of how a changing communication environment might influence the routine collection of data from the public in areas related to health behavior, attitudes, knowledge, and communication. Theoreticians were invited to discuss the advantages and limitations associated with the goal of connecting these dots across levels of analysis, with the scientific community looking to complete the bridge between basic and applied science in the area of health information delivery. Health disparity experts were brought in to discuss the role of communication, information systems, and education in helping to create equity in the delivery of health related knowledge and services among subpopulations within the United States. That group was especially mindful of the assertion, voiced by Friedman, that in a "world gone flat" it should be possible to create a "level playing field" for public consumers of health information and personal health decision making. Finally, program organizers invited visionary leaders in the areas of health care redesign, public health service delivery, and health information technology to help attendees gain a better understanding of where future changes in communications technology might be taking the field.

THE PURPOSE OF THIS BOOK

The purpose of this book is to bring together the insights of the May 2007 HINTS meeting into a format that is useful for the health communication community at large. Accordingly, each author begins with a tie-in to the NCI's HINTS program as a provocative starting point for their discussions on why and how to collect an evidence base to inform the science and practice of health communication at a time of unprecedented change. The authors were encouraged to go beyond the HINTS program to think more broadly about the role of data as a translational tool for monitoring and understanding the rapidly changing currents of a communication revolution that will most assuredly have a paradigm shifting impact on population health nationally and globally.

The book is divided into three major sections, each with its own assigned editor and content leader. The first section, led by Gordon Willis, tackles the methodological issues that are confronting administrators of scientific surveys during a time in which the communication technologies upon which these surveys depend are rapidly changing. Ironically, the standard RDD survey was introduced in the 1960s as a way of reaching more Americans, more efficiently, than door-to-door interviews or mail-based surveys. Telephones had reached a high point of penetration and the computer technology existed to create randomized lists of telephone numbers, so the next logical extension of the technology was to use telephony as a solution to the problem of studying the knowledge, attitudes, and behaviors of populations. Today, with so much change occurring in the telecommunications industry, the standard telephone survey has come under pressure to change. A profusion of telemarketers into the telephone call space has made it difficult to reach families, leading to the introduction of caller ID as a way of filtering out unknown callers. For many, the option of maintaining a mobile telephone number while foregoing a traditional landline number has become an attractive alternative. The first section tackles these problems head-on, leading the reader through some of the most critical thinking in the area from leaders in the field.

The second section deals with a moral imperative in health communication research, that of working together to solve issues of health disparities. Much has been written about the devastating impact that lack of knowledge can have on the ability of individuals to solve everyday problems, including problems related to health. As information technology moves knowledge into an electronic sphere, what will that do to the promise of equitable access to health information for all members of society? Are there solutions beyond the "digital divide": ways of extending the benefits of evidence-based health information well beyond the point at which the technology ends? The second section of the book, led by Erik Augustson, takes on the problem of information reach. This section illustrates how mining an evidence base of rigorously collected, scientifically sound data, can provide tools for addressing that part of the health disparities puzzle attributable to gaps in knowledge.

The third section, led by Lila Rutten, sets the stage for future considerations in health communication and informatics research. In his book *Get There Early*, futurist Bob Johansen (Johansen, 2007) makes a case for sensing the future to compete in the present. All businesses, he explained, must look beyond the immediate horizon to sense a path forward into new markets and new directions. The ones that do this thrive in a world of changing options and new technologies; the ones that do not whither and fail. The same can be applied to all areas of public endeavor. The best science is one that seizes the opportunities afforded by a rapidly changing knowledge base, and then focuses its resources on answering questions that were not even imagined in previous generations. Consider the impact that completion of the Human Genome project is having on the ways in which biomedical scientists explore solutions to cancer, neurological disease, birth defects, diabetes, and addiction. The third section of the book takes the reader ahead of the current state of evidence, to look at where new opportunities for investigation may be arising. In this final section, some of the best thinkers in health communication research offer their insights into what a future world could look like if built on a solid evidence base of empirical data.

Finally, Gary Kreps and Lila Finney Rutten offer their reflections on the lessons from three administrations of the HINTS program as a concluding chapter to the book. Dr. Kreps shares a special affinity to the HINTS program, as it was his branch at the NCI that commissioned work on the survey at the beginning of the decade. He remains a steadfast stakeholder in the outcomes of the program, and offers his thoughts as to how the HINTS experience in particular, and evidence collection in general, can be expanded to take full advantage of the extraordinary opportunity afforded to communication science at the turn of the millennium. Together, all of these chapters should provide grist for the mill to the earnest health communication scientist looking to assess the behavioral and social processes unfolding during the latest, and in some ways most pervasive, communication revolution.

CONCLUDING THOUGHTS: HEALTH RESEARCH 2.0

The revolutionary path from movable type to social reform may have seemed straightforward and seamless when considered in historical retrospect, but it was a path that took many twists and turns. It was a path in which individuals embraced the iconoclastic thinking of new philosophies and new science, and by so doing shattered the prevailing expectations of the time. It was a path marked by the belief that information and knowledge were power and that by sharing information the human condition would somehow improve; and such a path is commonly threatening to those in power, thus it was road marked with book burnings and censorship as well as free speech and ascendant thought.

So, too, the newest revolution in communications technology is leading its own tortuous path through misspent expectations and the gravity of the countervailing status quo. One need only think of the dot com implosion of 2001 to recall what the pundits were saying about the futility of business conducted on the Web, and then contrast that with the economic success of Google, Microsoft, Apple, and the others who persisted and succeeded along the way. Even these companies experienced failures, when the market was not quite ready for a new technology, or when the technologists failed to use the power of the new media to solve the right business problems (Hesse & Shneiderman, 2007; Shneiderman, 2002). For every step forward in health information technology, it seems, is another step backwards or to the side. Such is the legacy of conducting research in the quickly sifting sands of the health communication environment at the turn of the millennium.

A consoling thought is that as the information environment changes, as a new more sophisticated framework for "augmented intellect" (Engelbart, 1962) comes online, the practice and conduct of normal science should naturally change and evolve (Kuhn, 1996). Intuitively, the HINTS program reflects some of the evolutionary values to emerge from the paradigm-shifting capacities of the new infrastructure.

First, the HINTS program places a premium on community participation. Cancer is simply too big a problem for any one laboratory to solve alone. With the successful mapping of the more than 3 billion base pairs in the human genome, and with the successful archiving of terabytes of data from population-based surveys and disease registries, scientific discovery cannot proceed as usual. Efforts must be made to accelerate discovery by "crowd sourcing" the problem, by turning the data and the problems over to a larger community of dedicated scientists who can work together to solve the multifaceted issues of cancer and cancer communication (Surowiecki, 2004). The NCI is grateful to the scores of scientists who have already downloaded the HINTS data, and who are working tirelessly to contribute new knowledge to the community in the form of papers, posters, and talks. Without the combined effort of an incomparable community of health scientists, the program would not make progress.

The second value is to rely on the collective intelligence of the scientists and practitioners who contribute to the HINTS dialogue. Science has always been an accretive enterprise, with distant colleagues working in tandem to contribute knowledge within the "invisible college" of topic-oriented research (Crane, 1969). Collective intelligence in science emerges through contributions to the literature base and in the back-and-forth conversations occurring within working groups and conferences. That is one of the reasons why the HINTS Web site encourages users of the data to submit their publications for listing within the community. It is also the reason why conferences, and intellectual contributions to edited volumes such as this one, are so important to the program.

The third value is an unequivocal reliance on data. Certainly, most scientists are accustomed to statistical thinking (measures of central tendency, probabilities) in the ways in which they solve problems. Lay audiences and policy makers often are not, relying instead on stereotypes or emotionally appealing anecdotes. For this reason, the HINTS Web site was built to offer all visitors—public and professional—direct access to HINTS data with weighted population estimates generated dynamically for every question in the survey. The program is also considering ways of linking its data to the weighted estimates generated by other scientific surveys, a value on data sharing. A promising architecture for this type of data sharing is the NCI's own cancer Biomedical Informatics Grid (Buetow, 2005). Grid architectures represent a type of shared "cyberinfrastructure" allowing scientists to combine semantically equivalent, or interoperable, data sets in statistically integrative ways (Abbas, 2004). Weather maps represent a type of grid-enabled output as data from thousands of remote sensors are combined (often in real time) into very informative and predictive representations of underlying meteorological processes. The promise of grid-enabled population data, as illustrated in Fig. 1.2, is that complementary data can be combined to accelerate discovery. As datasets are combined through cyberinfrastructure, the result will be an new era of computational thinking that promises to alter the ways in which science and public discourse occur in ways yet unimagined (Atkins et al., 2003; Shneiderman, 2008).

Not coincidentally, the three core values of the HINTS program (architectures for participation, collective intelligence, and data as the new "Intel inside") are characteristic of a new generation of Web applications termed collectively Web 2.0. The facets are omnipresent in some of the most successful Web enterprises present today, from the "user data" presented to users selecting downloadable songs and videos from ITunes®, to the online social networks of FaceBook®, to the collective intelligence and knowledge management of Wikipedia®. Some economists have argued that these new facets represent a dramatically new way of thinking about intellectual property and business models (Tapscott & Williams, 2006). Whether that is true or not, they do appear to be part and parcel of a new augmentative intellectual environment for health science: a type of Health Science 2.0. Hopefully, HINTS and other efforts to build the evidence base in health communication will continue to take advantage of the best aspects of the new science to achieve true population impact.

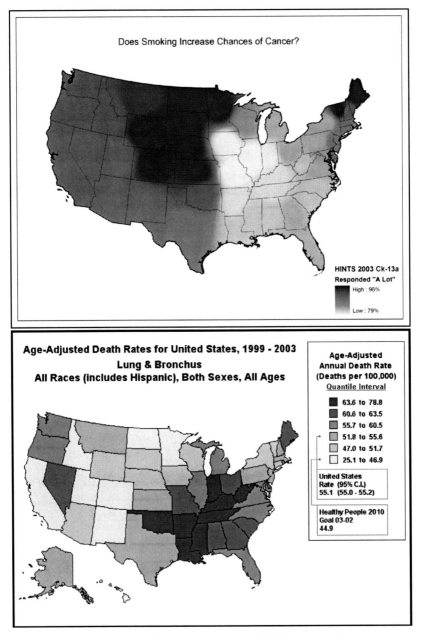

FIGURE 1.2. Juxtaposed data maps from HINTS 2003 (Does smoking increase chances of cancer?) and the SEER Cancer Mortality Registry (Age-Adjusted Death Rates). Notice the overlap between believe (deniers of cancer causation in HINTS) and cancer mortality along the Appalachian ridge.

REFERENCES

Abbas, A. (2004). *Grid computing: A practical guide to technology and applications.* Hingham, MA: Charles River Media.

Abrams, D. B. (2006). Applying transdisciplinary research strategies to understanding and eliminating health disparities. *Health Education Behavior, 33*(4), 515-531.

Atkins, D. E., Droegemeier, K. K., Feldman, S. I., Molina, H. G., Klein, M. L., Messerschmitt, D. G. et al. (2003). *Revolutionizing science and engineering through cyberinfrastructure: Report of the National Science Foundation Blue-Ribbon Advisory Panel on Cyberinfrastructure.* Ballston, VA: National Science Foundation.

Bardini, T., & Friedwald, M. (2002). Chronicle of the death of a laboratory: Douglas Engelbart and the failure of the knowledge workshop. *History of Technology, 23,* 193-212.

Berland, G. K., Elliott, M. N., Morales, L. S., Algazy, J. I., Kravitz, R. L., Broder, M. S. et al. (2001). Health information on the Internet: Accessibility, quality, and readability in English and Spanish. *Jama, 285*(20), 2612-2621.

Buetow, K. H. (2005). Cyberinfrastructure: Empowering a "third way" in biomedical research. *Science, 308*(5723), 821-824.

Cayton, H. (2006). The flat-pack patient? Creating health together. *Patient Education Counseling, 62*(3), 288-290.

Crane, D. (1969). Social structure in a group of scientists: A test of the "Invisible College" hypothesis. *American Sociological Review, 34*(3), 335-352.

Davis, R., Gilpin, E. A., Loken, B., Viswanath, K. V., & Wakefield, M. (Eds.). (2008). *The role of the media in promoting and reducing tobacco use* (Vol. 19). Washington, DC: U.S. Department of Health and Human Services.

Dillman, D. A. (2007). *Mail and internet surveys: The tailored design method* (2nd ed.). Hoboken, NJ: Wiley.

Donohue, G. A., Tichenor, P. J., & Olien, C. N. (1975). Mass media and knowledge-gap hypothesis reconsidered. *Communication Research, 2*(1), 3-23.

Edwards, B. K., Brown, M. L., Wingo, P. A., Howe, H. L., Ward, E., Ries, L. A. et al. (2005). Annual report to the nation on the status of cancer, 1975-2002, featuring population-based trends in cancer treatment. *Journal of the National Cancer Institute, 97*(19), 1407-1427.

Engelbart, D. C. (1962). *Augmenting human intellect: A conceptual framework* (Summary Report). Palo Alto, CA: Stanford Research Institute.

Federal Trade Commission. (2005). *Federal Trade Commission Cigarette Report for 2003.* Washington, DC: Author.

Fischer, C. S. (1992). *America calling: A social history of the telephone to 1940.* Berkeley: University of California Press.

Freimuth, V. S. (1993). Narrowing the cancer knowledge gap between whites and African Americans. *Journal of the National Cancer Institute Monograph, 14,* 81-91.

Friedman, T. L. (2007). *The world is flat: A brief history of the twenty-first century.* New York: Picador.

Frost, K., Frank, E., & Maibach, E. (1997). Relative risk in the news media: A quantification of misrepresentation. *American Journal of Public Health, 87*(5), 842-845.

Gore, A. (1991). Infrastructure for the global village. *Scientific American, 265,* 150-153.

Gustafson, D. H., Brennan, P. F., & Hawkins, R. (2007). *Investing in e-health: What it takes to sustain consumer health informatics.* New York: Springer.

Hertzfeld, A., & Capps, S. (2005). *Revolution in the valley* (1st ed.). Beijing; Sebastopol, CA: O'Reilly.

Hesse, B. W. (2005). Harnessing the power of an intelligent health environment in cancer control. *Studies in Health Technology Information, 118,* 159-176.

Hesse, B. W. (2008). Of mice and mentors: Developing cyberinfrastructure to support transdisciplinary scientific collaboration. *American Journal of Preventive Medicine, 35*(2S), S235-S239.

Hesse, B. W., Nelson, D. E., Kreps, G. L., Croyle, R. T., Arora, N. K., Rimer, B. K. et al. (2005). Trust and sources of health information: The impact of the Internet and its implications for health care providers: Findings from the first Health Information National Trends Survey. *Archives of Internal Medicine, 165*(22), 2618-2624.

Hesse, B. W., Shaikh, A. R., Toward, J. I., & Edgar, T. (2002). *Final report of the CDC main web site evaluation* (Prepared under contract to the Centers for Disease Control and Prevention). Rockville, MD: Westat.

Hesse, B. W., & Shneiderman, B. (2007). eHealth research from the user's perspective. *American Journal of Preventative Medicine, 32*(5 suppl), S97-103.

Hiatt, R. A., & Rimer, B. K. (1999). A new strategy for cancer control research. *Cancer Epidemiological Biomarkers Prevention, 8*(11), 957-964.

Hornik, R. C. (2002). *Public health communication: Evidence for behavior change.* Mahwah, NJ: Lawrence Erlbaum.

Institute of Medicine. (2001). *Crossing the quality chasm: A new health system for the 21st century.* Washington, DC: National Academy Press.

Johansen, R. (2007). *Get there early: Sensing the future to compete in the present* (1st ed.). San Francisco, CA: Berrett-Koehler.

Kemper, D. W., & Mettler, M. (2002). *Information therapy: Prescribed information as a reimbursable medical service* (1st ed.). Boise, ID: Healthwise, Inc.

Kerner, J. F., Guirguis-Blake, J., Hennessy, K. D., Brounstein, P. J., Vinson, C., Schwartz, R. H. et al. (2005). Translating research into improved outcomes in comprehensive cancer control. *Cancer Causes Control, 16*(suppl 1), 27-40.

Kreps, G. L., Gustafson, D., Salovey, P., Perocchia, R. S., Wilbright, W., Bright, M. A. et al. (2007). The NCI Digital Divide Pilot Projects: Implications for cancer education. *Journal of Cancer Education, 22*(1 suppl), S56-60.

Kreps, G. L., & Viswanath, K. (2001). Communication interventions and cancer control: A review of the National Cancer Institute's health communication intervention research initiative. *Family and Community Health, 24*(3), ix-xiii.

Kuhn, T. S. (1996). *The structure of scientific revolutions* (3rd ed.). Chicago, IL: University of Chicago Press.

Man, J. (2002). *Gutenberg: How one man remade the world with words.* New York: Wiley.

Marchionini, G., Hert, C., Liddy, L., & Schneiderman, B. (2000, November). *Extending understanding of federal statistics in tables.* Paper presented at the 2000 conference on Universal Usability, Arlington, VA.

Markoff, J. (2005). *What the dormouse said—How the sixties counterculture shaped the personal computer industry.* New York: Viking.

McLuhan, M. (1967). *Understanding media: The extensions of man.* London: Sphere Books.

Morra M. E., van Nevel J. P., Nealon E. O., Mazan K. D., & Thomsen C. (1993). History of the Cancer Information Service. *Journal of the National Cancer Institute Monographs, 14,* 7-33.

Nass, S. J., Stillman, B., National Cancer Policy Board (U.S.). Committee on Large-scale Science and Cancer Research., & National Research Council (U.S.). Division on Earth and Life Studies. (2003). *Large-scale biomedical science: Exploring strategies for future research.* Washington, DC: National Academies Press.

National Cancer Institute (Ed.). (1999). *Cancer risk communication: What we know and what we need to learn.* Bethesda, MD: Author.

Nelson, D. E., Kreps, G. L., Hesse, B. W., Croyle, R. T., Willis, G., Arora, N. K. et al. (2004). The Health Information National Trends Survey (HINTS): Development, design, and dissemination. *Journal of Health Communication, 9*(5), 443-460; discussion 481-444.

President's Cancer Panel. (2007). *Promoting healthy lifestyles: Policy, program, and personal recommendations for reducing cancer risk.* Washington, DC: U.S. Department of Health and Human Services.

Rheingold, H. (2000). *The virtual community: Homesteading on the electronic frontier* (rev. ed.). Cambridge, MA: MIT Press.

Rice, R. E. (2001). The Internet and health communication: A framework of experiences. In R. E. Rice & J. E. Katz (Eds.), *The Internet and health communication: Experiences and expectations* (pp. 5-46). Thousand Oaks, CA: Sage.

Robinson, S., Hesse, B. W., Shaikh, A. R., Coss, M., & Crawford, C. (2003). *Using converging methods across disciplines to guide the redesign of a large, information-rich web site.* CHI '03 extended abstracts on Human Factors in Computing Systems, April 5-10, 2003, Ft. Lauderdale, FL. Retrieved June 15, 2008, from http://portal.acm.org/citation.cfm?doid=765891.765912

Rutten, L. F., Moser, R. P., Beckjord, E. B., Hesse, B. W., & Croyle, R. T. (2007). *Cancer communication: Health Information National Trends Survey* (No. NIH Pub. No. 07-6214). Washington, DC: National Cancer Institute.

Shneiderman, B. (2002). *Leonardo's laptop: Human needs and the new computing technologies.* Cambridge, MA: MIT Press.

Shneiderman, B. (2008). COMPUTER SCIENCE: Science 2.0. *Science, 319*(5868), 1349-1350.

Smith, T. W., & Suls, J. (2004). Introduction to the special section on the future of health psychology. *Health Psychology, 23*(2), 115-118.

Surowiecki, J. (2004). *The wisdom of crowds: Why the many are smarter than the few and how collective wisdom shapes business, economies, societies, and nations* (1st ed.). New York: Doubleday.

Tapscott, D., & Williams, A. D. (2006). *Wikinomics: How mass collaboration changes everything.* New York: Portfolio.

The Royal Institution of Great Britain. (2001). *Guidelines on science and health communication*. London, England: Author.

U.S. Department of Health and Human Services. (2008). *The ONC-Coordinated Federal Health IT Strategic Plan: 2008-2012*. Washington, DC: U.S. Department of Health and Human Services.

U.S. Department of Health, Education, and Welfare. (1964). *Smoking and health: Report of the Advisory Committee to the Surgeon General of the Public Health Service*. Washington, DC: U.S. Department of Health, Education, and Welfare, Center for Disease Control.

Viswanath, K. (2005). Science and society: The communications revolution and cancer control. *National Review of Cancer, 5*(10), 828-835.

Viswanath, K., Breen, N., Meissner, H., Moser, R. P., Hesse, B., Steele, W. R. et al. (2006). Cancer knowledge and disparities in the information age. *Journal of Health Communication, 1*(1 suppl 1), 1-17.

Viswanath, K., & Kreuter, M. W. (2007). Health disparities, communication inequalities, and eHealth. *American Journal of Prevention Medicine, 32*(5 suppl), S131-133.

Wagner, E. H. (2004). Chronic disease care. *British Medical Journal, 328*(7433), 177-178.

I

SURVEY METHODOLOGY

2

THE MEANS TO AN END

Methodology in Surveys of Health Communication

Gordon Willis
National Cancer Institute, NIH

Abraham Lincoln once said that "If I had 8 hours to cut down a tree, I'd spend 6 hours sharpening my axe." This states well the value of a sharply focused methodology: To the extent that we expend effort in developing our methods, we make the task ahead of us all the more efficient and productive. For current purposes, a key question is whether population surveys focusing on the dynamics of health communication present unique methodological problems, or at the least, bring particular aspects of the methods universe to the forefront. In many ways, the methodological developments pertinent to the realm of health communication are identical to those that challenge health surveys (and perhaps all self-report surveys) generally, and that have been comprehensively covered by Aday and Cornelius (2006). Most broadly, the methodologist's job is to devise procedures for, in turn, (a) having a well-conceptualized set of guiding objective to work from; (b) developing questions that will satisfy those objectives, and that function effectively when administered to survey respondents; (c) developing a sampling frame—or set of individuals to be surveyed—that is appropriate and statistically valid; (d) organizing and administering the survey in such a way that sufficient respondent cooperation is obtained;

and (e) making effective use of the information obtained. Each of these facets presents a host of challenges and potential pitfalls, and demands careful attention to the balance of resource allocation and potential trade-offs, and ultimately results in a set of principled compromises (see Groves, 1989, for a discussion of survey errors vs. survey costs).

CONCEPTUALIZING THE SAMPLE-BASED POPULATION SURVEY

The chapters in this section endeavor to explicate the means by which health communication researchers can "sharpen the axe" with respect to questionnaire design, development, administration, and analysis. To start, health researchers must design survey-based investigations in such a way that critical research questions are well defined; and so that the survey serves as a meaningful vehicle for addressing those questions. Chapter 3, by Rakowski, Rothman, and Kobrin, introduces this area. It defines several key concepts and terms from population-survey science, and focuses on the manner in which health communication theory can be served by such surveys. Rakowski et al.'s main thesis is that population-based surveys have a role in the process of theory refinement; hence, health communication surveys should be used to develop theory in this area. They briefly review four major characteristics of sample surveys: (a) mode of data collection (in-person, telephone, mail, or Web-based); (b) geographical scope (local, county, state, regional multistate, national, or international); (c) sampling frame; and (d) random versus nonrandom nature of sampling. They stress two benefits of population-level surveys: generalizability, and large sample size for overall and subgroup analyses.

The authors then turn to a review of the potential—and limitations—associated with the use of population surveys for conducting theory-relevant research. They review *proactive* and *reactive* overall approaches; and describe two ways of representing such theories: A *structural* depiction, and a *process* depiction. Finally, they suggest the utility repeated cross-sectional surveys to examine trends in such a way that hypotheses can be developed and then investigated in later rounds of survey data collection. Overall, Rakowski et al. encourage investigators to consider how theory-relevant questions, and perhaps even those that allow theory testing, can be incorporated into the survey from the outset.

COGNITIVE AND COMMUNICATIVE PROCESSES RELATED TO SURVEYS OF HEALTH COMMUNICATION

A second major requirement of health communication surveys is that researchers adopt methods that accommodate the cognitive, social, and communicative demands presented by the administered survey instrument. First, the requirements must be balanced between comprehensive information, which is obtained by maximizing the scope and therefore length of the questionnaire—and the simultaneous requirement to avoid respondent fatigue and break-offs, which are facilitated by minimizing questionnaire length. More fundamentally, given that interviewer-administered, self-report survey participation is by definition based on a set of implicit or explicit communicative events among investigator, interviewer, and respondent, such surveys themselves can be described as communications *about* communication—and this presents something of a paradox. To the extent that the cognitive challenges to the meaningful uptake of health information itself overlaps with the demands of answering questions about such communications, we run the risk that some respondents have poor capacity for absorbing health communication. As such, these respondents may be least able to reveal this meaningfully through responses to survey questions that themselves may demand nontrivial communicative abilities.

This conundrum is exacerbated by the fact that health communication surveys, such as the Health Informational National Trends Survey (HINTS), put considerable demands on cognitive processes involving comprehension, memory, and mental sorting of events that are themselves often mundane (e.g., frequency and source of obtaining health information), and that are not normally enumerated in the course of everyday life, or especially memorable. For example, the typical health survey, in asking the number of times one has been to the doctor in the past 12 months, although itself problematic, at least inquires about events that are discrete and potentially remembered as countable units. In contrast, inquiring about frequency of use of various communication modalities, such as the Internet versus medical providers, not only requires an implicit quantification of these, but a comparison of magnitude that is unlikely to be something the respondent will have given much thought to. Hence, communication surveys must endeavor to administer items that are conceptually simple, easy to mentally incorporate as small "chunks," and that ask for information that can be reasonably generated on the spot. The methodological challenges of design of such questions are in large part addressed through empirical testing, in order to assess the spectrum of questions that the typical survey respondent can comfortably process. In Chapter 4, Kerwin and Willis examine the role of cognitive interviewing as a means to providing insights into this area, and in assisting researchers in fashioning a questionnaire that collects meaningful information.

ESTABLISHING A SAMPLE FRAME FOR THE SURVEY

Chapter 5 by Link, discusses a critical factor facing administrators of tele-phone surveys: the implications of the increasing prevalence of cellular tele-phones among members of the population one endeavors to survey. Link discusses (a) demographic differences in health-related variables between landline and cell-only populations; (b) operational considerations in includ-ing cell phone numbers, including response rate, cost, and degree of respon-dent motivation and attention, and; (c) statistical issues involving establish-ment of a sample frame, weighting, and combining telephone-based samples. To conclude, Link focuses specifically on the challenges of developing a coherent sample frame that includes cell-only households, and critically evaluates the option of reliance on a U.S. Postal Service mailing address sam-ple, rather than a telephone-based sample, for surveys that rely on telephone administration.

MEANS FOR REDUCING NONRESPONSE

Even the best-designed questionnaire and sampling plan has only potential value, however, until it is administered to willing survey respondents. As such, we must also consider the challenges of survey administration, and how to best entice sampled individuals to choose to become respondents rather than nonrespondents. This challenge is especially important given the serious problem of declining response rates, which now afflict surveys worldwide (as also discussed by Link, Chap. 5). Health communication sur-veys may be particularly vulnerable to unit nonresponse, to the extent that potential respondents may be disinclined to participate in a survey whose topic seems abstract, academic, and of little clear personal utility to them. Whereas surveys on many health topics (e.g., smoking, AIDS, cancer pre-vention) tap critical areas of health, and therefore are often viewed as impor-tant by the population at large, it is less clear that an introduction describing a survey concerning "where you get information about health" will carry sufficient heft, in this regard. Survey designers must be particularly careful to consider the way that survey packaging, advance letters, scripting of ini-tial telephone communications, or opening sections of self-administered questionnaires can be formulated to maximize respondent interest.

Chapter 6, by David Cantor, empirically examines nonresponse, in terms of both reducing its level and measuring its effects. Concerning the former, Cantor assesses the impact of respondent monetary incentives, and of administration mode (use of a Web survey platform)—in increasing response rates. With respect to the latter, he measures the effects of nonresponse through benchmarking of HINTS estimates to those of several large national surveys, and through conducting level-of-effort analyses that determine the effects of intensive efforts to reach and survey more difficult respondents.

ANALYSIS OF REPEATED CROSS-SECTIONAL SURVEYS

Finally, to address issues concerning the analysis of population survey data, Rizzo, Moser, Waldron, Wang, and Davis (Chap. 7) describe statistical methods for examining changes across years using repeated cross-sectional health surveys. Using the HINTS program as an example, they illustrate how Internet usage to seek cancer information changed over two survey cycles, and how to compute descriptive statistics and predictive models. This approach reiterates the proposal by Rakowski et al. in Chapter 3, related to the use of repeated surveys for establishment of hypotheses and theory-testing. The authors present the statistical approaches appropriate to three basic goals:

1. Estimating a change over time in a characteristic such as a mean or a percentage and testing the significance of that change.
2. Estimating a change in a characteristic while controlling for differences in the composition of the survey samples between administration cycles.
3. Combining across survey years to produce an overall average value for a characteristic, under the assumption that the mean has not changed between years.

The methods described within Chapter 7 can be extended to population health communication surveys more generally, and should be of interest to researchers who contemplate comparing or combining survey data.

In conjunction with the later sections of the volume, the chapters that focus on methodology will hopefully guide the way toward a set of approaches to the conduct of surveys of health communication that ultimately give rise to informative, high-quality data for use by theoreticians and practitioners in the area of health policy research, and in other relevant areas of the social sciences generally.

REFERENCES

Aday, L., & Cornelius, L. (2006). *Designing and conducting health surveys* (3rd ed.). San Francisco: Wiley.

Groves, R. (1989). *Survey errors and survey costs*. New York: Wiley.

3

OPPORTUNITIES FOR CONDUCTING THEORY-RELEVANT CANCER CONTROL RESEARCH USING POPULATION-LEVEL SURVEYS

William Rakowski
Brown University

Alexander Rothman
University of Minnesota

Sarah Kobrin
National Cancer Institute

Population-level surveys of health and health practices rarely have been designed to include questions that would allow testing hypotheses drawn from one or more theories of health behavior. Most surveys are cross-sectional and designed to provide snapshots of what people know, what behaviors they are and are not performing, health-related events in their recent past, and what health conditions they are coping with at the time of the survey. When aggregated over several years, the data from these surveys can provide descriptions of changes in health and health practices over time. But, what other pictures could these surveys take? And, what other information could they gather? In this chapter we examine the role that health behavior theory could play in answering these questions. Furthermore, we consider possible roles that population-level surveys can play in the testing and refinement of health behavior theories.

The Health Information National Trends Survey (HINTS) provides an opportunity to examine these issues. HINTS was designed to complement other national population-level surveys such as the Behavioral Risk Factor Surveillance System (BRFSS) and National Health Interview Survey (NHIS) by focusing on health communication practices and health information. HINTS routinely collects nationally representative data about the American public's use of cancer-related information. The leaders of the HINTS initiative have offered a compelling case for why it is critical to track people's communication practices and their associations with people's beliefs and behavior (Nelson et al., 2004), but the question of what specific practices and constructs to include in the survey and how to manage the selection process is a recurring issue. We suggest that theories of health behavior may be able to play a role to help address this issue, for HINTS and other population-level surveys. In particular, we address two questions: (a) To what extent should theory be used to guide the development and selection of survey items? and (b) To what extent should a survey be constructed to maximize opportunities for theory-testing and development?

Theories of health behavior generate predictions and hypotheses regarding the associations between two or more constructs. They delineate the processes—biological, psychological, and environmental—that underlie people's health practices and specify the individual- and structural-level factors that moderate those processes. For example, a theory may specify how perceptions of personal risk motivate people to take precautions and for whom the impact of risk on behavior is likely to be particularly strong (Weinstein et al., 2007). Where do theories of health behavior come from? Theories are the products of a continuous interaction between deductive logic and inductive reasoning. Initial concept development is followed by a cycle of studies for construct refinement, testing of hypothesized paths of association, and, when needed, a reorganization of the original conceptualization. At some point in this process, a theory captures the attention of the field through a seminal publication, and, if shown to be useful will continue to be employed by investigators. As Noar and Zimmerman (2005) showed, theories of health behavior such as the Theory of Planned Behavior (Ajzen, 1991), Social Cognitive Theory (Bandura, 1986), and the Transtheoretical Model (TTM; Prochaska, DiClemente, & Norcross, 1992) have motivated a tremendous amount of health behavior research. The volume of research is impressive, but it has had surprisingly limited impact on the theories that initially motivated the work (Rothman, 2004; Weinstein & Rothman, 2005). Although, over time, theories may fall in and out of favor, the predictions specified by the theories have proven to be remarkably stable (Rothman, 2004; Weinstein & Rothman, 2005). Despite the steady accumulation of findings that might suggest additions, deletions, or modifications to fit specific circumstances, the degree to which theories have been modified has been modest. To an important degree, this state of affairs reflects the fact that investigators have focused on opportunities to confirm hypotheses derived from theories and have tended not to take full advantage of opportunities to challenge or falsify predictions derived from the dominant theories.

To date, discussions regarding theory development and testing have primarily focused on the important role played by randomized controlled trials (RCTs), including both laboratory studies that test whether individual or small sets of constructs "behave" as expected and interventions designed to test the impact of constructs outside of the laboratory. Although experimental RCTs remain invaluable for testing causal associations, we believe that population-level surveys can also play an important, complementary role in the process of theory refinement. In particular, population-level surveys can provide investigators with the opportunity to examine predictions derived from a theory across a rich array of dimensions, including across behaviors, across samples, and across settings. For example, population-level surveys might afford the opportunity to test whether the predictive value of a model is consistent across a series of cancer-screening behaviors. Most studies conducted in- or outside the laboratory are unable to examine the degree to which predictions are robust across these dimensions because time and financial constraints prevent collecting the variety and quantity of data that allow for this type of comparison. Additionally, population-level surveys may provide an opportunity to examine the impact of factors that are *not* typically specified within psychological models of health behavior. For example, a national population survey conducted in the United States could afford the opportunity to examine whether predictions regarding the impact of risk perceptions on behavior are consistent across different geographic regions. Of course, the contributions that surveys can make to theory development are constrained by numerous factors. In the following sections, we examine in greater detail both the strengths and limitations of how surveys can contribute to theory development.

WHAT IS A "POPULATION-LEVEL SURVEY"?

Before proceeding further, it is helpful to review some of the features that characterize a "population-level survey." In that regard, there are four characteristics that might be used to define the sample for any given survey. These four characteristics are not necessarily orthogonal, so that all combinations may not be possible. Also, this chapter does not intend to imply that the specific examples used for each characteristic are exhaustive; they are intended to provide a heuristic for specifying types of survey databases.

One characteristic of a survey is its mode of data collection. Options can include in-person interviews, mailed questionnaires, telephone interviews, and Web-based data collection. Mode of data collection may affect the "population" nature of a survey by having an impact on who is willing (or not willing) to complete the survey, and/or it may have implications for the types or formats of questions people can be asked.

The second and third characteristics combine to define the source of the sample. The second characteristic of a sample is its recruitment scope, and can include the levels of local, county/parish, regional within-state, entire state, regional multistate, national, or international. The third feature is the sampling frame or context for recruitment, and can include a single site/setting/event, multiple but separate sites/settings/events, a central repository or registry of names, a central repository or registry of health events that are linked to people, and an entire neighborhood or geographic locale. The sampling frame can include everyone (universal) or can be purposive and designate people with certain characteristics.

The fourth characteristic is the random versus nonrandom nature of the sample, regardless of recruitment scope or sampling frame. A nonrandom sample would normally be considered a convenience sample, whereas the feature of a random sample is that it allows calculated probabilities of selection from a defined denominator. That denominator consists of an identifiable population, whose members can be enumerated.

In a population-level survey individual-level weights can be applied to the data to derive representative or generalizable results back to the defined denominator. State- and national-level population surveys such as the NHIS, BRFSS, and HINTS benefit from the nature of their samples. The survey design, sampling methods, and availability of "weights" that correct for various factors (e.g., nonresponse, oversampling) allow investigators to be confident that any findings are representative of the population that comprises the denominator. Results of analyses designed to test even relatively simple associations between questions in population-level surveys can, therefore, have substantial implications because of the "random" and "population" nature of the samples. For example, investigators have used population-level data on self-rated health to illustrate in a convincing manner its ability to predict morbidity and mortality (Idler & Benyamini, 1997; Rakowski, Mor, & Hiris, 1991).

A population-level survey is most often seen as referring to a sample that represents a geographic region such as a city, county, state, census region, or the country as a whole. However, a population-level survey also can be used to describe any group, even one that is geographically dispersed, that can be identified with sufficient specificity to constitute a denominator for valid calculations of indicators such as prevalence and incidence rates for that group (e.g., military veterans, roofers, taxi drivers, or roadside construction workers).

The properties of the survey sample provide investigators with unique opportunities to examine their theories. In many cases, the formative work that underlies most theories of health behavior has been conducted with convenience samples and has relied on sample sizes that constrain opportunities for comparisons across subgroups. Population-level surveys offer investigators access to subgroups within a population that they otherwise might not be able to reach in sufficient numbers. Although the populations that are targeted in any given survey may be driven by a broad range of factors and may, in fact, be unrelated to any *a priori* theoretical issue, investigators may be able to capitalize on the population that is reached to identify samples that are of relevance to their interests. In some cases, investigators may find that available samples are limited in size or scope, but the results from initial work with these samples might be a compelling basis for greater attention to those particular groups in future surveys (or intervention studies).

USING SURVEYS TO CONDUCT "THEORY-RELEVANT RESEARCH"

The term *theory-relevant research* is deliberately general in order to accommodate research that involves both testing predictions derived directly from a theory as well as analyses that are generative and address factors not currently specified in a theory. *Theory-testing* research is specific to analyses that investigate the validity of constructs and their relations in already proposed theories. Theory testing includes analyses to investigate the measurement properties of individual constructs or variables, including stratified analyses that compare those properties across subgroups of the total population or across different behavioral domains. Other analyses would examine associations among constructs, as hypothesized by a theory. These analyses require having data for two or more constructs from a theory, each with adequate measurement properties. Stratified analyses of these associations are also pertinent for theory-testing research.

Although theory-relevant research typically focuses on predictions derived from a single theory, it need not be limited in this manner. To the extent that there are adequate measures for constructs from more than one theory, predictions derived from different theories can be compared within a particular behavioral domain, or for a particular subgroup of people, as well as across different behavioral domains or different subgroups.

In addition to testing predictions directly derived from a specific theory, investigators may pursue opportunities to examine the impact of constructs not currently specified in the theory. For example, because HINTS provides a rich description of how and where people search for health information, it provides an opportunity to examine whether differences in people's communication practices are associated in the hypothesized effect of risk perceptions on precautionary behavior. Investigators also may find ways to use survey data to generate and test novel hypotheses or operationalize novel constructs that are not connected directly to any existing theory. In this case, survey data serve to stimulate a line of work and provide the initial findings needed to motivate the dedication of resources toward the experimental and measurement work that is needed to affirm the empirical validity of the initial findings.

TWO APPROACHES FOR USING SURVEYS TO TEST AND DEVELOP THEORY

As implied previously, surveys can provide opportunities to test theoretical questions, but those opportunities are strongly affected by whether the survey was designed to test a given theoretical question. Surveys can therefore provide either a proactive or a reactive setting for investigators to test theory.

The Proactive Approach

A proactive approach lets theory-relevant questions be posed prior to the development of the survey and, thus, allows those questions to guide the content and format of at least some of the survey. For example, in HINTS 2003, a question on intention for future screening was used that allowed investigators to examine operationalizations of stage-of-change as defined by the TTM. The HINTS 2003 also included a series of risk-related questions that allowed respondents to be staged, based on the Precaution Adoption Process Model (Weinstein, 1988). In the HINTS 2007, a set of questions was developed that will afford an opportunity to test the generalizability of predictions derived from initial laboratory research on Terror Management Theory (Arndt, Cook, Goldenberg, & Cox, 2007).

A proactive approach increases the likelihood that investigators will have access to all of the constructs needed to test their hypotheses and that the measures used to assess those constructs are as reliable and valid as possible. By specifying *a priori* what constructs are needed to test a given question, the investigators provide important information to the survey design team regarding the interdependence among different items within the survey. Additionally, when investigators are forced to specify what is needed to test their hypotheses, investigators are able to articulate not only why testing the hypothesis is important, but also how this effort can capitalize on the features of a particular survey. This proactive approach benefits other users of the survey as well, providing a better integrated and more coherent set of covariates that may relate to behaviors other than those of interest to the theory-testing investigator.

Although proactively structuring a survey to test particular theory-related questions should heighten the quality and strength of that test, it may also narrow the coverage of items included in the survey. This narrowing poses a challenge to survey developers. Because the total number of survey items is limited, prioritizing specific theoretical questions requires a clear articulation of the survey's priorities and the development and implementation of a decision process that can help ensure that those priorities are kept in mind as decisions are made. Realistically, population-level surveys are complex undertakings, that necessarily have sponsors and purposes that also have substantial influence on content. For example, population-based surveys such as the BRFSS and the NHIS provide surveillance data assessing adherence to guidelines for cancer screening. As a result, opportunities to add new questions are limited by the primary need to track responses to specific questions over time. There is a process for questions to be added to the BRFSS, particularly the optional modules, but doing so requires both approval by the BRFSS state coordinators, as well as the availability of resources to cover the specific cost-per-question for each one that is added in a given year. The HINTS was created to fill a particular niche, relative to health communication and health information, but even so, decisions must be made about what will and will not be asked in a given year.

Because of the time and space constraints posed by surveys, there are considerable costs associated with including an extended set of questions on a single topic. For example, in HINTS 2005, parallel sets of questions were developed to assess people's "mental models" for three different cancers: lung, colorectal, and skin. One of the original reasons for looking at several cancers was to examine the degree of similarity in people's mental models of cancer across the three types. However, when added together, the complete battery of items was too time-consuming and would have severely limited what else could be assessed in the survey. Therefore, the sample was divided into thirds and participants were randomly assigned to answer the questions for only one of the three cancers. This division still allowed for comparisons of mental models across cancers, but shifted these comparisons from a within-subject comparison to a between-subject comparison.

A proactive approach to theory testing can prove frustrating at times because it keeps attention on the pragmatic factors that constrain the content that can be included. In many cases, grand plans must be reconfigured into modest goals. Yet, a deliberate, proactive specification of the questions a population-level survey is designed to address will greatly enhance the quality of the theory-relevant analyses that investigators are able to conduct.

The Reactive Approach

Reactive theory-testing and theory-relevant research is the primary way investigators use population-level data sets. Investigators pursing opportunities for theory testing have to work with the questions that are included in the survey—questions that are often not designed with a given theoretical question in mind. Therefore, in a reactive context, investigators typically have to rely on using proxy measures for some constructs (e.g., Han, Moser,

& Klein, 2006). Although the limitations posed by proxy measures are clear, the process of developing a proxy measure may enrich an investigator's conceptual thinking about a construct by forcing her or him to articulate a construct's defining attributes (McGuire, 1989). The development of a new measurement strategy to employ within the survey database may even prove to be generative and prompt additional work designed to examine the psychometric properties of the new measure and its relation to more traditional measures of the construct. It is important to remember that each question is a unique data element, regardless of the original purpose for its inclusion in the survey. Creative, yet conceptually defensible combinations can be made. Also, users should review not only the questionnaire/interview itself, but also the final data codebook that may contain additional information. For example, the BRFSS logs the number of adults (male, female, total) in the household as part of the final codebook, although the information is asked as part of the household screener script for interviewers.

When considering opportunities for theory-relevant research, investigators may be able to integrate data from different data sets, beyond individual-level surveys. In particular, to the extent that investigators are interested in patterns of relations within or across geographic areas such as states, counties, or even census tracts, investigators may be able to capitalize on the complementary strengths of different data sets. For example, the Area Resource File can be linked to the BRFSS to add availability of county-level health services and sociodemographic indicators to serve as covariates of individual-level reports of cancer-related behaviors. Restrictions may exist on the data that can be extracted and on conditions of use, but investigators may be rewarded if they think creatively about how to pursue these linkages.

DEPICTIONS OF THEORY AND ASSOCIATED RESEARCH QUESTIONS FOR USING WITH DATA FROM POPULATION-LEVEL SURVEYS

The next sections of this chapter discuss ways of depicting theories, analyses appropriate for testing theory, and potentials and limitations of using population-level surveys for doing these analyses. The discussion is relevant both for the proactive and reactive approaches just described.

Two ways of depicting theories are reviewed. One way is a "structural" depiction, the second is a "process" depiction. Each way of depicting a theory implies its own theoretically relevant "language" or terminology. Each of these languages/terminologies in turn implies the types of theory-relevant, and even theory-testing, research that could be done. As noted later, structural and process depictions of theory can be integrated into a single diagram, but they are discussed separately here in order to highlight their specific features.

Structural Depiction of Theory

All theories are grounded in one or more "paradigms"—sets of general, highest-order principles about the factors that underlie behavior. Any given paradigm can be the source of several theories. For example, the "logico-rational, value-expectancy" approach to health behavior, which highlights the role of individual-level decision making, is represented in several commonly used theories of health behavior (e.g., Health Belief Model [HBM; Janz & Becker, 1984], Theory of Reasoned Action/Planned Behavior [Ajzen, 1991; Fishbein, 1979], the TTM [Prochaska et al., 1992], and the Precaution Adoption Process Model [Weinstein, 1988]).

There are also theories based on individual-level variables that propose constructs at a more general level than individual-level decision making (e.g., Self-Determination Theory [Deci & Ryan, 1985; Ryan & Deci, 2002], and the Theory of Salutogenesis [Antonovsky, 1979]). Their shared paradigm is based on principles of a qualitatively defined, personality-level integration of resources used for coping.

Structural diagrams show the "pieces" of a theory and perhaps also some of their interrelationships (e.g., nested constructs, proposed correlations). At the top of the diagram is the overarching paradigm used for understanding health behavior. One or more specific theories are then "grounded" in that philosophy, so there is a unique diagram for each theory. At the next level down, the core constructs of a particular theory are shown. These "latent constructs" are defined in turn by the specific variables that are proposed to represent them. "Variables" are then also defined in turn by the specific items that are used to operationalize them and create "scales." In effect, therefore, there is a hierarchy of elements. Figure 3.1 shows a heuristic, structural representation of the TTM, based on this set of levels.

The structural depiction of theory leads to a specific "language" for the types of theory-relevant research that can be done. Realistically, the validity of overarching paradigms cannot be tested in any population-level survey. Similarly, even the validity of any single theory cannot be tested in a single survey. Some would say that paradigms and theories can never be truly proven or disproven, but simply found to be more (or less) useful for particular situations. Surveys can therefore make contributions to theory at the "lower," more concrete or specific levels of a hierarchical representation of theory. At these levels, the relevant terminology includes constructs, variables, scales, goodness-of-fit, and typical strategies and indices for development of measures. Latent constructs can be investigated, if consistent with the composition of the theory.

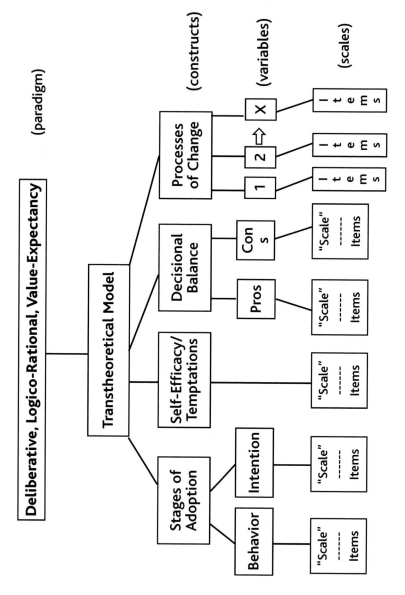

FIGURE 3.1. Depiction of the Transtheoretical Model of behavior change, showing a "structural" hierarchy of its key constructs and associated terminology.

Theory-relevant research questions (that can be tested using a population-level survey) include (a) What is the population-level distribution of a theory-relevant variable? (b) What are the psychometric properties of a theory-relevant variable? (c) What is the goodness-of-fit for the association between two or more variables? (d) Are psychometric properties robust across population subgroups? Health behavior can be used as a dependent variable in these analyses. Nonetheless, these analyses will still be based on cross-sectional data in most population-level surveys now used in cancer control.

Process Depiction of Theory

The process depiction of a theory places the constructs and/or variables of a theory into a "start-to-finish" casual chain that is proposed to lead to a behavior change. Figure 3.2 shows a heuristic, process-type causal diagram. The classic depiction of the Theory of Reasoned Action/Planned Behavior is an excellent example of a process-type diagram (Ajzen, 1991; Fishbein, 1979). The theory-relevant language of process depictions of theory includes exogenous, endogenous, and mediator variables; direct and indirect effects; proximal and distal variables; feedback loops of mutual influence; and as with structural diagrams, goodness-of-fit.

Several research questions can be addressed with survey-level process depictions of theory. For example, (a) Do direct and indirect paths between variables exist as predicted by the theory? (b) Are the hypothesized paths relevant across population subgroups? (c) Are the hypothesized paths relevant across different health behaviors? and (d) Is it possible to confirm hypothesized "feedback loops" or reciprocal effects?

Figure 3.2 is admittedly simple, relative to diagrams that might be proposed. Any of the exogenous and endogenous entries in the figure might also be "latent constructs," that would in turn have two or more variables (and their respective scales) that represent them. Process diagrams can therefore also include structural or hierarchical components, and are often analyzed by structural equation modeling or latent construct methods. The key issue is whether population-level surveys contain the necessary sets of questions for such analyses.

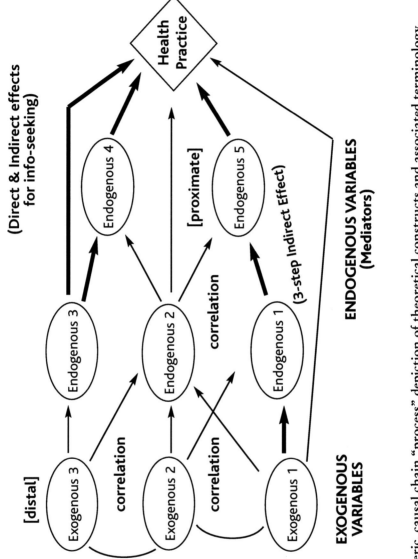

FIGURE 3.2. A generic, causal chain "process" depiction of theoretical constructs and associated terminology.

Conceptual Heuristic Versus Causal Diagrams

As a final point, it can be helpful to distinguish two types of diagrams. One of these is a heuristic diagram that presents a specific theory or even a general perspective from behavioral and social science. For example, the traditional depiction of the original HBM (Janz & Becker, 1984) shows the elements of the theory in a diagram that does not portray a time sequence among the variables. Some representations of the TTM show a circle or a spiral (McGuire, 1989) that refer to general premises of the model, rather than specific hypotheses about associations among its elements. More broadly, the typical portrayal of a socioecological perspective shows the nested levels of factors affecting health practices and health status per se. In some instances, sociodemographic variables are placed somewhere in a heuristic diagram, perhaps as left-most exogenous variables. The usual purpose of including them is to indicate that those contextual factors can somehow influence the primary elements of the theory (e.g., the content that defines the meaning of a construct).

A critical challenge posed by a heuristic diagram, however, is translating the general principles outlined in the figure into specific, testable hypotheses. This requires taking the broad class of constructs shown in the heuristic and deciding how to operationalize it in the context of the existing study and depict testable associations among variables.

Other theory-based diagrams are drawn to purposely specify a causal sequence. For example, the typical depiction of the Theory of Reasoned Action and Planned Behavior (Ajzen, 1991; Fishbein, 1979) presents a four-step sequence leading to behavior, with intention as the construct most proximate to behavior. Theories such as this provide a very clear set of testable predictions as well as guidance regarding how to operationalize the specified constructs. The structure afforded by these models also provides a framework for thinking about whether and how other factors might moderate the relations specified in the theory. Specifying moderator variables would allow investigators to capitalize on the diversity of groups who are usually embedded in population-level surveys.

TREND ANALYSES WITH CROSS-SECTIONAL POPULATION-LEVEL SURVEYS

Cross-sectional surveys like the NHIS, BRFSS, and HINTS can also be examined in sequence, using trends to create hypotheses that would be investigated in the next round of data collection (Rizzo et al., Chap. 7, this volume). For example, if HINTS 2003 and 2005 surveys showed that

Internet use for seeking health information were found to be increasing over time among persons aged 75 years and over, and if Internet use were also associated with less satisfaction with information given by one's primary care provider (a fabricated example for this chapter), then might it be hypothesized that in the next round of the HINTS, persons aged 75 years and over would report less satisfaction with provider-given information than in prior HINTS.

CONCLUDING COMMENTS

The issue is not whether population-level surveys can contribute to theory-relevant cancer control research. Surveys of various types have always contributed to theories of health behavior. There are two bottom-line questions. The first is "How can the content of an existing survey be used to do theory-relevant analyses?" Such research is a type of "output" from the database, and relies on having a pool of theory-relevant questions as the "inputs." To date, most such research will come from a "reactive" approach, and will rely on investigators being as creative as possible with the data they inherit for secondary analyses. Expectations need to be modest from a reactive situation. Making population-level survey data public that had no deliberate up-front, theory-based contributions, and then letting investigators "have at it" in their analyses relies largely on what amounts to the serendipity of investigators finding "gems" for analysis.

The second question is, "How can health behavior theory be used to improve the theory-relevant potential of population-level surveys?" The proactive approach offers the opportunity to increase the potential for population-level surveys to inform theory development. As we look ahead to population-level surveys still to be designed, careful consideration will need to be given to the overarching goals of each survey. The selection of theory-based constructs for inclusion in a survey carries an element of risk, and requires deliberate forethought. Types of theory-relevant analyses that might be conducted should be considered in advance. The risk is putting one's "eggs" in a necessarily restricted number of conceptual "baskets." For example, should question content come from a new theory that offers the opportunity to address a gap in the current literature or should content come from an established theory that could still benefit from refinement? Can a population-level survey build both into its data collection? Even so, there are many candidate theories from which to choose. Although theory can inform the design and implementation of surveys, it is also important to recognize that theory is but one of a range of factors that must be dealt with as planners delineate the primary aims of population-level surveys. How to balance the frequently competing demands that these factors place on surveys has been and will likely continue to be an on-going challenge for teams charged with the design and implementation of the survey. However difficult these questions are to deliberate and resolve, if there is an objective of doing theory-relevant research, persons with theory-relevant expertise should be consulted for input to survey content.

REFERENCES

Ajzen, I. (1991). The theory of planned behavior. *Organizational Behavior and Human Decision Processes, 50*, 179-211.

Antonovsky, A. (1979). *Health, stress and coping.* San Francisco, CA: Jossey-Bass.

Arndt, J., Cook, A., Goldenberg, J. L., & Cox, C. R. (2007). Cancer and the threat of death: The cognitive dynamics of death-thought suppression and its impact on behavioral health intentions. *Journal of Personality and Social Psychology, 92*, 12-29

Bandura, A. (1986). *Social foundations of thought and action: A social cognitive theory.* Englewood Cliffs, NJ: Prentice Hall.

Deci, E. L., & Ryan, R. M. (1985). *Intrinsic motivation and self-determination in human behavior.* New York: Plenum.

Fishbein, M. (1979). Theory of reasoned action: Some applications and implications. In H. Howe & M. Page (Eds.), *Nebraska Symposium on Motivation* (pp. 65-116). Lincoln: University of Nebraska Press.

Han, P. K., Moser, R. P., & Klein, W. M. (2006). Perceived ambiguity about cancer prevention recommendations: Relationship to perceptions of cancer preventability, risk, and worry. *Journal of Health Communication, 11*(suppl 1), 51-69.

Idler, E. L., & Benyamini, Y. (1997). Self-rated health and mortality: A review of twenty-seven community studies. *Journal of Health and Social Behavior, 38*(1), 21-37.

Janz, N. K., & Becker, M. H. (1984). The health belief model: A decade later. *Health Education Quarterly, 11*, 1-47.

McGuire, W. J. (1989). A perspectivist approach to the strategic planning of programmatic scientific research. In B. Gholson, W.R. Shadish, Jr., R.A. Neimeyer, & A.C. Houts (Eds.), *Psychology of science: Contributions to metascience* (pp. 214-245). New York: Cambridge University Press.

Nelson, D. E., Kreps, G. L., Hesse, B. W., Croyle, R. T., Willis, G., Arora, N. K., Rimer, B. K., Viswanath, K. V., Weinstein, N., & Alden, S. (2004). The Health Information National Trends Survey (HINTS): Development, design, and dissemination. *Journal of Health Communication, 9*(5), 443-460; discussion 81-84.

Noar, S. M., & Zimmerman, R. S. (2005). Health Behavior Theory and cumulative knowledge regarding health behaviors: Are we moving in the right direction? *Health Education Research, 20*(3), 275-290.

Prochaska, J. O., DiClemente, C. C., & Norcross, J. C. (1992). In search of how people change: Applications to addictive behaviors. *American Psychologist, 47*, 1102-1114.

Rakowski, W., Mor, V., & Hiris, J. (1991). The association of self-rated health with mortality in a sample of well-elderly from the Longitudinal Study of Aging (1984-1986). *Journal of Aging and Health, 3*(4), 527-545.

Rothman, A. J. (2004). "Is there nothing more practical than a good theory?": Why innovations and advances in health behavior change will arise if interventions are used to test and refine theory. *International Journal of Behavioral Nutrition and Physical Activity, 27*(1), 11.

Ryan, R. M., & Deci, E. L. (2002). An overview of self-determination theory. In E. L. Deci & R. M. Ryan (Eds.), *Handbook of self-determination research* (pp. 3-33). Rochester, NY: University of Rochester Press.

Weinstein, N. D. (1988). The precaution adoption process. *Health Psychology, 7*, 355-386.

Weinstein, N. D., Kwitel, A., McCaul, K. D., Magnan, R.E., Gerrard, M., & Gibbons, F. X. (2007). Risk perceptions: Assessment and relationship to influenza vaccination. *Health Psychology, 26*(2), 146-151.

Weinstein, N.D., & Rothman, A.J. (2005). Revitalizing research on health behavior theories. *Health Education Research, 20*, 294-297.

4

COGNITIVE INTERVIEW PRETESTING OF A HEALTH INFORMATION SURVEY

Lessons Learned

Jeffrey Kerwin
Westat Inc.

Gordon Willis
National Cancer Institute

COGNITIVE INTERVIEWING AND QUESTIONNAIRE DESIGN

Since the early 1980s, survey researchers and cognitive psychologists have joined forces to develop and promote the interdisciplinary science, cognitive aspects of survey methodology (CASM; Tourangeau, Rips, & Rasinski, 2000). CASM is predicated on the assertion that the act of answering a survey question requires the successful operation of a series of cognitive functions, including comprehending the question posed, retrieving relevant information from memory, perhaps engaging in a self-evaluation of the accuracy of the information retrieved, and then assembling and reporting this information in a form that is consistent with the requirements of the data collector (e.g., selecting the best match from a set of provided response categories). For example, answering the survey question: "In the past week, on how many days did you go on the Internet" requires comprehension of the key elements "past week" and "go on the Internet." The respondent must also recall relevant memories, and may make a judgment concerning the adequacy of the response (e.g., the individual may have been unable to access a computer all week, but decides to report "usual" behavior nonetheless). Finally, to provide an answer, the respondent may or may not select the format desired by the investigator (e.g., "I use it all the time;" "Every day;" "Not much"). The cognitive model presumes that survey questions may exhibit features that preclude successful cognitive processing, and that may result in survey response error (i.e., answers that are inaccurate; Conrad & Blair, 2004; DeMaio & Rothgeb, 1996; Jobe & Mingay, 1991; Willis, 2005a, 2005b). Furthermore, respondents must be motivated enough to enact these steps, rather than shortcutting them (Krosnick, 1991). In the proceeding example, the question may contain vague elements ("past week";"go on the Internet") that create divergent interpretations across respondents; or it may induce biased responding (e.g., the desire to provide a non-zero response).

To study this information-processing chain in an applied environment—that is, when pretesting or otherwise evaluating survey questions—researchers have relied mainly on the use of the *cognitive interview*, a method specifically designed to assess the cognitive processes underlying individuals' answers to draft survey questions, in order to determine where questions may pose cognitive demands that lead to error. Additionally, given a more recent focus by psycholinguists, sociologists, and anthropologists on the sociocultural nature of survey responding, especially under interviewer-based administration (as opposed to self-administration), the cognitive interview also endeavors to assess interpersonal and sociocultural factors that influence responses (e.g., the potential influence of demand characteristics relating to socially desirable responding; or the tendency to avoid extreme response categories. Hippler, Schwarz, & Sudman, 1987; Tourangeau et al., 2000).

Operationally, cognitive interviewing involves a series of individual (as opposed to group) interviews in which a specially trained interviewer administers the tested questionnaire to specially recruited volunteers. In addition to requesting answers, as in a usual survey interview, the cognitive interviewer assesses functioning of the items through the use of two verbal report procedures: *verbal probing* and *think-aloud*. Think-aloud is the older of the procedures, and requires verbalization of one's thoughts while engaged in the act of answering survey questions. The interviewer mainly encourages the respondent to "Tell me what you are thinking." Investigators then analyze the resulting think-aloud *protocol* to identify problems in answering the tested questions that have a cognitive basis. There are drawbacks to think-aloud procedures, however; in particular, some respondents find thinking aloud to be difficult or unnatural and the process can be somewhat inefficient and meandering in nature.

Therefore, an alternative procedure—*verbal probing*—has come into prominence, either in place of or in addition to the think-aloud procedure. Probing involves the administration of targeted probe questions, by the interviewer—"questions about the questions"—that delve further into the respondent's reactions to the evaluated. Under *concurrent probing*, immediately after the respondent responds to the tested question, the interviewer asks probes such as "Tell me more about that"; and "What does the phrase 'health information' make you think of?" Probes may investigate a specific cognitive process (e.g., comprehension probes assess understanding of key terms, whereas retrieval probes address memory for key items of information). *Elaborative probes*, on the other hand, request that the respondent provide further information or explanation, and strive to determine whether the answer provided to the tested question matches the situation that emerged through elaborated discussion (Beatty, 2004; Willis, 2005b).

An alternative to concurrent probing is *retrospective probing* (also called *cognitive debriefing*), in which probes are administered subsequent to the interview, rather than as a part of it. Waiting until after the interview to probe avoids potential reactive effects of probing that may contaminate the interview; but has the distinct disadvantage of delay, such that respondents may no longer be able to recall the thoughts associated with responses to particular questions. For interviewer-administered questionnaires, investigators therefore are more likely to adopt some form of concurrent probing.

Cognitive interviews are normally conducted in one or more small *rounds* of 8–12 individual interviews. Respondents are recruited who are suitable for the tested instrument (e.g., for a general population survey of adults, a range of individuals aged 18 years or older are sought). After a round of testing, interview- and question-specific reports are typically written, aggregated across interviews and interviewers, and reviewed by the questionnaire design team. On the basis of these qualitative findings, investigators make recommendations concerning question wording modification, ordering, or addition/deletion of items.

Cognitive interview testing has the advantage of very intensively investigating the functioning of survey questions from a number of perspectives, nominally cognitive, but also including elements of sociology, anthropology, and linguistics. Because of its probing nature, cognitive interviewing allows investigators to observe and appreciate the existence of "silent misunderstandings" (DeMaio & Rothgeb, 1996) between investigators and survey respondents that may not otherwise emerge. As for limitations, cognitive interviewing is qualitative, somewhat judgmental and even impressionistic in nature (in both conduct and analysis), and relies on small samples that may not be fully representative of the larger population. Furthermore, cognitive testing may underestimate problems, as laboratory-based respondents may be more motivated than field survey respondents (e.g., they may engage in less "satisficing," as discussed by Krosnick, 1991). As such, cognitive interviewing is most useful when it is included as one component of a comprehensive pretesting strategy that also makes use of expert review, and further empirical field-based pretesting.

COGNITIVE INTERVIEWING PROCEDURES FOR HINTS 2003, 2005, AND 2007

Extensive cognitive interview pretesting has been conducted prior to each cycle of HINTS administration. For the first HINTS (2003), two iterative rounds of interviews were conducted, each with nine participants. We also conducted two rounds of interviews for HINTS 2005, with similar numbers of participants. Given the substantial methodological changes implemented for HINTS 2007 (moving from strictly random-digit dial to mixed-mode administration; see Cantor, Chap. 6, this volume), we conducted five rounds: three devoted to testing questions for telephone administration, followed by two rounds of testing draft versions of a mail survey instrument. Although the HINTS questionnaire has been translated into Spanish, cognitive testing was only conducted in English.

For all of the cycles of HINTS cognitive testing, participants were recruited within the Washington, DC area. Most volunteered in response to ads placed in weekly newspapers or on the Internet (e.g., Craigslist, neighborhood e-mail listservs). For any given round of interviews, we sought to recruit and schedule participants reflecting a variety of ages (18 years or older), racial/ethnic backgrounds, and education levels, as the HINTS is a general survey of the adult U.S. noninstitutionalized household population. In some rounds, there was a focus on recruiting a greater than usual number of persons over age 45 or 50 because several different sections of HINTS questions were designed strictly for people who should be receiving particular cancer-screening tests. Regardless, demographic diversity was generally achieved, although participants tended to have graduated from high school and attended college to a greater degree than is true for the population as a whole. This is common among cognitive testing projects, however (Willis, 2005b), and in our experience, individuals of relatively low levels of education (especially those not completing high school) seem to have much less interest in participating in cognitive interview studies than individuals who have completed higher levels of education.

Participants met with HINTS project staff members for one-on-one interviews in the contractor's qualitative interviewing facility. For each round, the first author conducted at least half of the interviews, with the remaining interviews being conducted by one or two staff members with varying levels of experience in cognitive interviewing. In each interview, project staff administered draft sections of the HINTS instrument, and probed participants for their interpretations of key terms in the questions (e.g., "cancer screening"), or other issues of concern and interest to the HINTS management teams. Participants often were asked to elaborate on the basis of their answers, so that judgments could be made as to whether their answers were consistent with the intent of the questions, or whether the questions and corresponding response options adequately captured participants' experiences or opinions. Probing was generally conducted using a *concurrent* manner (i.e., immediately upon receiving an answer to a test question). In a number of instances, however, probing was done only after a set of related draft questions had been answered (i.e., as a debriefing, or *retrospective* interview). Much of the probing was planned in advance of the cognitive interviews (*anticipated probing*, as termed by Willis, 2005b), but interviewers also probed any observations (e.g., provocative utterances or hesitations on the part of a respondent) suggesting a potential problem with a question—that is, Emergent probing (Willis, 2005b). The interviews typically lasted from 40 to 60 minutes, and participants were generally paid $40 to $50 for their time.

ANALYSIS OF COGNITIVE INTERVIEWS

Results of cognitive interviews consisted of text-based comments made by the interviewers, on a question-by-question basis, for each interview. These comments described in detail a participant's response and the basis for it. The comments typically described one or more of four cognitive processes discussed earlier: how the participant interpreted a question of interest, what sort of information was recalled, how the recalled information was judged and integrated, and how a response was ultimately chosen. After each testing round of interviews was completed (typically nine subjects per round), comments were reviewed by the first author and summarized in a report for the HINTS questionnaire design team. In some cases, counts were kept of the frequency with which particular problems emerged. Mainly, problems were detected according to the judgment of the analyst, who determined from the written summaries whether the question objectives were being satisfied, and whether the participants' behaviors suggested questionnaire design flaws that should be addressed by the management team.

ILLUSTRATIVE FINDINGS FROM HINTS COGNITIVE INTERVIEWS

Asking Survey Respondents About Their Beliefs and Perceptions of Cancer

A major goal of HINTS is to measure and track over time the American population's perceptions and knowledge regarding cancer. For example,

HINTS has asked respondents about their perceived risk and fear of developing cancer, the factors associated with the risk for cancer, and the likelihood of a patient surviving cancer. One issue that has arisen when developing these questions stems from the fact that cancer is not one disease, but rather a class of conditions that affect varying parts of the body. Some HINTS questions ask about issues related to a specific cancer site (e.g., breast, prostate, lung), but the National Cancer Institute (NCI) is also interested in the public's views about "cancer in general." Further complicating matters, survey respondents have widely varying levels of sophistication regarding the topic. Some see cancer as a nebulous and very general health concept, and possess little appreciation for the distinctions between different types or sites of cancer. Others are much more aware of the distinctions, and still others have a high degree of knowledge about one or two particular types of cancer as a result of personal or family experience.

In the questionnaire design phase leading to HINTS 2005, there was an interest in developing scales to capture a respondent's "mental model" of cancer; that is, the belief system that underlies perceptions of cancer and which may affect behaviors that one might take related to prevention, in particular. These scales included items such as:

Cancer is an illness that when detected can typically be cured.

Strongly agree
Somewhat agree
Somewhat disagree
Strongly disagree

How long will the average person who has developed cancer live?
Would you say . . .

Less than a year,
One to 5 years,
Five to 10 years, or
More than 10 years?

In an initial round of cognitive interviews for HINTS 2005, some participants repeatedly indicated that "it depends." Some even expressed frustration, as they perceived these to be overly simplistic questions: "*I believe some cancers are incurable and others are curable!*"

Other participants appeared to have little or no trouble reporting a view of "cancer" in such general terms. However, when we probed these participants as to what they were thinking about when answering, many mentioned the cancers for which they viewed themselves at greatest personal risk based on family history, or the cancers that had afflicted close family members or friends. As one put it, *"When you talk about cancer, I can only think about something I've had, or . . . concerns me."* As another example, one participant discussed how his views fell into "two extremes," in that a sister had overcome leukemia through a bone marrow transplant years before, whereas a cousin who had been diagnosed with brain cancer had recently died. He said he dealt with this dilemma by "taking the optimistic approach" when answering the questions, thus giving much greater weight to his sister's experience than to that of his cousin.

In another round of interviews, we examined the possibility of asking the questions more than once (i.e., asking the same questions about at least two types of cancer). Although this appeared to make the questions more straightforward and easier to answer for some participants, others still noted that this depends, in that there are other unspecified factors to be considered in order to generate an answer, namely how early the cancer is detected and treated (e.g., *"If it is detected early enough, then I would 'strongly agree'"*).

Furthermore, a new problem arose when asking these items about multiple cancers: The approach understandably made such questions more tedious and burdensome for those with relatively little knowledge of various cancers. For such persons, answering this section of the HINTS interview may have seemed similar to taking a test. It was ultimately decided that HINTS 2005 would administer this set of questions only once to each respondent, focusing on a particular cancer (randomly chosen among colon, lung, or skin cancer).

ASKING ABOUT AWARENESS AND EXPOSURE TO HEALTH COMMUNICATION MESSAGES

Many Americans are incidentally (i.e., passively) exposed to health communications, if not every day then at least intermittently. With respect to cancer, various organizations (including the NCI) sponsor major media campaigns designed to educate the public about the risks of smoking, the importance of cancer screenings, the associated benefits of early detection, and so on. Of course, people are exposed to health information through sources beyond the media as well, such as family members, friends in the workplace, and health care providers. HINTS seeks to determine the sources or channels through which the public has been exposed to messages about cancer, and there has been a corresponding interest in assessing the content of these messages.

Our cognitive interviews have shown that capturing such information from survey respondents can be a challenge. Not surprisingly perhaps, much of the challenge stems from normal limitations with attention and recall. For example, one version of a question tested for HINTS 2005 was:

Thinking about the past year only, have you heard anything about preventing cancer. . . .

> *From a doctor or other health care professional? (yes/no)*
> *From family or friends? (yes/no)*
> *In newspapers? (yes/no)*
> *In magazines? (yes/no)*
> *On the radio? (yes/no)*
> *On the Internet? (yes/no)*
> *On television? (yes/no)*

Most respondents readily answered "yes" or "no" for each potential source. In our probing, we asked cognitive interview participants to describe in their own words some recollections of what they had seen or heard about preventing cancer. Although some could point out specific stories they had heard on television or read in the newspaper about the benefits of cancer screening, or of eating foods believed to reduce the risk of cancer, other participants had replied "yes" more on the general impression that such health messages are commonplace:

> *(1) "It's a little difficult to dredge up where and when various bits and pieces fell into place . . . 40 years ago we learned that you need roughage in the diet . . . so to ask [whether I've seen] anything about roughage in the diet preventing cancer within the last year, maybe I did and maybe I didn't . . . it just didn't make an impression because it's old news."*

> *(2) "I can't remember, like, specifics . . . you know, the information just runs together when you hear it in the news or read it in the newspaper, and you read it online . . . they're all saying the same thing."*

The questionnaire design team decided not to ask these questions in the actual administration of the 2005 HINTS.

The difficulties respondents have with recall have also been observed with HINTS questions that attempt to collect information on the content of salient messages to which they have been exposed. For example, a series of items tested for HINTS 2007 was as follows:

> *In the past year, have you seen or heard or read anything about preventing cancer? (yes/no)*

> *(If "yes") Thinking about the past year only, what have you seen or heard or read about preventing cancer? (open-ended response)*

Many participants reported at the first item having been exposed to cancer prevention information, yet seemed unable to recall and report anything specific in the second item (which itself served as a type of cognitive probe). They frequently gave only very general answers, some of which had no clear connection to issues of prevention:

> *"Diet, exercise, supplements that can help."*
> *"Different foods to eat that are good against cancer."*
> *"Something on HPV (human papillomavirus), and various cancers."*
> *"Cigarettes and smoking."*

Based on these observations, we revised the question wording and reduced the reference period from 1 year to 1 month, as follows:

> *Do you recall any specific topic that you have heard or seen in the past month about preventing cancer? (yes/no)*
>
> *(If "yes") What was the topic?*

Although in further cognitive testing these changes appeared to reduce somewhat the tendency for respondents to report "yes" at the first item when in fact they could not recall anything specific, they were judged to be only minimally effective. It seems that many respondents believe that they must have been exposed to cancer prevention messages and want to report this, yet recalling specific instances and the nature of the communication is a more significant challenge. Ultimately, these questions were dropped from consideration for inclusion in the 2007 HINTS.

ASKING SURVEY RESPONDENTS ABOUT COMMUNICATIONS WITH THEIR HEALTH CARE PROVIDERS

Another area of interest for HINTS concerns respondents' communications and interactions with their health care providers. For example, the survey asked respondents whether or not their doctors have recommended certain cancer-screening tests. The 2007 HINTS also assessed how actively involved respondents are in decisions regarding their health care and how they perceive relationships with their doctors. In the cognitive interviews conducted with such questions, several key issues were observed. One particular interest that the NCI has had in this area is whether or not doctors encourage patients to ask questions or express any concerns when making recommendations to be screened for cancer. For example, a question concerning colon cancer screening asked:

> *Thinking about the last time a health care provider talked to you about being checked for colon cancer, did your health care provider encourage you to ask questions or express any concerns you had about colon cancer testing? Would you say yes—definitely, yes—somewhat, or no, not at all?*

A common reaction on the part of cognitive interview participants is a feeling that the "no, not at all" response to this question could be taken as a criticism of their doctors. Such a reaction is evident by a comment from one participant who answered the question by stating, "*He didn't encourage it, but he's open to my questions.*"

These participants are perhaps reacting to the fact that the question, as worded, does not anticipate that a patient may be completely comfortable asking questions or expressing concerns without the doctor explicitly encouraging them to do so. It is easy to imagine that someone who has a great deal of trust in a doctor they have relied on for many years would be reluctant to report in a survey that this doctor does not actively encourage open expression by the patient.

Such a question also may pose a problem related to recall of information. For example, it presumably would be challenging to consider and answer this question if a doctor discussed the cancer screening test a number of years ago. Another potential difficulty, which became evident only when encountering it in the cognitive interviewing, stems from the possibility that the discussion of the cancer-screening test may have occurred within the context of a health care visit with a much broader purpose, such as an annual physical. It is possible that the doctor encouraged the respondent to "*ask questions or express any concerns*" during the visit, but that this explicit encouragement did not occur precisely when the discussion about cancer screening took place. As a result of problems noted, the team decided not to ask this question in the 2007 HINTS.

Furthermore, a series of questions in the 2007 HINTS asked respondents how they view the communications they have had with their health care providers over the past year. For example:

> *During the past 12 months, how often did doctors, nurses, or other health professionals involve you in decisions about your health care as much as you wanted? Would you say always, usually, sometimes, or never?*

> *How often did they help you deal with feelings of uncertainty about your health or health care? Would you say always, usually, sometimes, or never?*

In cognitive interviews of the 2007 instrument, participants almost always easily provided answers to this series of items. However, probing revealed that answers were not always consistent with the intent of the question. For example, answers sometimes reflected a more general satisfaction with one's health care provider, rather than any actual communications that occurred between the respondent and his or her providers. When probed, participants sometimes could recall no specific occurrence in which they felt their doctor had involved them in their health care decisions, even though they had readily answered that this "always" or "usually" occurred. Furthermore, in some instances there had not been any real decisions to be made regarding one's health care, or with respect to the second item above, the participants were unable to report any "feelings of uncertainty" about their care.

With some participants, the reluctance to criticize one's doctor seemed to come into play as well. Interestingly, when participants did recall a specific occurrence that seemingly contributed to their answer, it sometimes was revealed to have occurred prior to the 12-month reference period. For example, some participants had experienced relatively few doctor visits in the past 12 months, and so thought further back in time (perhaps without even realizing they were doing so) for experiences on which to base their answer. Others recalled occurrences more than 12 months old that remained highly salient. One participant, for example, thought back to an event more than 2 years prior in which she had been upset that her doctor refused her request to be referred to a specialist. Finally, at least one participant in our cognitive testing inadvertently answered not on the basis of communications regarding her own health and health care, but that of her children. Nevertheless, the questionnaire design team felt these questions would be a useful addition to the HINTS 2007 questionnaire, and they were retained.

DISCUSSION

In this chapter we discussed what cognitive interviewing procedures and highlighted selected findings from the HINTS questionnaire development process we felt might be of interest to researchers in the field of health communication. It is important to emphasize a major benefit of the application of cognitive interviewing techniques to the pretesting of survey instruments: the detection of "silent misunderstandings" that all too frequently occur between researchers and survey respondents (DeMaio & Rothgeb, 1996). Survey respondents within a field environment[1] typically accede to the perceived demands of the survey interview's question and response format. For example, they quickly realize that their role is to choose from a small set of fixed response categories the one that best represents their *true* answer.

---

[1]By "field" we refer to telephone as well as in-person survey administration.

Many times they appear do so without any apparent difficulty. The problem, however, is that observing a smooth question–response process between an interviewer and respondent may hide serious issues of concern for the researcher. Effective probing of respondents' thought processes, and the basis for their answers, can reveal questionnaire design flaws that would be otherwise difficult or impossible to detect. Often the question flaws are entirely unanticipated by the questionnaire design team.

The HINTS cognitive interviewing experience has shown how challenging it can be to craft survey questions meeting measurement goals that may be important in the health communications arena. Within the U.S. household population, many people are bombarded with health-related messages in the form of recommendations (from both legitimate and non-legitimate sources), anecdotal stories of experiences with a disease from family members and friends, and perhaps most of all, advertising. Health communications researchers are understandably interested in the messages to which people have been exposed, and the channels through which this exposure occurred, and this is one of the reason that HINTS was created. Unfortunately, much of this exposure occurs in a passive manner, where individuals are not seeking this information, and thus much of it does not remain salient in memory over time (see Benware & Deci, 1984). Of course, this is compounded by the possibility the individual may never have paid much attention to the message in the first place. On the other hand, HINTS does devote many questions to individual experiences with active seeking of health information (in particular, cancer information). Cognitive interviews on such questions have suggested that people have much less difficulty recalling and reporting details concerning these experiences, such as where and how they sought the information, and how they used it. Our remaining challenge, therefore, is to develop procedures for developing items that function effectively across the full range of the active–passive continuum.

OVERALL RECOMMENDATIONS BASED ON COGNITIVE TESTING RESULTS

Given what was learned while performing cognitive interviewing for the HINTS, what follows are some "lessons learned" that could be applicable to other similar types of health surveys:

1. Avoid questions about overarching concepts (i.e, "cancer in general") that are more general than the level at which respondents are prone to think. This effect cuts both ways, however, such that it is

also possible to ask too specifically. Overall, we need to strike an appropriate balance with respect to specificity of item content.

2. Avoid questions concerning mundane events that require recall over a long time period (in particular, "ever"), as this puts unreasonable demands on recall processes. For many items, the past 12 months is likely the longest possible temporal interval that will function effectively.

3. Accept that health-related communications with care providers, in particular, may be characterized by indirect features (e.g., "He always made me comfortable asking questions, though he didn't direct me to ask any"). Therefore, it may be best to ask about respondents' perceptions (e.g., how comfortable they felt asking questions), as opposed to particular events (i.e., whether they were explicitly told to ask them).

4. Given the vagaries and subtleties of questions on very abstract survey response processes linked to queries about communication and knowledge, and because we lack a set of design principles that will allow researchers to script or select questions confidently, we suggest that for any new survey being developed, empirical investigation in the form of qualitative and cognitive interviewing will be valuable.

REFERENCES

Beatty, P. (2004). The dynamics of cognitive interviewing. In S. Presser, J. Rothgeb, M. Couper, J. Lessler, E. Martin, J. Martin, & E. Singer (Eds.), *Methods for testing and evaluating survey questionnaires* (pp. 45-66). Hoboken, NJ: Wiley.

Benware, C. A., & Deci, E. L. (1984). Quality of learning with an active versus passive motivational set. *American Educational Research Journal, 21*(4), 755-765.

Conrad, F., & Blair, J. (2004). Data quality in cognitive interviews: The case for verbal reports. In S. Presser, J. Rothgeb, M. Couper, J. Lessler, E. Martin, J. Martin, & E. Singer (Eds.), *Questionnaire development evaluation and testing methods* (pp. 67-87). Hoboken, NJ: Wiley.

DeMaio T. J., & Rothgeb J. M. (1996). Cognitive interviewing techniques: In the lab and in the field. In N. Schwarz & S. Sudman (Eds.), *Answering questions: Methodology for determining cognitive and communicative processes in survey research* (pp. 175-195). San Francisco: Jossey-Bass.

Hippler, H., Schwarz, N., & Sudman, S. (Eds.). (1987). *Social information processing and survey methodology.* New York: Springer-Verlag.

Jobe, J. B., & Mingay, D. J. (1991). Cognition and survey measurement: History and overview. *Applied Cognitive Psychology, 5,* 175–192.

Krosnick, J. (1991). Response strategies for coping with the cognitive demands of attitude measures in surveys. *Applied Cognitive Psychology, 5,* 213-236.

Tourangeau, R., Rips, L. J., & Rasinski, K. (2000). *The psychology of survey response.* Cambridge: Cambridge University Press.

Willis, G. B. (2005a). Cognitive interviewing. In S. Best & B. Radcliff (Eds.), *Polling America: An encyclopedia of public opinion* (pp. 92-98). Westport, CT: Greenwood Press.

Willis, G. B. (2005b). *Cognitive interviewing: A tool for improving questionnaire design.* Thousand Oaks, CA: Sage.

5

IMPLICATIONS OF CELL PHONE USAGE IN SURVEY RESEARCH FOR INFORMING

Communication Research and Practice

Michael W. Link
The Nielsen Company

Survey research in health communications is at a crossroads. The challenges facing the industry, such as declining participation, falling coverage of land-line telephone frames, and growing diversification of the U.S. society are forcing researchers to look in new directions for solutions. Although nearly every approach or mode used in survey research has seen significant declines in participation rates over the past 10 years, none has been more hard-hit than telephone-based research—the methodology on which most studies in health communications, including the Health Information National Trends Survey (HINTS), are based. Perhaps no problem has become more vexing than that of reaching households that have discarded the use of traditional landline telephones in favor of cell phones as their sole form of telecommunications. This chapter focuses on the challenges to survey research posed by "cell phone-only households" and the potential new approaches for reaching these individuals.

THE CHALLENGE OF CELL PHONES

For the past three decades, random-digit dial (RDD) telephone surveys have been the primary means of collecting survey data for measuring health-related knowledge, attitudes, and behaviors. However, the past decade has witnessed significant declines in participation rates for RDD surveys as a result of factors such as call-screening technologies, heightened privacy concern, and a general malaise (if not outright hostility) toward unsolicited calls to the home (Curtin, Presser, & Singer, 2005; Steeh, Krigis, Cannor, & DeWitt, 2001). Yet, although researchers have long focused on the growing problem of nonresponse in telephone surveys, it is actually the remarkable decline in sample frame coverage that poses the most serious threat to this mode (i.e., through challenges to the representativeness of the population reachable through telephone). Between 2000 and 2007, telephone frame coverage dropped from 97% to approximately 85% (Blumberg, Luke, Cynamon, & Frankel, 2007). The primary cause of this erosion of coverage is the dramatic increase in cell phone-only households.[1]

Cell phones are indispensable in today's society, but cause major challenges for survey researchers. In particular, the growing trend of "cord-cutting"—whereby households drop their landline telephone service in favor of exclusive use of their cell phone for telecommunications—has made many households difficult, if not impossible, to reach. According to The Nielsen Company's National People Meter sample, 17.5% of households had no landline telephone as of September 2007. Of those, approximately 15% were cell phone-only households, and the remainder had no type of telephone in the household. Cell phone-only households tend to fall into two distinct groups: the "economically motivated," consisting of lower income households (renters/movers/students) and the "on-the-go lifestyle" group, who tend to have relatively higher incomes and are more tech savvy and/or professional people. More than half of all adults living with unrelated roommates and one-in-four adults aged 18-34 years live in cell phone–only households (Blumberg & Luke 2007). These are some of the same groups that are increasingly under-represented in current RDD landline telephone surveys (Mokdad, Link, & Hu 2007; Lambries, Oldendick, Link, & Williams, 2007). As a result, population coverage provided by landline telephones has eroded to pre-1970s levels, raising concerns about how represen-

---

[1]A secondary concern with landline-based RDD samples is that the geographic specificity of numbers in such sampling frames is declining with the advent of number portability, whereby a person can chose to "port" their landline telephone number to a cell phone or vice versa (Link, Town, & Mokdad, 2007). This allows individuals, within certain limits, to take their number from one geographic area to another; however, from an RDD sampling perspective, the number would remain in its original area code-exchange bank. The geographic mobility inherent in cell phones only exacerbates this problem as more people adopt these devices as their only means of telecommunications. There is similar concern with the growth of Voice over Internet Protocol (VoIP) as a communication medium. Although many users of VoIP telephones are accessible using standard RDD methods, a small but growing number are using VoIP for long-distance communications whereby the telephone number may be assigned to one geographic area, but the call terminates at a household outside of that area.

tative traditional telephone surveys and other data collection efforts conducted using landline telephone samples are. With the growing popularity of cell phones, this trend is expected to continue.

Differences Between Groups Based on Household Telephone Type

The growing cell phone population is of concern primarily because in a growing number of areas these individuals differ behaviorally from those in households with landlines. Based on their analysis of a February 2004 supplement to the Current Population Survey (CPS), Tucker, Brick and Meekins (2007) warned that there was a high potential for bias in telephone survey estimates that only sample from landlines and exclude cell phones. Demographic characteristics of respondents differed significantly by type of household telephone access with cell phone-only respondents being more likely to be younger, not married, and Hispanic. These differences in demographic characteristics of respondents are similar to those reported elsewhere (Blumberg, Luke, & Cynamon, 2006; Brick, Dipko, Presser, Tucker, & Yuan, 2006). Brick et al. (2006) found that topic salience and household inaccessibility resulted in substantial nonresponse bias in estimates of households by type of telephone service (landline, cell phone, or both), with topic salience (their survey focused on uses of new technologies—in particular cellular telephones) being a larger factor for households selected from a landline frame and inaccessibility being a greater concern for those sampled from a cell phone frame. Additionally, for the cell phone sample, a higher than expected proportion of respondents were from cell phone-only households. On further investigation, the researchers found differential nonresponse rates among those who use their cell phone often versus those who use their cell phone less frequently, with the latter group appearing to be more willing to complete a survey.

In a survey conducted with a sample drawn from a cell phone frame, Link, Battaglia, Frankel, Osborn, and Mokdad (2007) found that the cell phone-only households differed significantly from those with landlines in terms of key health-related behaviors (smoking, binge drinking of alcohol, and ever having had an HIV test). These differences persisted even when controls were added for other potential confounders (e.g., age, sex, race, education, marital status, children in households, and state of residence), indicating that current weighting practices in most landline surveys are insufficient to account for these differences. The unfortunate conclusion they draw is that although most landline surveys post-stratify by factors such as sex, age, race, and education, it appears that many of those in cell phone-only households are significantly different in at least some of their health problems and behaviors despite controlling for these characteristics, and that weighting to these factors does not account fully for the differences. Such differences extend to other behaviors as well, such as use of media. For example, researchers at Nielsen found that cell phone-only households watch television less frequently than do households that have a landline telephone (Link, 2007). Even when looking within certain segments of the sample, such as homes with young adults, or with residents at similar life stages, they found that households that do not have a landline telephone still watch less television than their landline counterparts.

Operational Considerations When Conducting Interviews Via Cell Phones

It may seem simple to resolve cell phone-related sampling problems by including cell phone–only homes in a research sample, but this is not a simple task. Steeh (2004) conducted one of the first survey pilot studies in 2003, attempting to sample and interview respondents by cell phone. The study focused primary on the practicability of conducting such interviews and delineating some of the operational considerations that must be addressed in such surveys, including the willingness of approximately one-in-five cell phone respondents to complete interviews of 15-minute duration over their cell phones, the requirement of developing calling rules and protocols that account for respondent safety when reached in their car or other situations in which interviewing may have been hazardous or distracting, and the need to expand the number and type of final disposition codes beyond those specified by the American Association for Public Opinion Research (AAPOR) for landline telephone surveys (AAPOR, 2008). Brick et al. (2007) reported that although conducting surveys with sampled cell phone numbers was feasible, the approach produces lower response rates than landline surveys, higher refusal rates, and lower refusal conversion rates. Moreover, they noted that although use of incentives can boost response rates, sending text messages did not improve participation.

Unfortunately, contacting and interviewing respondents via their cell phones also involves a number of operational considerations that differ from contacting and interviewing a person over a landline. Concerns include *place-shifting*, where respondents are no longer reached only in their homes, but may be located outside of the home as well, possibly driving a vehicle, which leads to concerns for the respondent's safety. There could also be an increased financial burden for respondents depending on their particular cellular plan. Although many cell phone users appear very willing to talk in all kinds of locations—including public and semiprivate places in which they are seemingly oblivious of those around them—a question of data reliability can also come into play. A survey respondent reached on a cell phone may consciously or unconsciously limit the candor and openness (and thus the accuracy) of the responses given, depending on the sensitivity of the questions being asked.

Another issue is the degree to which persons interviewed by cell phone are "cognitively engaged" in the activity. Cell phones are one of many modern tools that facilitate the "multitasking" so prominent in today's society. Not only do researchers need to be concerned about questions of safety with regard to potentially interviewing someone who is driving, but they need to be concerned as well with how respondents answer questions while engaged in other activities, such as shopping, being outdoors, or dining in a restaurant. Ideally, researchers would like respondents to be "fully engaged" mentally in the interview process and not distracted by other activities or stimuli. We know very little, however, about the conditions in which respondents find themselves when they are taking part in an interview by cell phone.

Problems associated with combining and weighting cell phone surveys extend as well to that portion of the population that has both a cell phone and a landline. Respondents who have both types of telephones and were sampled based on their landline phone differed significantly across a number of demographic characteristics from those sampled based on their cell phone number (Link et al., 2007). There also appears to be differential nonresponse among this group depending on the type of telephone on which they make and receive most of their telephone calls (Brick et al., 2006). Those sampled from a landline telephone frame are more likely to report relying more on their landline than their cell phone, whereas this finding is reversed for those sampled according to their cell phone number. As a result, for a study to be fully representative it is necessary for researchers to sample from both landline and cell phone exchanges, interviewing all cell phone households (regardless of whether they have a landline) without screening for cell-only households.

Current federal guidelines also make it impractical to conduct large-scale data-collection efforts over a cell phone. Under the federal Telemarketing Consumer Protection Act of 1991 (TCPA, 47 U.S.C. 227), which is enforced by the Federal Communications Commission, automatic telephone dialing systems cannot be used to contact a cell phone without the user's "prior express consent." This restriction applies to all forms of autodialers and predictive dialers, and applies to intrastate calls, interstate calls, and calls from outside the United States. There is also no "good faith" exception for inadvertent or accidental calls to cell phones.

Several studies have noted that even if conducting surveys by sampling cell phone numbers may be technically feasible, it is costly (Brick et al., 2006; Fleeman, 2005; Link et al., 2007; Steeh, 2004) relative to landline telephone surveys (the costs of which are already high because of the need for increased effort to achieve acceptable response rates). As a result, researchers will likely want to conduct as few cell phone interviews as possible and simply weight these responses accordingly. The difficulty at this point, however, is that there is currently no good population standard denoting telephone access below the national level (i.e., state, county, or city levels). Currently, the National Health Interview Survey provides the only external standard against which to adjust data by type of household telephone access; however, this survey only provides data down to the census region level, not the state, local, or other subnational levels (Blumberg et al., 2006). Researchers are therefore left unable to account for this factor in their weighting schemes using the internal survey data (a potentially problematic approach), or to assume that the national estimates fit equally at the subnational level and make adjustments accordingly (a dubious assumption). Neither is therefore likely to be a good solution.

Another brutal fact facing researchers is that the consistent decline in landline telephone survey response rates is a testament to the fact that a substantial percentage of the population does not want to partake in survey efforts, regardless of a study's goals. There is no reason to think that respondents on cell phones should be any different. Researchers who decide to conduct interviews by cell phone need, therefore, to tread cautiously in this area, balancing the desire to obtain valid and reliable data with the need to minimize, however possible, burden on respondents.

Testing a Revolutionary New Sampling Approach

Probability sample design alternatives to landline RDD surveys that are of comparable speed, efficiency, and cost are scarce. Face-to-face area probability surveys tend to achieve higher response rates, but the costs associated with traditional counting and listing procedures (i.e., those based on in-person methods rather than mail lists) and conducting in-person interviews are often prohibitive. Conversely, mail surveys have tended to provide a less expensive means of collecting information, yet this approach until recently has been hampered by the lack of address-based sampling frames with sufficient coverage of the general population. Likewise, Internet penetration, although fairly high (as of December 2008, an estimated 74% of American adults reported using the Internet), does not provide sufficient coverage for conducting surveys of the general adult population (Pew Internet, 2009).

Given the problems associated with cell phone sampling, interviewing, and weighting, along with the limitations of other more traditional approaches, some have chosen to take a very different path to tackling the cell phone–only problem, moving away from a reliance on telephone samples and taking advantage of the availability of large-scale address databases. Address-based sampling (ABS) is a new approach that involves the selection of a random sample of addresses from a frame of residential addresses. ABS provides researchers with a sampling methodology for surveys of the general public with comparable costs and improved coverage to RDD methodologies. Most importantly, ABS includes cell phone–only homes without having to actually call the cell phone.

In the United States, the U.S. Postal Service (USPS) has made available its Delivery Sequence File (DSF), an address file that contains all delivery addresses serviced by the USPS. Coverage assessments have found that 97% to 98% of the households in the United States have usable addresses. This list includes addresses for Post Office (PO) boxes as well as single-unit, multiunit, and other types of housing structures. Furthermore, these addresses can be reverse-matched to commercially available databases to identify a relatively large proportion of telephone numbers. Initial evaluations of the USPS address files as a means of reducing the costs associated with enumeration of primarily urban households in area probability surveys have proven to be promising (Iannacchione, Staab, & Redden, 2003; O'Muircheartaigh, Eckman, & Weiss, 2003; Staab & Iannacchione, 2004). The frame's standardized format also facilitates geocoding of addresses and linkage to other external data sources, such as the census zip code tabulation areas data. These data can be used to stratify the frame for sampling target populations.

Use of an ABS approach does have some drawbacks. Researchers cannot obtain DSF information directly from the USPS, but rather must purchase the information through a nonexclusive license agreement with private list vendors. The quality and completeness of the address information obtained from these vendors can vary significantly based on how frequently the company updates the listings, the degree to which the listings are augmented with information from other available databases, and if the company purges records based on requests from householders to not release their information (Link et al., 2005). Moreover, vendors differ in their experience with and ability to draw probability samples from the DSF list. This can be problematic for researchers who do not wish to draw their own samples and tend to rely on vendor expertise for this task. DSF coverage in rural areas also tends to be lower than in urban areas (Link et al., 2005). Additionally, in some rural areas the DSF contains simplified (i.e., city, state, and zip code–only) listings, rather than full street addresses. The percentage of these types of addresses in the database is declining, however, as local governments adopt emergency 911 protocols, which require that all households be identified with a street address. The DSF contains PO boxes and multidrop addresses (i.e., multiple persons associated with the same address), which may be problematic for in-person and telephone surveys where a street address is required to locate the household or an associated telephone number. Such addresses may be less of an issue for mail surveys.

Finally, households with multiple mailing addresses (e.g., a street address and a residential PO box) induce selection multiplicities in mail surveys. Iannacchione et al. (2003) provided some evidence that a large percentage of households with residential PO boxes in their Dallas County study also have mail delivered to their street address. In a national sample based on the DSF, however, Staab and Iannacchione (2004) were not able to develop a reliable estimate of the percent of households with a PO box that also received home mail delivery. It is likely that in some areas households with a PO box do not receive home mail delivery. This may be more likely to occur in rural areas where a PO box is provided at no cost and no home mail delivery is made. Thus, including PO boxes may be necessary to ensure coverage of all households. Despite these limitations, the DSF appears to be a promising source of information for developing sampling frames of residential addresses.

Initial evaluations of ABS as an alternative to RDD for general population surveys were conducted by the Centers for Disease Control and Prevention for use on the Behavioral Risk Factor Surveillance System (BRFSS), one of the world's largest RDD health surveys (Link et al., 2006; Link, Battaglia, Frankel, Osborne, & Mokdad, 2008). Two rounds of testing during 2005 and 2006 were conducted with households sampled from the USPS address frame, first using mail surveys, and then later utilizing mail surveys with telephone survey follow-up of nonrespondents (a mixed-mode approach). In both instances, the mail survey and mixed-mode approaches produced significantly higher response rates than those obtained in the RDD surveys in states where the RDD response rate was below 40%. For states with higher response rates, only the mixed-mode approach (and not the mail-only survey) produced higher response rates than the traditional RDD method. The ABS approach also provided access to households with only cell phones, and to a smaller degree, to households with no telephone coverage. The percentage of cell phone only households across the six states examined here was similar to the percentage reported at the national level (Blumberg et al., 2006). Respondents to the mail survey tended to be older and more educated than those interviewed in the RDD version of BRFSS; however, there tended to be few differences in the estimates obtained when the mail and telephone surveys were compared.

Nonetheless, the ABS mail survey approach had some limitations when used to conduct the BRFSS. First, improvement in response rates were obtained only in those states where the RDD response rates were low (i.e., below 40%). In North Carolina, where the RDD response rate was above 45%, the mail survey response rate was significantly lower than the telephone response rate, even when two questionnaire mailings were sent. Second, the mail survey obtained responses from a much higher percentage of non-Hispanic Whites and people who had at least some college education and from a significantly lower percentage of persons who do not live in a metropolitan statistical area (MSA) than did either the RDD survey or the CPS. This skewed distribution across these key demographic groups raises some concerns about potential bias in the estimates (see Link, Battaglia, Frankel, Osborne, & Mokdad, 2006, for more detailed analysis of this issue). Third, use of the mail survey approach would likely force some fundamental changes in the way in which a surveillance system, such as BRFSS, currently operates. Mail surveys require a longer fielding period (typically 8 weeks or more) than the current monthly schedule for the BRFSS telephone survey. Use of a mail survey would also reduce the length and flexibility of the BRFSS questionnaire. The telephone version of the BRFSS contains a core survey of 70 to 75 questions (asked in all states), optional modules of 1 to 20 questions (standardized topic modules that can be adopted by the states), and state-added question modules of 1 to 50 questions (typically unique to each state, focusing on state-specific health issues). The 2005 mail survey pilot tested only the core questionnaire. Lengthening the mail questionnaire could increase respondents' reluctance to complete the survey, and customizing each state survey to include the optional or state-added modules would significantly increase the operational complexity of administering the survey.

The study also highlighted areas where data collection efficiencies using an ABS approach may be gained. In addition to city-style addresses, it appears that inclusion of PO boxes, "throwback" addresses (i.e., city-style address where the resident has requested delivery to their PO box) and "drop-point units" (i.e., an address with multiple units) is important for both coverage and the nonignorable number of completed interviews obtained from these types of addresses. The same does not appear to apply, however, to addresses identified as vacant or seasonal by the UPSP. More than 60% of the addresses identified as vacant units were confirmed to be ineligible addresses. Although the percentage of vacant units resulting in a completed interview was relatively high in some states (20% in Washington), the number of completed interviews from this address type as a percentage of the total number of completed interviews was quite small (8 of 532 in Washington). Exclusion of vacant units from an ABS sample design is unlikely, therefore, to have a significant negative effect on coverage bias. Likewise the extremely small number of addresses designated as seasonal units argues for their exclusion as well.

Although the DSF appears to be an effective frame for conducting address-based sampling of the general population, its true potential may be in facilitating mixed-mode surveys. Cross-referencing addresses with other public data bases yielded telephone numbers for 50% to 66% of the addresses, depending on the state. Moreover, among the subset of nonrespondent cases with unknown eligibility that received two mail questionnaires, more than 60% had identifiable telephone numbers. Although additional research will be required to determine how accurately these telephone numbers match with the addresses, early indications are that conducting a telephone survey follow-up to the mail survey is quite feasible. Moreover, address-based sampling may facilitate the more cost-effective use of other interviewing modes, such as Web surveys or interactive voice response (IVR; Fricker, Galesic, Tourangeau, & Yan, 2005). Households could be sampled through an address-based frame, such as the DSF, then provided a link to a Web site, given the telephone number for an IVR survey, mailed a hardcopy questionnaire, or any combination of these approaches. For example, drawing from the work of BRFSS, the HINTS 2007 survey used a dual-frame multimode approach based on address-based sampling in an attempt to increase response rates. Like the BRFSS pilot study, the HINTS design used a telephone follow-up (when numbers were available) for mail households that did not return surveys. Additionally, the survey included some embedded experiments for mail respondents who did not initially respond including sending mail surveys in a Federal Express envelope versus a plain envelope and follow-up using either IVR, a live call, or no call.

Extending potential ABS designs further, recent studies have shown that combining telephone surveys with either Web or mail survey options can produce higher response rates in general population surveys than use of telephone alone (Link & Mokdad, 2006). Resources permitting, face-to-face surveys could also be added to this mix, particularly because use of the DSF was initially tested as a means of identifying households for such surveys (Iannacchione et al., 2003; O'Muircheartaigh et al., 2003; Staab & Iannacchione, 2004). The DSF, therefore, has the potential to serve as a sampling base for a wide variety of single or multimode survey designs.

Future research efforts should continue to evaluate the expansion of address-based coverage as more rural areas adopt city-style addresses that conform to 911 emergency number rules. Use of the DSF in particular as an ABS frame for the conduct of surveys via other modes (telephone, Web, IVR, face-to-face, etc.) as well as combinations of modes needs to be explored more fully as complements to RDD designs. Given the continued decline in RDD response rates and the increased use of cell phones it seems clear that an alternative design is needed to fill a growing gap as the new mainstay for health communication research.

CONCLUSION

Survey research conducted by telephone is at a point of transformation. The declines in coverage for the landline telephone frame, number portability, and a host of other issues lead to the inevitable conclusion that traditional RDD surveys as we know them are coming to an end. At the same time, however, the need for survey data has never been greater, with a desire for subnational or local-level data being in high demand but short supply. To meet this need, researchers will need to find alternative, cost-effective ways of sampling from the general public. This may involve sampling of cell phones along side landline telephone numbers in a dual-frame solution. Or it could mean abandoning the sampling of telephone numbers altogether and moving to an ABS solution. Either approach is complex and not without its drawbacks. Approaches are available or being forged that will help shape the future of survey research in this regard, ensuring that timely, cost-effective, scientifically valid data continue to be collected to further our understanding of public health concerns.

REFERENCES

American Association for Public Opinion Research. (2008). *Standard definitions: Final dispositions of case codes and outcome rates for surveys* (5th ed.). Lenexa, KS: Author.

Brick, J. M., Dipko, S., Presser, S., Tucker, C., & Yuan, Y. (2006). Nonresponse bias in a dual frame sample of cell and landline numbers. *Public Opinion Quarterly, 70,* 780-793.

Brick, J. M., Brick, P. D., Dipko, S., Presser, S., Tucker, C., & Yuan, Y. (2007). Cell phone survey feasibility in the U.S.: Sampling and calling cell numbers versus landline numbers. *Public Opinion Quarterly, 71,* 23-39.

Blumberg, S., & Luke, J. V. (2007). Wireless substitution: Early release of estimates based on data from the National Health Interview Survey, July–December 2006. Retrieved July 24, 2009, from http://www.cdc.gov/nchs/data/nhis/earlyrelease/wireless200705.pdf.

Blumberg, S., Luke J. V., & Cynamon, M. L. (2006). Telephone coverage and health survey estimates: Evaluating the need for concern about wireless substitution. *American Journal of Public Health, 96,* 926–931.

Blumberg, S., Luke J. V., Cynamon, M. L., & Frankel, M. (2007). Recent trends in household telephone coverage in the United States. In J. Lepkowski, C. Tucker, M. Brick, E. De Leeuw, L. Japec, P. Lavrakas, M. Link, & R. Sangster (Eds.), *Advances in telephone survey methodology* (pp. 56-86). Hoboken, NJ: Wiley.

Curtin, R., Presser, S., & Singer, E. (2005). Changes in telephone survey nonresponse over the past quarter century. *Public Opinion Quarterly, 69,* 87-98.

Fleeman, A. (2006). *Merging cellular and landline RDD sample frames: A series of three cell phone studies.* Paper presented at the second International Conference on Telephone Survey Methodology, Miami, FL.

Fricker, S., Galesic, M., Tourangeau, R., & Yan, T. (2005). An experimental comparison of web and telephone surveys. *Public Opinion Quarterly, 69,* 370-392.

Iannacchione, V. G., Staab, J. M., & Redden, D. T. (2003). Evaluating the use of residential mailing addresses in a metropolitan household survey. *Public Opinion Quarterly, 76,* 202-210.

Lambries, D., Oldendick, R. W., Link, M. W., & Williams, L. (2007). *Young people may not be in jail, but most are in cells: Cross-time impact of changes in phone use on telephone survey representativeness.* Paper presented at the 62nd annual conference of the American Association for Public Opinion Research, Anaheim, CA.

Link, M. W. (2007). Cutting the cord: Reaching the cell phone-only household. *Nielsen Consumer Insight*. Retrieved November 20, 2007, from http://www.nielsen. com/consumer_insight/ci_story5.html

Link, M. W., Battaglia, M., Frankel, M., Osborn, L., & Mokdad, A. (2006). Address-based versus random-digit dialed surveys: Comparison of key health and risk indicators. *American Journal of Epidemiology, 164*, 1019-1025.

Link, M. W., Battaglia, M., Frankel, M., Osborn, L., & Mokdad, M. W. (2007). Reaching the cell phone generation: Comparison of U.S. cell phone survey results with an ongoing landline telephone survey. *Public Opinion Quarterly, 71*, 814-839.

Link, M. W., Battaglia, M., Frankel, M., Osborn, L., & Mokdad, A. (2008). Comparison of address based sampling (ABS) versus random-digit dialing (RDD) for general population surveys. *Public Opinion Quarterly, 72*, 6-27.

Link, M. W., Battaglia, M., Giambo, P., Frankel, M., Mokdad, A., & Rao, R. S. (2005). *Assessment of address frame replacements for RDD sampling frames.* Paper presented at the 2005 annual conference of the American Association for Public Opinion Research, Miami Beach, FL.

Link, M., and Mokdad, A. (2006). "Can Web and Mail Survey Modes Improve Participation in an RDD-based National Health Surveillance?" *Journal of Official Statistics, 22*, 293-312.

Link, M. W., Town, M., Mokdad, A. (2007). Telephone number portability and the prevalence of cell phone numbers in random digit-dialed survey samples. *International Journal of Public Opinion Research, 19*, 504-511.

Mokdad, A., Link, M. W., & Hu, S. (2007). *Where are we losing respondents? Trends in survey eligibility and participation.* Paper presented at the 62nd annual conference of the American Association for Public Opinion Research, Anaheim, CA.

O'Muircheartaigh, C., Eckman, S., & Weiss, C. (2003). Traditional and enhanced field listing for probability sampling. In *Proceedings of the American Statistical Association, Survey Methodology Section* (CD-ROM) (2563-2567). Alexandria, VA: American Statistical Association.

Pew Internet (2009). Generational differences in online activities. Pew Internet & American Life Project. Retrieved July 24, 2009, from http://www.pewinternet.org/Infographics/Generational-differences-in-online-activities.aspx

Staab, J. M., & Iannacchione, V. G. (2004). Evaluating the use of residential mailing addresses in a national household survey. In *Proceedings of the American Statistical Association, Survey Methodology Section* (CD-ROM). Alexandria, VA: American Statistical Association.

Steeh, C. (2004). *A new era for telephone surveys.* Paper presented at the annual meeting of the American Association for Public Opinion Research, Phoenix, AZ.

Steeh, C., Krigis, N., Cannon, B., & DeWitt, J. (2001). Are they really as bad as they seem? Nonresponse rates at the end of the twentieth century. *Journal of Official Statistics, 17*, 227-247.

Tucker, C.J., Brick, J.M., & Meekins, B. (2007). Household telephone service and usage patterns in the United States in 2004: Implications for telephone samples. *Public Opinion Quarterly, 71*, 3-22.

6

TWO APPROACHES TO ADDRESS NONRESPONSE

A Case Study With the Health Information National Trends Survey

David Cantor
Westat and Joint Program
for Survey Methodology

The Health Information National Trends Survey (HINTS) is a random-digit dial (RDD) survey that was administered in 2003, 2005, and 2007. This time period spans a dramatic change in the climate of conducting general population surveys, especially those using an RDD sample frame. Response rates for RDD surveys began a steady decline in the 1990s and continued to drop through 2008 (e.g., Battaglia et al., 2007; Curtin et al., 2005). This has threatened the quality of RDD surveys, while at the same time increasing the level of effort needed to implement these surveys.

This chapter illustrates two different strategies that can be used to address nonresponse. One strategy is to minimize the nonresponse. This is the traditional approach and attempts to reduce the possibility of error. The second strategy is to assess the effects of nonresponse on survey estimates. This approach emphasizes the idea that nonresponse error occurs only when the mechanisms for nonresponse are related to the phenomena being studied. It is therefore important to understand this relationship when interpreting the implications of nonresponse.

The goal of the chapter is to illustrate why it is important to use both strategies. This is achieved by illustrating how these two strategies were applied for use in the HINTS. When combined, these strategies provide information on not only what error might be associated with the estimates, but what survey procedures might be leading to nonresponse error.

The nonresponse-related research for HINTS includes several experiments that were used to guide the survey design. Unlike larger surveys, the HINTS does not have the resources to conduct pilot studies to test new methodologies. It was possible, however, to develop and embed studies within the early stages of the HINTS production samples. The information from these studies was used to guide decisions for later sample waves, as well as the design for subsequent collection periods. Using this strategy, several new methodologies were developed and tested. These included the use of incentives and the use of multiple modes of interviewing.

In addition to trying to minimize nonresponse, research also included an analysis of response rates and its implications on nonresponse bias for the HINTS estimates. Between 2003 and 2005, there was a significant drop in the HINTS response rate. Low response rates increase the likelihood that an estimate is significantly biased. However, response rates are not directly correlated with nonresponse bias (see, e.g., Groves, 2006); it depends on the extent the propensity to respond is correlated with the estimates of interest. In order to understand the effects of nonresponse for HINTS, it was necessary to assess how it affects the specific estimates that are of interest to the survey.

This chapter describes the research just discussed, along with the changes that were made in light of the research in developing the third survey cycle.

METHODS TO REDUCE NONRESPONSE: INCENTIVES

As just noted, a direct response to declining response rates is to try to reduce nonresponse. There are many ways to do this (Groves et al., 2004). One of the most reliable methods is to use incentives to increase respondent motivation. During the late 1990s, a number of RDD surveys experimented with incentives. The results were somewhat mixed, depending on the type of incentive offered. The major complications relate to how the incentive is offered (pre-paid vs. promised) and the amount offered.

Prior research has found that an incentive that is pre-paid at the time the survey request is made is consistently more effective than an incentive that is contingent on the respondent completing a survey (Singer, 2002). However, an RDD survey is constrained in how an incentive can be introduced. A pre-paid incentive is possible when trying to complete the initial screening interview. The incentive can be provided in the advance letter, which is sent to the household prior to making the initial call to the unit. Once the screening interview is completed and a respondent is selected, the interviewer then tries to complete the main interview with the person who was randomly selected as the respondent. Because there is no natural break in the administration process, it is not possible to provide an incentive to the selected individual prior to the request to do the main survey. It is only possible to offer a promised incentive that is contingent on the respondent completing the questionnaire.

Based on prior research, HINTS 2003 tested an incentive that pre-paid sampled households a token amount of money prior to making any telephone contact. HINTS 2005 tested an incentive that promised sampled respondents money if they completed the main HINTS interview.[1] Both of these tests were completed during each respective data-collection effort. The results from these experiments were used to design the incentive strategies at later points in time.

Pre-Paid Incentives at the Screening Interview

The incentive experiment in 2003 tested a $2 pre-paid incentive to complete the screening interview. In order to send the incentive, it was first necessary to match the sampled telephone numbers to a database that was linked to an address. This address was used to send out an advance letter to the household. This letter included the $2 incentive. It was not possible to match all telephone numbers in the sample to an address. As discussed in Cantor, O'Hare, and O'Connor (2007), the matching process cannot be completed for approximately 20% to 30% of the residential addresses in an RDD sample. The results described here provide response rates for that portion of the sample that had a matched address.

The experimental design included sending an incentive at both the initial mailing and at refusal conversion. Refusal conversion is a procedure that involves calling back households that initially refuse to do the interview. When making the call, the interviewer asks the person answering the phone to reconsider his or her decision. The call is made after waiting a short period of time (e.g., 2 weeks) and is preceded by a letter that provides the household with more information about the study. The incentive for refusal conversion was included in this second letter.

If successful, an incentive at refusal conversion is more efficient, because it does not go to those who initially agree to do the interview. The procedure is somewhat controversial, as it seemingly rewards those who engage in negative behavior (i.e., refusing). Nonetheless, it is consistent with theories related to respondent behavior (e.g., Groves, Singer, & Corning, 2000), which point to differences across respondents for reasons to participate in a survey. With two different incentive levels ($0 and $2), this resulted in four experimental groups:

---

[1]Hereafter referred to as the "extended interview."

1. $0 at initial contact, $0 at refusal conversion
2. $2 at initial contact, $0 at refusal conversion
3. $0 at initial contact, $2 at refusal conversion
4. $2 at initial contact, $2 at refusal conversion

The response rates for both the screener and extended interview are provided in Table 6.1. There is a statistically significant ($p < .05$) effect of the incentive at the initial contact on screener response rates (top panel, 57.6 vs. 62.3). The difference for the incentive at refusal conversion is not statistically significant. The second panel provides the effects of these treatments on the extended interview response rates. This tests the possibility that the effects of the incentives provided at the screener carry over to increasing the cooperation at the extended level. This did seem to occur for the incentives sent prior to the initial contact. The extended rate was increased from 59% to 64.5% ($p < .05$). The overall effect was to increase the response rate by approximately 6 percentage points (34% vs. 40.2%).

One reason to increase response rates is to minimize the threat of nonresponse bias. The assumption is that the lower the response rate, the greater the chance of significant bias. To evaluate if the incentive had a significant

TABLE 6.1. Response Rates by Experimental Group

	No Incentive	$2 Incentive	Difference	Standard error	Lower Bound CI	Upper Bound CI
Screener						
Initial contact	57.6%	62.3%	4.7%	1.6%	1.5%	7.8%
Refusal conversion	59.0%	60.9%	2.0%	1.3%	−0.7%	4.6%
Interaction			1.1%	1.4%	−1.6%	3.9%
Extended interview						
Initial contact	59.0%	64.5%	5.5%	2.1%	1.2%	9.8%
Refusal conversion	60.7%	63.0%	2.3%	2.3%	−2.3%	6.8%
Interaction			−1.0%	1.8%	−4.7%	2.6%
Overall no—advance to advance	34.0%	40.2%	6.2%	1.7%	2.9%	9.5%
Overall no— refusal to refusal	35.8%	38.4%	2.6%	2.6%	−2.6%	7.7%
Overall interaction			0.1%	1.4%	−2.7%	2.8%

CI, confidence interval
Source. Rizzo, Park, Hesse, and Willis (2004)

effect on nonresponse bias, the analysis compared a large number of survey outcomes of interest to HINTS across the experimental groups. With a few exceptions, this analysis did not find significant differences. Given the effect of the incentive was only about 6 percentage points, this finding is not surprising (e.g., Groves, 2006).

Promised Incentives

Following the 2003 experiment, an incentive experiment was conducted within HINTS 2005 that promised an incentive to respondents selected to complete the main interview. As noted previously, a promised incentive has not been found to be as effective as a pre-paid incentive. According to Dillman (2000), once promised an incentive, the respondent begins to view the offer as an economic exchange, rather than a token expression of appreciation. Once it shifts in this way, the amount of money that is promised will likely have to be higher than what one would offer with a pre-paid incentive. On the telephone, this promise may also introduce questions about the credibility of the survey. For example, it might be difficult to distinguish between a promise of money to complete a survey from a marketing solicitation (which often gets attention by offering prizes and money).

Promised incentives do have several advantages. One is that it is the only way to provide an incentive to respondents to complete the extended interview. As noted earlier, the sequencing of the survey is such that there isn't an opportunity to send money in advance of requesting to do the extended interview. There should also be an increased chance that a promise would work at the extended interview (vis-à-vis the screener) given that, at this point, someone in the household has already completed the screening interview and there is some rapport built up with the interviewer. There is a greater opportunity to explain the study and provide a rationale for offering money. Another advantage of a promised incentive is that it can be offered to all respondents. A pre-paid incentive requires an address, which is only available for a portion of the RDD sample.

HINTS 2005 experimented with three different promised incentive groups—$0, $5, and $15. At the time of the experiment, there had not been a great deal of research on this type of incentive. Of the research that had been conducted, $15 seemed to be the minimum amount needed to measure a significant effect. At least one experiment had shown that this amount may not be high enough. Nonetheless, the amount of research in this area was limited. In combination with the financial constraints on the HINTS budget, it was decided to test a $15 incentive and to evaluate whether amounts less than $15 would be effective.

The results of this experiment were promising after the initial contacts with respondents were made. The response rate after the initial contact for those in the $15 group was 55% compared with 49% for the $0 and $5 groups ($p < .05$). However, after refusal conversion was carried out, this difference disappeared. The final response rates were 62%, 60%, and 61% for the $0, $5, and $15 groups, respectively. The incentive provided some additional motivation to respondents who might otherwise be nonrespondents at the initial contact. After going through refusal conversion, these individuals eventually agreed to complete the interview without an incentive.

Design Decisions on Incentives and Implications

The research described here on pre-paid and promised incentives was used in the plans for HINTS 2005 and 2007. The success of a pre-paid incentive in 2003 led to decisions to use it in 2005 and 2007. The anticipated increase in response rates at the screener, as well as the possibility of a carry-over effect at the extended interview was the primary reason to adopt the procedure. A pre-paid incentive for refusal conversion was not adopted. The projected gain in response rate did not seem worth the added expense. It was also unclear whether this type of incentive could be implemented on a federal survey, as it might be perceived as being inequitable.

The results from the experiment on promised incentives were used to recommend that it not be used for HINTS 2007. It was decided that if the amount was $15 or less an incentive would not significantly increase response rates. However, if $20 or more was offered, the question of using a promised incentive could be reconsidered, perhaps by including experimental manipulations that tested larger amounts (e.g., $25, $30).

The experiments described here illustrate the traditional approach when addressing problems of nonresponse. Namely, by trying to reduce nonresponse, it may be possible to limit the possibility of nonresponse error. This also provides a way to implement a more efficient survey process. By boosting the response rate, interviewers will make fewer calls to collect data and less time will be spent in the field. On the other hand, this study illustrates the difficulty in trying to reduce nonresponse in a meaningful way. According to the experiments, pre-paid incentives were effective, but they only raised response rates by around 5 percentage points. Although this boost is welcome, it was not enough to prevent continued decline in response rates over the first two administrations of HINTS.

Furthermore, the pre-paid incentive did not have effects on the estimates made from HINTS. The recommendation to implement the pre-paid incentive was based largely on the desire to reduce or halt the drop in response rates. However, as researchers have increasingly become aware, it is important to consider not only the level of the response rate, but also how rates are related to the reasons for nonresponse. In the section on assessing the effects of nonresponse, this point is discussed in more detail and an analysis of nonresponse bias is provided.

Methods to Reduce Nonresponse: Use of a Web Survey

Another method that might reduce nonresponse is to give more flexibility on how one can respond to the survey. Of particular interest was determining whether it was possible to give respondents an opportunity to fill out the survey on the Web. Access to the Web was steadily increasing over this time period and it was the hope that some individuals would prefer to complete the survey online rather than by telephone. The Web also offers some advantages from a data-quality perspective. For example, completing the survey online would enable respondents to provide better data on items that are considered sensitive or are subject to social desirability bias (de Leeuw, 2005). Finally, if a large number of people fill out the survey online, significant amounts of money could be saved.

In HINTS 2005 an experiment was conducted that gave respondents the option to fill out a Web survey, rather than completing a telephone survey. The intent of this procedure was to provide respondents with more flexibility in how they could respond to the survey. The hypothesis was that more flexibility would lead to a higher response rate, especially for respondents in the younger age groups who are more accustomed to using the Web. Prior attempts to conduct general population surveys using the Web had not been particularly successful. For example, experiments with the American Community Survey (ACS; Griffin, Fischer, & Morgan, 2002) and Census 2000 (Schneider et al., 2005) found it difficult to get a significant proportion of the sample to use the Web. These studies had been conducted as part of the mail procedures that are used on the ACS and Census 2000. With HINTS, the plan was to recruit individuals when making the call into the household. In combination with the growth of access to the Web, it was decided to try offering the Web as a means of completing the HINTS 2005 survey.

Conducting a general population survey using the Web has a number of challenges. One of the most important is that it is restricted to those who have access to this mode of interview. At the time of HINTS 2005, this was estimated to be approximately 65% to 70% of the population. Sampling those who have access to the Web also is a challenge. There is no list of households or individuals from which to sample (Link, Chap. 5, this volume). The invitation to participate in the survey has to be done through another mode, such as through the mail or over the telephone.

HINTS 2005 was designed to initially use the telephone to recruit respondents to use the Web. Using the RDD sample frame, the household was contacted using the same methods as for the telephone interview. When contacted, respondents were asked if they had access to the Web. If they did, they were then asked if they wanted to complete the survey online or by telephone. Those choosing Web were given the material needed to access the survey. A follow-up letter also was sent with the contact information. After waiting several weeks, if a response was not received via the Web, the respondent was called back and the survey was administered over the telephone.

Other approaches were considered. One was to mail households a request to complete the survey online. There were two significant issues with this approach. First, it left the respondent selection procedure in the control of the respondent. Unless all household members were asked to fill out the survey, this could result in significant bias to the study. Second, this method relied on the ability to conduct nonrespondent follow-up by telephone. However, as noted earlier, for a significant percentage of households no telephone number was available. Perhaps the most important reason for rejecting this approach was that it was not expected to yield a large number of individuals filling out the survey online. Prior experiments asking persons to fill out a survey online via a mail solicitation had not been particularly successful (Griffin et al., 2002; Schneider et al., 2005).

In HINTS 2005, we experimented with the Web procedure using two groups. One group was given the option to use the Web, if they had access. The second group was administered the normal procedures using the telephone. The experiment was conducted during the first part of the survey field period. A decision to continue the experiment during the second part of the field period was made as the results were analyzed.

As noted above, respondents were first screened as to whether they had access to the Web. The experiment found that of those who had access, approximately 50% who were given the choice said they would complete the survey online. The main reasons respondents reported for using the Web (Table 6.2) are consistent with the intent of giving respondents the choice. They preferred the convenience of the Web, as well as the possibility that it would take less time. Those who chose not to use the Web had some privacy concerns, but some experienced logistical problems related to the computer and its location.

Response rates for the Web group were significantly below the rates for those who were asked to complete the survey by telephone. The lower rate for the choice group was due to those individuals who stated they would complete the survey on the Web, but never completed an interview. Approximately 41% of those who selected the Web completed it in this mode. The remainder had to be called back, with only 20% completing it by telephone. The remaining 39% did not complete at all. As might be expected from this result, the cost of completing a Web survey was higher than

TABLE 6.2. Reasons Respondents Gave for Choosing Web or Telephone

CHOOSING THE WEB	CHOOSING THE TELEPHONE
• Convenience	• Privacy concerns with the Web
• Less time	• Slow computer connection
• Too long on the phone	• Computer is at work
	• Like doing the survey with a person
	• Would not end up doing the survey

expected. Most of this cost was related to the need to call back respondents who said they would complete the interview by the Web.

One explanation for these results is that many of those who chose the Web may have postponed the task of actually completing the survey. Once postponing it, many eventually neglected it entirely. Data from the Web survey indicated that most respondents who logged onto the Web survey did complete an interview. The drop off of response seemed to be from respondents who never visited the Web site. It may also have been the case that agreeing to fill out the survey online was a form of passive refusal. Respondents could avoid doing the survey without having to explain to the interviewer that they did not want to participate in the study.

The results from this experiment are consistent with several other experiments that were conducted around the same time as the HINTS. In a survey conducted by the Centers for Disease Control and Prevention (Link et al., 2005), approximately 15% of households responded by Web when sent a solicitation by mail.[2] This was well below the response achieved by a comparable mail survey. Fricker et al. (2005) used a similar design to HINTS 2005 and found it was very difficult to recruit persons to use the Web, even when a significant incentive was offered to do it in this mode.

Based on the HINTS and other experiences just cited, there are significant barriers to convert the flexibility afforded by the Web to motivating respondents to carry out the task using this mode. The latest research shows that currently mail and even telephone surveys seem to work better for a general population. One difference between the methods is the extent respondents have to take the initiative to complete the survey. To use the Web, respondents have to go to the computer, log onto the computer, get to the correct Web site, and put in an identification number. Problems at any of these steps will result in nonresponse. For a mail survey, the respondent needs to open and fill out the survey and mail it back. By virtue of opening the mail, the respondent has at least completed the first of these steps.

---

[2]This survey allowed anyone in the household to fill out the Web survey.

There are, of course, many other potential virtues of a Web survey. In comparison to a mail survey, a Web survey allows automation of the flow of the instrument. Perhaps more importantly, it is less expensive than a mail survey, especially as sample sizes get larger. Consequently it is in the interest of future surveys to investigate methods of integrating the Web as it becomes a larger part of everyday communication.

This experiment provided much useful information on practical issues with using the Web to implement a general population survey. However, in terms of reducing nonresponse, the experiment was not informative. This underscores the point made in the previous section: Implementing methods to increase the response rate may have limited effects. This last point is driven home by the fact that despite all of the efforts, the continuing erosion of response rates associated with RDD surveys was reflected on HINTS 2003 and 2005. The HINTS 2003 response rate was 33%, which was within the range of many other RDD surveys completed in the same time period. Nonetheless, this is significantly less than response rates for surveys conducted in the early 1990s. The overall HINTS 2005 response rate dropped 13 percentage points to around 20%, despite the use of a $2 pre-paid incentive. The implication is that it would have been even lower if the incentive had not been used. Regardless, this trend raises a concern for the quality of the estimates. The issue faced by analysts of HINTS, and similar RDD surveys, is assessing the implications these response rates have for data quality —in particular nonresponse bias.

ASSESSING THE EFFECTS OF NONRESPONSE

The second strategy to address nonresponse is to try to estimate the extent that it is leading to error in the estimates of interest. The response rate is not a direct indicator of nonresponse error. The size of the error depends on the level of nonresponse, and the extent that respondents differ from non-respondents for the outcome measures of interest. It is important to consider the effects of nonresponse for each survey outcome. Groves (2006) provide a summary of a series of nonresponse bias studies that show a number of outcomes with minimal bias and high nonresponse, as well as high bias and low nonresponse. Nonetheless, this analysis does show that as the response rate decreases, the number of measures that exhibit high bias increases.

In this section, I discuss nonresponse bias analysis conducted for HINTS. Two types of analyses were conducted: (a) comparing estimates to a "benchmark"—an external data source with better and/or different error properties; and (b) examining variation in measures by the level of effort (LOE) used to complete an interview.

Benchmarking Analysis

For the benchmarking analysis, selected estimates from HINTS 2005 were compared with estimates from the 2005 Current Population Survey (CPS) and the 2005 National Health Interview Survey (NHIS). The CPS has a response rate above 90% and is used as the benchmark for estimates of population totals for different demographic groups. NHIS has a response rate of 69% for the adult sample. Because the NHIS data are collected through a personal household interview, the survey also has better coverage relative to HINTS, especially of younger age groups, minority groups, and those without landline telephones.

Table 6.3 provides the age, sex, and race-ethnicity distributions for HINTS 2005 and the CPS. The HINTS overrepresents the older age groups relative to the younger age groups. For example, 22% of the HINTS 2005 respondents were 18 to 34 years old compared with 31% for the CPS. Similarly, the HINTS 2005 underrepresents males (36% vs. 48%) and slightly underrepresents Blacks.

These differentials reflect both failure in survey coverage (i.e., failure of the initial sample to fully represent the intended population), and nonresponse. In 2005, a significant proportion of the national population relied exclusively on cell phones. The RDD frame does not include telephone numbers for cell phones. Consequently, the HINTS survey underrepresents those who exclusively rely on cell phones. This underrepresentation is most dramatic for the younger age groups. Blumberg and Luke (2007) estimated that by the end of 2005, 7.7% of adults were living in households with only wireless service. However, this percentage is much higher for adults aged 18 to 24 (17.5%) and adults aged 25 to 29 (19.8%).

TABLE 6.3. Demographic Comparison of HINTS 2005 and CPS

	HINTS 2005	CPS
AGE		
18-34	22%	31%
65+	23%	16%
Gender		
Male	36%	48%
Ethnicity-Race		
Non-Hispanic White	74%	70%
Non-Hispanic Black	8%	11%

Discrepancies by age are important for HINTS because health and concerns related to health are correlated with age. The older the person, the more likely he or she will have some type of health-related problem. To compensate for the demographic differences just illustrated, the final survey weights for HINTS were adjusted to bring the final population totals in line with the CPS. The adjusted survey estimates will be biased to the extent that this adjustment does not capture differences between respondents and non-respondents within the demographic groups. For example, if 18- to 24-year-olds who responded to the survey access health information about cancer in a different way than those within that age range who did not respond, then the adjustment would not fully compensate for the underrepresentation of this age group on the survey.

A more direct measure of bias compares the fully weighted HINTS 2005 estimates to the NHIS for survey outcomes that are common between the two surveys. The NHIS included a number of health-related measures that also were included on HINTS 2005. When comparing estimates for the two surveys, there are several differences of note (Table 6.4). As one might expect from the demographic comparisons, HINTS respondents were generally less healthy than respondents to the NHIS. Compared with the NHIS, the proportion of people who self-reported to have good or excellent health in HINTS is approximately 11 percentage points lower. In all the measures about negative emotions, the HINTS estimates are significantly higher. The HINTS survey also appears to have included relatively more smokers and more people with cancer.

TABLE 6.4. Comparison of HINTS 2005 and NHIS Estimates on Health and Health Service Measures

HEALTH AND HEALTH SERVICE MEASURES	HINTS 2005 ESTIMATES (%)	NHIS ESTIMATES (%)	HINTS– NHIS (%)
In good or excellent health	76.3	87.6	−11.3
Feeling sad some, most, or all of the time	19.4	11.4	8.0
Feeling nervous some, most, or all the time	30.3	15.6	14.7
Smoked 100+ cigarettes in life time	47.2	42.1	5.1
Ever had cancer	11.3	7.3	4.0
Having access to health insurance	83.5	84.9	−1.4
Never visited a doctor in the past 12 months	16.4	18.6	−2.2

Level of Effort Analysis

The benchmarking analysis sheds light on the demographic and health-related characteristics of nonrespondents on the HINTS. However, the key outcome variables on HINTS are related to information-seeking behavior, for which no external data can be used as a benchmark. One way to target the analysis to these more important variables is through an analysis by the LOE needed to complete an interview. The basis of this type of analysis is the assumption that those who require more effort to be contacted and interviewed are more likely to resemble those who are not interviewed at all. Using this logic, if there is a difference in outcome measures by the effort expended to complete the interview, there is evidence of bias in the estimates.

The analysis uses two measures of LOE. One is the length of time the sampled case was in the field. The second measure of LOE is the respondent's willingness to cooperate, once contacted. The first is a measure of the effects of nonresponse that is due to not being able to contact the respondent. The second is a measure of the effects of nonresponse that is due to direct refusals. It is useful to separate these two sources of nonresponse because they are due to different processes. Noncontact is largely a function of how difficult it is to reach an individual (e.g., how often at home; whether the respondent answers his or her telephone). Refusal is a function of the respondents' attitudes to doing surveys, as well as their interest in the particular topic of the survey.

Analysis by Length of Field Period. During the field period for HINTS 2005, sample cases were released in batches. Each batch was a cross-section of the total sample. As the field period progressed, yield from the initial sample was significantly lower than expected. In order to collect the desired number of completed interviews, some of the batch groups were released relatively late in the field period. Batch groups released late in the field period were not subject to as many callbacks as those released early. This had a significant effect on the screener level response rate and accounts for some of the drop in response rate between HINTS 2003 and HINTS 2005.

To analyze outcomes by the effort to contact the respondent, three groups were formed according to how long the sample was in the field. The longer the case was in the field, the more effort (and attempts to contact) was made to complete an interview. In the discussion here, these three groups are referred to as the high (Group 1), middle (Group 2), and low (Group 3) groups. The high group corresponds to the cases where the most effort was expended. The other two groups correspond to the middle and lowest levels of effort expended, respectively. Each of these groups represents a random sample of the total sample released for interviewing.

A case in Group 3 received an average of five calls at the screener level, whereas Group 1 received, on average, approximately seven calls. As expected, the screener level response rates were positively associated with the length of field period, as indicated by the difference of 8.6 percentage points between Groups 1 and 3. The response rates at the extended interview level were not noticeably different.

In the analysis of LOE to contact respondents, estimates from the groups were compared using the base weights.[3] Thirty-five communication and health communication variables were selected for the analysis. There were few significant differences between the batch groups representing different LOE. For many of those that were significant, the differences were not large. When comparing Group 1 and Group 3, 6 of the 35 variables were statistically significant at the 0.05 level (Table 6.5). These six variables represent four different questionnaire items. Group 3 members were more likely to read the newspaper, less likely to use the Web to search for cancer information, and more likely to ask their provider about cancer.

TABLE 6.5. Significant Differences in Communication Variables by Length of Field Period

	HIGH	LOW	HIGH–LOW
Number of days reads newspaper	3.8	4.1	-0.3
Read newspaper 7 days a week (%)	36.3	43.0	-6.7
Most recent search for cancer information —printed material (%)	18.2	14.6	3.6
Cancer information was too hard to understand (mean)+	2.7	2.0	0.7
Where would you first go for cancer information—Internet (%)	25.7	31.1	-5.4
Where would you first go for cancer information—provider (%)	58.7	55.3	3.4

+1 = *strongly agree*, 2 = *agree*, 3 = *disagree*, 4 = *strongly disagree*

[3]Comparisons using the final weights were also done. There were no significant differences for the communication-related variables between the base and fully adjusted weights.

Analysis of Level of Cooperation. A second measure of LOE was whether respondents initially refused to do the interview. As noted earlier, the reasons why someone refuses are typically different from why an individual cannot be contacted (Groves et al., 2004). Consequently, it is useful to use the level of cooperation by respondents as a second measure of LOE. This is done by comparing estimates of those who completed the interview after initially refusing with those who initially cooperated (i.e., who never refused).

Approximately 30% of the respondents who were interviewed had initially refused the interview. Nonresponse was highest for the respondent screening process. Among the converted refusers to either the screener or the main interview, approximately 66% had initially refused the screener. The remainder of the converted cases refused extended interviews. There were very few cases that initially refused both the screener and the extended interview.

When comparing key measures for those who initially refused to those who never refused reveals a large number of differences (Table 6.6). Of the 62 communication, health communication, and health-related variables that were examined, 28 were statistically significant ($p < .05$). The differences are also generally larger than those related to the length of the field period. A number of the differences between the ever-refused and the never-refused are greater than 10%. Those who refused are generally less likely to be looking for cancer information; less likely to be looking on the Web; and less likely to have had a pap smear, hysterectomy, or ever heard of human papillomavirus (HPV).

There is a pattern of larger differences for those who refused the extended interview relative to those who refused the screening interview. For example, 54% of those who never refused either the screener or the extended interview reported seeking cancer information, compared with 50% for those who refused the screening interview and 42% who refused to do the extended interview. We speculate that these differences are related to the amount of information provided to respondents at each stage of the process. There is generally not enough time to provide detail about the survey when administering the screening interview. Respondents generally refuse within the first few seconds of the call without knowing much about the content of the survey. In contrast, when administering the extended interview, interviewers have time to explain the survey. With survey-specific knowledge, respondents' attitudes toward the topic may influence cooperation. Those who are least concerned or interested in cancer and/or health-related communications may be the least motivated to cooperate. This is consistent with Leverage-Salience theory (Groves et al., 2000), which predicts that topic salience will influence the decision to participate, such that respondents will be more likely to participate when the topic is personally salient.

TABLE 6.6 Survey Measures by Refusal Status

DEMOGRAPHICS
Percent age 18-34
Percent age 65+
Percent non-Hispanic Black
Percent non-Hispanic White
Percent with income $100K or more
Percent retired
Percent employed
Tenure
Percent in single-person household

COMMUNICATION
Percent with Internet
Number of days/week read newspaper
Percent read newspaper 7 days/week
Number of days watch national news
Number of days/week watch local news

HEALTH COMMUNICATION
Percent trust doctor a lot[a]
Percent trust health information in magazines a lot
Percent seeking cancer information for self
Percent who had self or someone else seeking cancer information
Percent someone else seeks cancer information for respondent
Of those seeking cancer information, percent using the Internet
Percent who would first go to the Internet to seek cancer information
Percent who would first go to their provider to seek cancer information

HEALTH CARE AND SERVICES
Number of times/day eat fruit (average)
Percent that had a papsmear[b]
Percent that had a hysterectomy[b]
Percent with health insurance
Percent that did not see a provider in last 12 months
Percent that have heard of HPV

HPV, human papillomavirus
[a]Percent difference between Never refused and ever refused.
 Computed as [(ever-never)/never] x 100
[b]Difference between ever refused and never refused is not statistically significant
 at .05. Difference between of never refused and either refusal at screener or refusal
 at extended is significant at $p < .05$

NEVER REFUSED	REFUSED			PERCENT DIFFERENCE[a]
	SCREENER	EXTENDED	EVER	
24%	22%	15%	20%	-16%
20%	25%	31%	27%	34%
9%	7%	3%	6%	-33%
73%	75%	82%	77%	5%
28%	31%	32%	31%	12%
19%	22%	26%	23%	23%
48%	43%	44%	44%	-9%
71%	73%	80%	75%	6%
16%	13%	13%	13%	-18%
62%	29%	59%	57%	-7%
3.8	4.2	4.2	4.2	9%
39%	43%	43%	43%	11%
4.3	4.6	4.5	4.6	5%
4.5	4.9	4.7	4.9	7%
70%	69%	63%	63%	-4%
21%	20%	15%	18%	-14%
54%	50%	42%	48%	-12%
57%	54%	45%	51%	-10%
32%	28%	22%	26%	-20%
41%	28%	43%	33%	-21%
31%	28%	23%	26%	-14%
55%	59%	62%	60%	-10%
1.3	0.9	1.1	1.0	-23%
67%	67%	57%	64%	-5%
26%	22%	27%	23%	-11%
85%	88%	86%	88%	3%
14%	11%	11%	11%	-25%
40%	37%	29%	34%	-15%

Those least likely to respond also seem to be more likely to rely on traditional media. They are slightly more likely to read the newspaper, watch TV news, and less likely to use the Internet. With respect to health communications, they are less likely to use the Internet to look for cancer information and more likely to visit a traditional provider.

Effects of Nonresponse on HINTS Trend Analysis

The LOE analyses just provided indicate that HINTS 2005 may have overestimated communication and health-seeking behavior within the general population. In particular, those least likely to seek health information are less likely to respond to the HINTS. This is consistent with the benchmarking analysis, which found that older, less healthy individuals are more likely to respond to the survey, and that these individuals also are more likely to seek health information. Given the drop in response rate between HINTS cycles, one natural question is whether the measures of change between these were adversely affected. Unfortunately, it is difficult to directly address this issue, as it is not possible to conduct a LOE analysis across HINTS 2003 and 2005. However, it is possible to compare the two HINTS surveys to similar measures from the NHIS for a limited number of health-related variables (Table 6.7). Although this is not directly related to the primary outcomes of interest to HINTS, it does provide some perspective on the magnitude of possible biases in measures of change.

For the NHIS, the largest changes are for smoking cigarettes and health insurance, which dropped in 2005 by 1.3 and 2 percentage points, respectively. These changes are mirrored by the comparable HINTS measures, which dropped by similar amounts. In several cases, the HINTS does exhibit some change, whereas the NHIS is stable. Two of the HINTS measures of emotional well-being increased in 2005 (sad, 1.6%; nervous, 1.7%) and fewer people went to the doctor (drop of 1.9%), whereas the NHIS trend shows no change. The HINTS differences are not large, but they border on statistical significance ($p < .10$). Proportionally, the largest changes on the HINTS that are not reflected on NHIS are reports of breast and prostate cancers. The prevalence of these diseases, however, is very low and the sample sizes are also quite small because they are specific to each sex. It should be noted that the total number of persons reporting ever having cancer does track closely with the NHIS.

Overall, there are few differences in trends between HINTS and NHIS. Of the differences just highlighted, the HINTS results tend to be consistent with the nonresponse patterns found in the earlier analyses. Those who were healthier were more likely to be nonrespondents with HINTS 2005. In comparison to HINTS 2003, this may be indicative of a slight upward bias in trends that are related to health status (e.g., looking for health information).

TABLE 6.7. Comparison of HINTS and NHIS Estimates (percents)

		2003	2005	DIFFERENCE
General health: Good	HINTS	76.7	76.3	−0.4
	NHIS	87.8	87.6	−0.2
Smoked 100+ cigarettes	HINTS	48.3	47.2	−1.1
	NHIS	43.4	42.1	−1.3
Feeling sad sometimes	HINTS	17.8	19.4	1.6
	NHIS	11.5	11.4	−0.1
Feeling hopeless sometimes	HINTS	11.7	11.3	−0.4
	NHIS	6.4	6.1	−0.3
Feeling worthless sometimes	HINTS	11.1	10.6	−0.5
	NHIS	5.4	4.9	−0.5
Feeling everything is an effort sometimes	HINTS	31.5	32.3	0.8
	NHIS	13.4	13.6	0.2
Feeling nervous sometimes	HINTS	28.6	30.3	1.7
	NHIS	15.5	15.6	0.1
Feeling restless sometimes	HINTS	36.5	36.2	−0.3
	NHIS	16.7	17.5	0.8
Have health insurance	HINTS	84.9	83.5	−1.4
	NHIS	86.4	84.4	−2.0
Never went to a doctor	HINTS	18.3	16.4	−1.9
	NHIS	18.4	18.6	0.2
Ever had cancer	HINTS	10.7	11.3	0.6
	NHIS	6.6	7.4	0.8
Ever had breast cancer (among female)	HINTS	3.1	5.2	2.1
	NHIS	2.1	2.2	0.1
Ever had cervical cancer (among female)	HINTS	2.5	2	−0.5
	NHIS	1	1.1	0.1
Ever had prostate cancer (among male)	HINTS	2.3	4.6	2.3
	NHIS	1.5	1.8	0.3

Summary of Nonresponse Bias Analyses

The analyses presented here provide evidence that HINTS 2005 does contain some bias as a result of nonresponse The benchmarking analysis indicates that the HINTS 2005 was more likely to survey older, less healthy individuals. This is evident from the larger percentages of persons in older age groups, as well as those who report being less healthy along several different indicators. The LOE analysis reinforced this conclusion by finding that those who were more likely to refuse the survey were less likely to be looking for cancer information; less likely to be looking on the Internet; and less likely to have had a pap smear, hysterectomy, or to have heard of HPV. It also found that those who refuse the interview are more likely to rely on more traditional forms of media (e.g., newspapers and television).

The LOE analysis subdivided the sources of nonresponse into refusals and noncontact. This analysis indicated that the source of nonresponse that had the biggest effect on the estimates was from refusals. Nonresponse due to noncontact did not seem to be systematically related to outcome variables. Among those who had refused the interview at some point, the largest differences were for those who initially refused to do the extended interview. Refusal to do the screening interview was not as highly associated with the outcome variables. This is consistent with the idea that an important source of nonresponse is from the salience of the survey. At the screening interview, respondents were less likely to know specifically about what the research entailed. Consequently, nonresponse was a bit more random relative to the measures of interest. At the extended interview, the interviewer was able to explain the purpose of the survey in more detail. This may have increased the likelihood that refusal was related to lack of interest in health and health communications (e.g., younger people, healthier, have not had cancer).

The results of the comparison of trends of HINTS and NHIS did not uncover significant bias. Trends in many of the health outcomes from HINTs seemed to coincide closely with trends in the NHIS. There was some indication that for particular types of emotional health and particular types of cancer, there was a difference in trends. These differences, however, were not large or consistent across measures. Some measures of emotional health did not show differences in trends, whereas others did. Similarly, measures of particular cancers (e.g., prostate) were different, whereas total cancer was not. This may indicate that there is a small bias for certain types of health-related phenomena, with HINTS 2005 overestimating health problems relative to HINTS 2003.

As with trying to directly reduce nonresponse, estimation of nonresponse error has several limitations. The LOE analysis is limited because it does not provide a measure of key outcomes for nonrespondents. It assumes that those who refused initially, but later cooperated, are similar to those who did not cooperate at all. As shown by several studies (e.g., Olsen, 2006), this assumption may not hold. We have argued that the differences that are found make theoretical sense because the patterns are related to the topic of the survey. However, the analysis has no way of verifying either that the direction of the bias or that the magnitude of the bias is correct.

The benchmarking and trend analyses are limited in several ways. Perhaps most importantly, they are limited in the types of estimates that can be compared. For the analysis presented here, for example, the estimates were limited to what was common to both the CPS, NHIS, and HINTS.

These happen to be measures related to demographics, health, and health services. This does not directly address error in the primary measures of health communication on the HINTS. A second problem with these analyses is that they assume that the only source of the differences between the surveys is from nonresponse. There are, of course, many other differences among the CPS, NHIS, and HINTS (e.g., mode of interview, coverage properties, and respondent selection).

DISCUSSION AND INTEGRATION FOR FUTURE ACTIONS

By using both strategies of minimizing and analyzing nonresponse, it is possible to develop a more informed strategy for designing future surveys. This is illustrated in the plans made for HINTS 2007, which introduced two changes to address the challenge of nonresponse. Some of these changes were made in direct response to the experiments and nonresponse analysis described earlier.[4]

Changing the Message to Respondents

Based on the continuing decline in the HINTS response rate, the survey administrators endeavored to improve communication of the reasons for conducting the survey to potential respondents. The significant drop in the screener response rate in HINTS 2005, despite the use of a $2 incentive, suggested that improving the message was needed. Conveying the importance of HINTS (or of health communication in general) to the public is not a simple task. Although the notion of having strategies and treatments to reduce cancer is very salient for many people, the inherent importance in obtaining information about how individuals learn about these strategies is not easy to communicate. In the absence of an effective message concerning this issue, advance letters may not be as effective as they could be. Furthermore, when interviewers attempt to explain the nature of the study, they may not be armed with material that is convincing. In fact, the nonresponse bias analysis seems to suggest that some of these materials may be highlighting features that introduce bias into the final sample.

Toward this end, HINTS 2007 conducted research to assess the public's understanding of the communication material used on the study. This was

---

[4]At the time of writing this chapter, HINTS 2007 was in the field. Consequently, we cannot report on the effects of the changes discussed in this section.

done through a series of focus groups that asked participants to react to different types of messages. For example, there is uncertainty around the use of the terms "National Cancer Institute" or "Cancer" within lead introductions. Both may leave the impression that the call is asking for money, as the former may be mistaken for a charitable organization, and the latter is a common cause of many charitable organizations. The use of the word "cancer" may also lead to people to think that the call is not relevant to them, if they have not had personal experience with that condition. On the other hand, both of these terms, if understood in the right context, should present clear strengths in convincing respondents to participate.

As a result of this research, the communication material for the survey was designed with three general goals in mind. The first was to have a set of talking points that provided specific information on the importance of the survey. The talking points provided concrete examples of the types of results that the survey produces. These were tested and refined by getting reactions from a series of focus groups. These points were then incorporated into the advance letters and the information interviewers used when trying to persuade respondents to do the survey. A second goal was to associate the survey with a government sponsor that the general public would readily recognize. Prior surveys had relied on the National Cancer Institute (NCI) as the primary sponsor. Focus groups indicated that this was not an organization that was readily recognized by the general public. In fact some mistook it as a private group asking for donations. Reference to the NCI was replaced with an agency that the general public would recognize, the Department of Health and Human Services. The third goal was to avoid characterizing the survey as being strictly related to cancer. Rather, the communications referred to a health information survey. This was done partly because of results of the nonresponse bias analysis that found that the survey was more likely to include persons who have had cancer. Confirming this result were reactions from focus groups that characterized early communication materials as being too focused on cancer as a topic.

Dual-Frame–Dual-Mode Survey Design

The continued decline of the response rate in 2005 suggested more radical changes to the design were needed. Given the well-established problems with telephone-only mode, a further change for HINTS 2007 was to implement a dual-frame design that mixes modes in a complementary way. One frame was RDD, and the second a national listing of addresses available from the U.S. Postal Service (USPS; see also Link, Chap. 5, this volume). This is a relatively comprehensive list (Iannacchione, Staab, & Redden, 2003) that includes both telephone and nontelephone households. This dual-frame design was used to administer a mail survey, with a subsample of nonrespondents followed up by telephone. Research by Link and colleagues (2004, 2005) suggested that use of a mail survey, with appropriate follow-up, can achieve a comparable or higher response rate than RDD alone. One experiment (Link & Mokdad, 2004) found a mail survey led to significantly more responses than a Web survey (15% vs. 43%) and that a mail survey with a telephone follow-up produced a significantly higher response rate than an RDD telephone survey (40.1% vs. 60%). The experiment allowed anyone in the household to fill out the mail/Web survey. Consequently, the respondents from the Web and mail were significantly different from those selected over the telephone. The results across key survey measures were also significantly different.

Additionally, the USPS frame provides access to populations who do not have a landline telephone. In 2007, this was approximately 12% of the adult population in the United States, with approximately 30% of those aged 18 to 24 years who reported not having a landline. These individuals are not currently part of the RDD sample frame and can only be reached by making special efforts.

The HINTS 2007 mail survey asked all adult household members to complete a HINTS questionnaire. This practice avoided asking respondents themselves to select a respondent within the household. Link et al. (2005) reported encouraging results related to this methodology. The overall mail response rate they achieved using standard follow-up procedures for six states was comparable or higher than HINTS 2005. Additionally, the demographics associated with the respondents to the survey were more reflective of a general population sample, in comparison with other respondent selection methods.

Overall, we expect that a mail survey may be a more flexible mode for future applications of HINTS and other population health surveys. It is less expensive to administer than a telephone survey, especially given that the cost of using the telephone has been increasing due to the increased labor costs involved in obtaining a completed interview. One would not expect a mail survey to increase in cost in the same way. Moving to an address-based frame leaves open the opportunity to implement other modes if they are found to be appropriate. For example, it would be possible to conduct in-person follow-up, if at some point this was something the survey administrators found appropriate. Sampled persons could also take a Web version of the HINTS, if that is found to be more convenient than doing a mail survey.

Of course, a mail survey also has a number of potential drawbacks. In particular, paper-based self-administration requires that respondents navigate the questionnaire (e.g., complicated skips and filters). A mail survey also may introduce mode differences, relative to a telephone-based mode. For example, a mail survey typically has lower response rates from respondents with less education (Hauser, 2005). There may also be differences in how respondents interpret and respond to individual items (Dillman, 2000).

The dual-frame design provides a way to assess the implications of the two modes, by comparing survey outcomes between modes. Although this is not a formal experiment, it can functionally serve as one because households have a chance of being selected for either the mail or the RDD survey. The only exception to this is for households without a landline telephone, which are on the USPS frame but not on the RDD frame. The design, therefore, is conducive to doing a mode analysis. Response rates, and their potential for introducing bias into the estimates, can be compared across the two sample frames. Similarly, important survey outcomes can be compared across modes. These analyses will provide a way to evaluate and, if necessary, adjust responses if that is appropriate.

SUMMARY

This chapter has illustrated two different methods of addressing the growing concerns with nonresponse. One method attempts to reduce nonresponse, whereas the other attempts to analyze the implications of nonresponse on key estimates. As illustrated in the application to HINTS, both approaches are important for addressing the problem. By minimizing nonresponse, the effects on data quality should be reduced. Nonresponse bias analysis provides indications of the direction and magnitude of error.

This point was discussed within the context of research conducted as part of the HINTS. This research was motivated by the changing survey environment. It included methods to increase response rates in two ways — the use of incentives and offering options to use alternative interview modes. The use of a pre-paid incentive successfully raised the response rate by about 5 percentage points. Neither the use of a promised incentive nor offering respondents a choice to use the Web were effective in increasing response rates. A nonresponse bias analysis found that respondents to HINTS tended to be older, more likely to have cancer, less healthy, and more likely to be looking for information about cancer. To some extent, this may lead to over-estimates of persons seeking information about cancer. There was also some evidence that nonrespondents are more likely to rely on more traditional modes of communication.

The designers of the HINTS used the research presented here to modify the design for HINTS 2007. There was a concerted effort to improve the communication material the survey used when contacting potential respondents The objective of the new material was to not only convince more individuals on the importance of the survey at the screening stage, but to also reach healthier individuals who may not initially be interested in a survey related to cancer. HINTS 2007 will also begin using a second mode of interviewing (mail survey). This was based on the acknowledged difficulties in stemming the decline of response rates for RDD surveys, as well as the promise of better rates when using a mail survey.

Once the HINTS 2007 data are collected, analysis will focus on assessing the optimal mix of frame modes for future HINTS surveys. The dual-frame design of HINTS 2007 provides the flexibility to implement related designs in the future. The trend in the HINTS data could be preserved if it is decided to use only a mail survey for the next round, use only the telephone, or mix the two modes *again* For example, if there are significant mode effects found in HINTS 2007 or the telephone survey response rates continue to decline, it may be decided to use a mail-only survey in the next round. If this is done, then trend analysis could be conducted by comparing the mail survey results in HINTS 2007 to the subsequent mail-only survey. It would also be possible to introduce a new mode (e.g., Web survey), if that is seen as appropriate. Which one of these designs are eventually adopted will be a function of the results of HINTS 2007, as well as the ongoing evolution of the survey environment. At least part of this decision will be based on the success the mail survey has with increasing response rates, as well as the extent it can address the nonresponse error issues of prior HINTS waves.

REFERENCES

Blumberg, S. J., & Luke, J. V. (2007). Wireless substitution: Early release of estimates based on data from the National Health Interview Survey, July–December 2006. National Center for Health Statistics. Retrieved August 22, 2009, from http://www. cdc.gov/nchs/data/nhis/earlyrelease/wireless200705.pdf

Cantor., D., O'Hare, B., & O'Connor, K. (2007). The use of monetary incentives to reduce nonresponse in random digit dial telephone surveys. In J.M. Lepkowski, C. Tucker, J.M. Brick, E. De Leeuw, L. Japec, P.J. Lavrakas, M.W. Link, & R.L. Sangster. (Eds.), *Advances in telephone survey methodology* (pp. 471-498). Hoboken, NJ: Wiley.

Curtin, R., Presser, S., & Singer, E. (2005). Changes in the telephone survey nonresponse over the past quarter century. *Public Opinion Quarterly, 69*, 87–98.

Dillman, D. A. (2000). *Mail and internet surveys: The tailored design method* (2nd Ed.). Hoboken, NJ: Wiley.

Fricker, S., Tourangeau, R., Galesic, M., & Yan, T. (2005). An experimental comparison of web and telephone surveys. *Public Opinion Quarterly, 69*, 370-392.

Griffin, D. H., Fischer, D. P., & Morgan, M. T. (2001). *Testing an internet response option for the American Community Survey.* Paper presented at the annual meeting of the American Association for Public Opinion Research, Montreal, Canada.

Groves, R. (2006). Nonresponse rates and nonresponse bias in household surveys. *Public Opinion Quarterly, 5*, 646-675.

Groves, R. M., Fowler, F. J., Couper, M. P., Lepkowski, J. M., Singer, E., & Tourangeau, R. (2004). *Survey methodology*. Hoboken, NJ: Wiley.

Groves, R. M., Singer, E., & Corning, A. (2000). Leverage-saliency theory of survey participation. *Public Opinion Quarterly, 64*, 299-308.

Hauser, R. M. (2005). Survey response in the long run: The Wisconsin longitudinal study. *Field Methods, 17*, 3-29.

Iannacchione, V., Staab, J. M., & Redden, D. T. (2003). Evaluating the use of residential mailing addresses in a metropolitan household survey. *Public Opinion Quarterly, 67*, 202- 210.

de Leeuw, E. D. (2005). To mix or not to mix data collection modes in surveys. *Journal of Official Statistics, 21*, 233-255.

Link, M., Battaglia, M. P., Frankel, M. R., Osborn, L., Mokdad, A. H., & Rao, S. R. (2005). *Effectiveness of an address-based sampling frame alternative to RDD: 2005 BRFSS mail survey pilot results*. American Statistical Association Proceedings of the Section of Survey Research Methods. Retrieved August 22, 2009, from http://www.amstat.org/sections/srms/Proceedings/

Link, M., & Mokdad, A. (2004). *Are web and mail modes feasible options for the behavioral risk factor surveillance system?* Paper presented at the Eighth Health Survey Research Methods Conference, Peachtree City, GA.

Olsen, K. (2006). Survey participation, Nonresponse bias, measurement error bias, and total bias. *Public Opinion Quarterly, 70*, 737-758.

Rizzo, L., Park, I., Hesse, B., & Willis, G. (2004). *Effect of incentives on survey response and survey quality: A designed experiment within the HINTS I RDD sample*. Paper presented at the annual meeting of the American Association for Public Opinion Research, Phoenix, AZ.

Schneider, S., Cantor, D., Malakhoff, L., Arieira, C., Segel, P., Nguyen, L., & Tancreto, J.G. (2005). Telephone, internet and paper data collection modes for the census 2000 short form. *Journal of Official Statistics, 21*, 89-101.

Singer, E. (2002). The use of incentives to reduce nonresponse in household surveys. In R. Groves, D. Dillman, J. Eltinge, & R. Little (Eds.), *Survey nonresponse* (pp. 163-177). New York: Wiley.

7

EXAMINING CHANGES ACROSS YEARS USING REPEATED CROSS-SECTIONAL HEALTH SURVEYS

Louis Rizzo
Westat Inc.

Richard P. Moser
National Cancer Institute

William Waldron
Information Management Services

Zhuoqiao Wang
Information Management Services

William W. Davis
Westat Inc.

The field of health communications is rapidly evolving. Its study is truly the study of "change." As the Internet penetration rate in this country continues to grow and as more people use the Internet to access health information, it is critical to understand changes in use over time to identify those who are taking advantage of this important resource, and just as importantly, what groups are not taking advantage of this resource and are perhaps falling into what has been called the "digital divide."

This chapter demonstrates the latest statistical methodology for examining changes over time using multiple cross-sectional surveys. Using the National Cancer Institute (NCI) Health Information National Trends Survey (HINTS) as an exemplar, we show how internet usage to seek cancer information has changed over two iterations of HINTS (2003 and 2005), and demonstrate how to compute both descriptive statistics and predictive models. We also explain how the methods can generalize to other surveys that employ a complex sampling design such as the National Health Interview Survey (NHIS) and the California Health Interview Survey (CHIS), as well as surveys with more than two iterations. This chapter originates with a HINTS data user's guide, which itself is based on a methodology paper written for the CHIS (Lee et al. 2006). This chapter is meant for the researcher seeking an understanding of conceptual issues; for those seeking more detailed procedural information, the HINTS user's guide (http://hints.cancer.gov) provides technical details concerning how to carry out these analyses in practice. The CHIS methodology paper is available on http://www.chis.ucla.edu. For those who are interested in the analysis of longitudinal (also called panel) surveys, an extensive literature already exists on this subject (one recent citation for example is Fitzmaurice, Laird, & Ware, 2004).

THREE TYPES OF ANALYSIS USING MULTIPLE BIENNIAL HINTS SURVEYS

Throughout this chapter, we use, as our primary outcome, estimates from HINTS of the percentage of respondents who ever looked for cancer information using the Internet. Most of the research variables of interest from the HINTS surveys are either dichotomous or can be analyzed as ordinal categorical variables.

This chapter focuses on three general goals as a simple categorization of the many types of analysis that can be done with multiple cross-sectional surveys like HINTS:

- Goal 1: Estimating a change over time in a characteristic such as a mean or a percentage, and testing the significance of the change:
  - Example 1: Has the percentage of persons who have ever looked for cancer information on the Internet changed between 2003 and 2005? What is the estimate of the amount of change? How can this change be tested with three survey iterations?
  - Example 2: Has the percentage of Black individuals who have ever looked for cancer information on the Internet changed between 2003 and 2005? What is the estimate of the amount of change? Is this level of change the same or different from other racial/ethnic groups?
- Goal 2: Estimating a change in a characteristic while controlling for compositional differences:
  - Example 1: Has the percentage of persons who have ever looked for cancer information on the Internet changed in the last 2 (or 4) years, after controlling for age, education level, and sex?

- Example 2: Has the percentage of college graduates who have ever looked for cancer information on the Internet changed in 2 (or 4) years, after controlling for age and sex?
- Goal 3: Estimating the average using data from multiple survey years, under the assumption that the mean has not changed between those years:
  - What is the average percentage of persons who have ever looked for cancer information on the Internet over the period 2003 to 2005? Over the period 2003 to 2007?

Note that Goals 1 and 2 illustrate the procedure to test for differences between items that are identical (or comparable) across years, whereas Goal 3 would be used to combine across years to obtain one larger sample size.

GOAL 1: ESTIMATING CHANGE WITHOUT CONTROLLING FOR OTHER FACTORS

The simplest example is the case of comparing national and subgroup means across 2 years, and we illustrate this kind of analysis using the (sequential) HINTS 2003 and HINTS 2005 surveys (these surveys are used throughout this chapter). We refer to the HINTS 2003 as *Year 0*, and the HINTS 2005 as *Year 2*, and consider estimating a characteristic such as a mean, percentage, regression coefficient, population standard deviation, etc.) in any particular year. The HINTS survey public-use databases provide jackknife replicate weights that can be used to generate consistent variance estimators (as does CHIS). For each of the first two HINTS surveys, 50 replicate weights have been provided that are used to generate correct variance estimates. For national-level estimates, variance estimates with up to 50 degrees of freedom can be generated for each HINTS survey year estimate. The http://hints. cancer.gov site provides links to technical reports for each survey, with details on the development of the replicate weights.

The true change between years is simply the difference between values of a characteristic (e.g., mean); because the samples are independent, the variance is the sum of the two variances. Table 7.1 provides a summary of this information.

A hypothesis test for the null hypothesis of no change (i.e., mean at Time 1 = mean at Time 2) can be evaluated via a one-tail test. The one-sided alternative may be more appropriate when any change that occurs is expected to be positive change (such as in the degree of Internet usage). Determining the correct degrees of freedom is not a trivial task, and the

TABLE 7.1.   Summary of Estimating Changes Using Two Independent Surveys

Year	True Value	Estimated Value	Variance of Estimate
0	θ_0	$\hat{\theta}_0$	$v(\hat{\theta}_0)$
2	θ_2	$\hat{\theta}_2$	$v(\hat{\theta}_2)$
Change	$\Delta = \theta_0 - \theta_2$	$\hat{\Delta} = \hat{\theta}_0 - \hat{\theta}_2$	$v(\hat{\Delta}) = v(\hat{\theta}_0) - v(\hat{\theta}_2)$

interested reader should consult the appendix at the end of this chapter for more information.

Table 7.2 presents estimated differences and confidence intervals for change between 2003 and 2005 in the percentages of adults who looked for cancer information online, for all adults, and for a number of socioeconomic subgroups. The degrees of freedom are estimated using the Satterthwaite approximation (see appendix for formula). The percentages and standard errors can be computed using a program, such as SUDAAN that is used to analyze surveys with complex sampling designs like HINTS, NHIS, and CHIS (for information on SUDAAN see e.g., Research Triangle Institute, 2004).

TABLE 7.2. Estimated Differences, and Confidence Intervals for Differences, in the Percentage of Adults Who Have Ever Looked for Cancer Information Online Between 2003 and 2005

Subgroup	2003 Weighted Percentage %	2003 Standard Error %	2005 Weighted Percentage %	2005 Standard Error %	Estimated Difference %	Standard Error of Difference %	Satterthwaite Degrees of Freedom	Lower Bound; 95% CI %	Upper Bound 95% CI %
All	19.7	0.6	28.3	0.7	8.6	0.9	95.3	6.8	10.4
AGE									
18–34	23.5	1.3	32.6	1.5	9.1	2.0	94.8	5.2	13.1
35–49	23.3	1.2	32.5	1.6	9.2	2.0	91.2	5.2	13.2
50–64	20.6	1.2	30.0	1.4	9.4	1.8	97.2	5.8	13.1
65+	4.2	0.5	9.6	0.8	5.4	0.9	83.4	3.6	7.2
EDUCATION LEVEL									
Less than High School grad	6.5	1.4	6.4	1.1	-0.1	1.7	92.5	-3.5	3.4
High school grad	12.0	0.9	19.9	1.6	8.0	1.8	79.6	4.3	11.6
Some college	23.9	1.3	34.7	1.9	10.7	2.4	86.7	6.1	15.4
College grad or more	36.0	1.3	46.5	1.6	10.5	2.1	93.0	6.4	14.5
RACE									
Non-Hispanic White	23.1	0.8	33.3	1.1	10.2	1.3	88.2	7.6	12.7
Non-Hispanic Black	13.6	1.7	23.3	3.4	9.6	3.8	72.4	2.1	17.2
Hispanic	7.2	1.0	11.2	2.0	4.1	2.2	71.9	-0.4	8.5
Non-Hispanic Other	22.1	2.4	28.2	3.7	6.1	4.4	83.8	-2.6	14.8

TABLE 7.2. Estimated Differences, and Confidence Intervals for Differences, in the Percentage of Adults Who Have Ever Looked for Cancer Information Online Between 2003 and 2005 (*continued*)

Subgroup	2003 Weighted Percentage %	Standard Error %	2005 Weighted Percentage %	Standard Error %	Estimated Difference %	Standard Error of Difference %	Satterth-waite Degrees of Freedom	Lower Bound; 95% CI %	Upper Bound 95% CI %
GENDER									
Male	16.7	0.8	25.3	1.4	8.6	1.7	77.2	5.3	11.9
Female	22.4	0.9	31.0	0.9	8.6	1.2	97.9	6.1	11.1
ANNUAL INCOME									
Less than $25,000	10.1	0.9	18.0	1.5	7.9	1.8	80.7	4.4	11.5
$25,000–$50,000	16.6	1.2	25.6	1.9	9.0	2.2	84.4	4.6	13.4
$50,000–$75,000	27.3	1.6	30.4	2.0	3.1	2.5	95.0	–2.0	8.1
More than $75,000	36.3	1.8	44.6	2.1	8.3	2.8	94.8	2.8	13.7

CI, confidence interval

For estimating changes with more than two data points, an obvious approach would involve a linear trend. In this case, one would estimate the intercept and slope parameters in a regression model, with the individual survey estimates as dependent variable, and time (t=0, t=2, t=4, etc.) as the predictor variable. The correct degrees of freedom for development of tests and confidence intervals can again be obtained from the Satterthwaite approximation given in the appendix.

From examining Table 7.2, it can be seen that there was an overall significant increase in the percentage of people in the United States who had ever looked for cancer information online, between 2003 and 2005, and that this increase was also significant for most demographic subgroups. The exceptions to this are those with less than a high school education, Hispanics, non-Hispanic others, and those having an income between $50,000 and $75,000.

It can be noted then that the analysis summarized in Table 7.2 provides answers for both examples 1 and 2 under Goal 1. The ease of this Goal 1 analysis is that it does not require any "connection" between the two data sets: It can be done running simple analyses on each semiannual data file. The downside of this analysis is that it only measures "marginal" changes. For example, suppose 20% of Hispanics (who are 15% of the population) and 30% of non-Hispanics used the Internet to collect cancer information in 2006. The overall percentage of Internet users is 28.5% in 2006. Suppose both of these Internet-user percentages remain the same through 2016, but Hispanics increase to 18% of the population. Then the overall percentage of Internet users will drop to 28.2% for 2016. No real change in behavior has resulted, but a compositional change has resulted: The distribution of subgroups has altered. A Goal 1 analysis will confound compositional changes and true "behavioral" changes (a particular part of the population changing its Internet behavior). The Goal 2 and 3 analyses can "unconfound" this confounding, but it requires combining the data files together and running more complex analyses.

COMBINING THE DATA FILES

For Goal 1, it is only necessary to obtain the separate data sets, compute the estimates and standard errors, compute differences by subtracting the two sets of estimates, and compute standard errors for those differences by adding the two variances. The degrees of freedom can then be approximated to generate tests and confidence intervals. For Goals 2 and 3, and for more sophisticated analyses, it will be necessary to combine the data files.

The main purpose of Goal 3 is to allow an augmented sample size: Many years can be combined, substantially expanding the available sample. This will considerably improve precision for those characteristics which do not change appreciably over time.

To create a combined data file, one can concatenate each year's public use file so that the number of respondents in the combined data file is the sum of the respondents from the individual data files. Two main tasks are required to combine data files. First, variables used in the analyses should have the same name and values or categories in all data files. Second, for HINTS and other surveys that supply replicate weights (e.g., CHIS), a set of new replicate weights need to be constructed. The number of replicate weights in this file will be the sum of the numbers of replicate weights for each individual data file, plus 1 (the full sample weight). The final weight in the combined file (referred to as NFWGT in our HINTS examples) is created by selecting the final weight (FWGT) from each respective survey.

For the HINTS surveys, there are 50 replicate weights for each survey. As an example, in Table 7.3 we consider three survey years (e.g., 2003, 2005, 2007). For the first 50 replicate weights (NFWGT1, . . . , NFWGT50), we use replicate weights FWGT1, . . . , FWGT50 for all sample persons represented in the HINTS 2003 survey, and the final weight FWGT (for all 50 replicates) for sample persons from the HINTS 2005 and HINTS 2007 sur-

TABLE 7.3. Construction of Statistical Weights for the Combined Data File

	FINAL SAMPLE WEIGHTS	REPLICATE WEIGHTS 1-50	REPLICATE WEIGHTS 51-100	REPLICATE WEIGHTS 101-150
HINTS 2003	2003 final weights (FWGT)	2003 replicate weights (FWGT1-FWGT50)	2003 final weight (FWGT)	2003 final weight (FWGT)
HINTS 2005	2005 final weight (FWGT)	2005 final weight (FWGT)	2005 replicate weights (FWGT1-FWGT50)	2005 final weight (FWGT)
HINTS 2007	2007 final weight (FWGT)	2007 final weight (FWGT)	2007 final weight (FWGT)	2007 replicate weights (FWGT1-FWGT50)
Combined data	Final weight (NFWGT)	Final replicate weights (NFWGT1-NFWGT50)	Final replicate weights (NFWGT51-NFWGT100)	Final replicate weights (NFWGT101-NFWGT150)

veys. For the first 50 replicate weights, only the HINTS 2003 survey contributes variance. For the next 50 replicate weights (NFWGT51, . . . , NFWGT100), we use replicate weights FWGT1, . . . , FWGT50 from the sample persons from the HINTS 2005 survey, and we use the final weight FWGT (for all 50 replicates) for sample persons from the HINTS 2003 survey and the HINTS 2007 survey. For replicate weights 51 through 100, only the HINTS 2005 survey contributes variance. For the remaining 50 replicate weights (NFWGT101, . . . , NFWGT150), we select replicate weights FWGT1, . . . , FWGT50 from the sample persons from the HINTS 2007 survey, and we use the final weight FWGT (for all 100 replicates) for sample persons from the HINTS 2003 survey and the HINTS 2005 survey. As such, for replicate weights 101 through 150, only the HINTS 2007 survey contributes variance. When the sums of squares for all 150 replicates are combined, the result is a sum of HINTS 2003, HINTS 2005, and HINTS 2007 variances, as desired (as the surveys are in fact independent). One can see how this method can be extended to data sets that have four or more sets of data and replicate weights.

It is also necessary to define a "Year" field equal to 0 for 2003 for HINTS 2003 sample members, equal to 2 for HINTS 2005 sample members, and equal to 4 for HINTS 2007 sample members. Goal 1, involving testing for changes over time with corresponding standard errors, test statistics, and confidence intervals, can be easily (and correctly) estimated from this combined data set using a contrast with the YEAR field (e.g., including +1 for HINTS 2007 records, 0 for HINTS 2005 records, and −1 for HINTS 2003 records will test for a linear trend over the three time points). The HINTS users guide (at http://hints.cancer.gov) provides SAS/SUDAAN and STATA software for generating replicate weights for combining two years (HINTS 2003 and HINTS 2005). Generalizing this code for multiple years is straightforward.

GOAL 2: ESTIMATING CHANGES, CONTROLLING FOR OTHER FACTORS

The estimated changes described previously are marginal changes: that is, they are composites that combine changes in Internet usage within specified subgroups and changes in the size of those subgroups. As a hypothetical example, an increase in 2005 in Internet usage for those with a college degree or more could be entirely because this group has increased in size and is now a larger percentage of the population—that is, within those groups, there may have been no change in the frequency of Internet usage. In general, analysts strive to separate these compositional changes from true secular trends in the characteristic of interest.

In this section, we explore how to conduct analyses that search for "true" non-compositional changes in HINTS data across years, by controlling for a set of covariates. For example, Table 7.4 presents results from checking for 2003 to 2005 differences using logistic regression (with binary dependent variable equal to 1, if the Internet was searched for health information, and 0 otherwise). The beta coefficients represent effects on a log-odds scale (as appropriate for a dichotomous dependent variable): the estimated odds ratios are also given (the transformed beta coefficients). Age, education level, and sex are also treated as main effects in this model, so the listed beta coefficient can be interpreted as a year-to-year change, after adjusting for changes in composition by age group, education level, and sex, between the two years. The odds ratio for the 2005 to 2003 difference for all subjects is 1.66: Fixing these other factors, the odds are 66% higher of using the Internet to search for cancer information in 2005 as compared with 2003 (with a 95% confidence interval ranging from 48% to 87% higher). It should be noted that this "answers" the question posed under Goal 2, Example 1. Examples of SAS/SUDAAN and STATA code to carry out these calculations are given in the HINTS user's guide available on http://hints.cancer.gov.

The model underlying Table 7.4 imposes a structure in which year-to-year differences only affect the intercept, and do not also show differences in the slopes for the other covariates in the model. But what if one wanted to test for differential effects of education by year on internet usage (i.e., an education–year interaction)?

For example, the odds ratio of 1.60 for 2005 versus 2003 should be read in this case as the ratio of percentages for college graduates or more (the base level). The corresponding ratio for "some college" is 1.6*(1.09) = 1.75, for "less than high school" 1.6*(0.6) = 0.96. Table 7.5 allows one to "answer" the question under Goal 2, Example 2. One can also extend the interactions between education level and the other predictors by doing separate analyses using education level as a subgroup. This allows for a more comprehensive answer to Goal 2, Example 2. The slope coefficients are individual to that education-level subgroup. Tables 7.6–7.9 present these results.

The analyses in Tables 7.6–7.9 present a full-scale interaction between education level and the other variables survey year, age, and sex, whereas in Table 7.5, only survey year is interacted with education level. The analyses in Tables 7.6–7.9 allow for clear presentation of odds ratios for each level of the education interaction variable, but comparing what is happening for each education level is more difficult than in Table 7.5. Note, for example, that the odds ratios seen in Tables 7.6 and 7.8 for the 2005 to 2003 main effects are very close to the odds ratios computed in the paragraph below Table 7.5: They represent the same parameter. In Tables 7.6–7.9 the estimates are "immediate"—as there is no need for supplemental hand calculations. The presentations in Tables 7.6–7.9, on the other hand, make comparisons between the four educational subgroups more difficult. Additionally, in the analyses in Tables 7.6–7.9, the number of estimated parameters is higher, which reduces the precision for all parameter estimates. There are many analyses that can answer the basic questions under Goal 2, with differing assumptions, and that focus on differing aspects. None is difficult to accomplish if the combined data set is created in advance and the same solutions can be applied to the analysis of similar cross-sectional surveys.

For three or more cross-sectional survey years, a linear trend can be tested by converting survey year from a categorical variable to a continuous variable (e.g., 2003 = -2, 2005 = 0, 2007 = +2), and estimating and testing the regression parameter corresponding to this variable within a logistic regression model that controls for other characteristics. The HINTS user's guide contains examples of SAS/SUDAAN and STATA code to carry out these calculations.

TABLE 7.4. Changes in Percentages of Adults Who Have Ever Looked for Cancer Information on the Internet between 2003 and 2005 Controlling for Age, Education Level, and Sex

	Beta Coefficient	Standard Error Beta Coefficient	Odds Ratio	Lower Bound; 95% CI Odds Ratio	Upper Bound; 95% CI Odds Ratio
Intercept	−1.74	0.11	0.17	0.14	0.22
Survey year					
2003	0.00	0.00	1.00	1.00	1.00
2005	0.51	0.06	1.66	1.48	1.87
Age					
18-34	1.57	0.10	4.78	3.93	5.83
35-49	1.45	0.09	4.27	3.57	5.13
50-64	1.32	0.10	3.75	3.06	4.60
65+	0.00	0.00	1.00	1.00	1.00
Gender					
Male	−0.36	0.07	0.70	0.60	0.81
Female	0.00	0.00	1.00	1.00	1.00
Education level					
Less than high school	−2.24	0.16	0.11	0.08	0.15
High school graduate	−1.31	0.09	0.27	0.23	0.32
Some college	−0.59	0.08	0.55	0.47	0.64
College graduate or more	0.00	0.00	1.00	1.00	1.00

CI, confidence interval

TABLE 7.5. Changes in Percentages of Adults Who Have Ever Looked for Cancer Information Online between 2003 and 2005, Controlling for Age, Education Level, and Sex; With a Year by Education Level Interaction

Subgroup	Beta Coefficient	Standard Error Beta Coefficient	Odds Ratio	Lower Bound; 95% CI Odds Ratio	Upper Bound; 95% CI Odds Ratio
Intercept	−1.73	0.10	0.18	0.15	0.22
Survey year					
2003	0.00	0.00	1.00	1.00	1.00
2005	0.47	0.09	1.60	1.34	1.91
Age					
18-34	1.57	0.10	4.80	3.94	5.84
35-49	1.45	0.09	4.29	3.58	5.14
50-64	1.32	0.10	3.75	3.06	4.60
65+	0.00	0.00	1.00	1.00	1.00
Gender					
Male	−0.36	0.07	0.70	0.60	0.81
Female	0.00	0.00	1.00	1.00	1.00
Education level 2003					
Less than high school	−1.97	0.25	0.14	0.09	0.23
High school graduate	−1.40	0.11	0.25	0.20	0.31
Some college	−0.64	0.09	0.53	0.44	0.64
College graduate or more	0.00	0.00	1.00	1.00	1.00
Education level 2005 vs 2003					
Less than high school	−0.52	0.32	0.60	0.32	1.13
High school graduate	0.16	0.17	1.17	0.83	1.65
Some college	0.08	0.15	1.09	0.81	1.46
College graduate or more	0.00	0.00	1.00	1.00	1.00

CI, confidence interval

TABLE 7.6. Changes in Percentages of Adults Who Have Ever Looked for Cancer Information Online between 2003 and 2005, Controlling for Age and Sex in the Education-Level Subgroup "Less than High School"

Subgroup	Beta Coefficient	Standard Error Beta Coefficient	Odds Ratio	Lower Bound; 95% CI Odds Ratio	Upper Bound; 95% CI Odds Ratio
Intercept	−4.41	0.44	0.01	0.01	0.03
Survey year					
2003	0.00	0.00	1.00	1.00	1.00
2005	−0.07	0.30	0.93	0.51	1.68
Age					
18-34	2.53	0.48	12.61	4.91	32.41
35-49	1.76	0.50	5.84	2.17	15.72
50-64	1.33	0.57	3.78	1.22	11.77
65+	0.00	0.00	1.00	1.00	1.00
Gender					
Male	−0.08	0.33	0.92	0.48	1.76
Female	0.00	0.00	1.00	1.00	1.00

CI, confidence interval

TABLE 7.7. Changes in Percentages of Adults Who Have Ever Looked for Cancer Information Online between 2003 and 2005, Controlling for Age and Sex in the Education-Level Subgroup "High School Graduate Only"

Subgroup	Beta Coefficient	Standard Error Beta Coefficient	Odds Ratio	Lower Bound; 95% CI Odds Ratio	Upper Bound; 95% CI Odds Ratio
Intercept	−3.43	0.24	0.03	0.02	0.05
Survey year					
2003	0.00	0.00	1.00	1.00	1.00
2005	0.64	0.14	1.90	1.45	2.49
Age					
18-34	1.97	0.23	7.15	4.55	11.25
35-49	1.91	0.22	6.76	4.33	10.55
50-64	1.62	0.25	5.03	3.04	8.34
65+	0.00	0.00	1.00	1.00	1.00
Gender					
Male	−0.55	0.18	0.58	0.40	0.82
Female	0.00	0.00	1.00	1.00	1.00

CI, confidence interval

TABLE 7.8. Changes in Percentages of Adults Who Have Ever Looked for Cancer Information Online between 2003 and 2005, Controlling for Age and Sex in the Education-Level Subgroup "Some College Only"

Subgroup	Beta Coefficient	Standard Error Beta Coefficient	Odds Ratio	Lower Bound; 95% CI Odds Ratio	Upper Bound; 95% CI Odds Ratio
Intercept	−2.28	0.16	0.10	0.07	0.14
Survey year					
2003	0.00	0.00	1.00	1.00	1.00
2005	0.56	0.12	1.74	1.38	2.20
Age					
18-34	1.49	0.17	4.44	3.15	6.26
35-49	1.46	0.17	4.33	3.09	6.06
50-64	1.31	0.18	3.72	2.61	5.29
65+	0.00	0.00	1.00	1.00	1.00
Gender					
Male	−0.50	0.13	0.61	0.47	0.78
Female	0.00	0.00	1.00	1.00	1.00

CI, confidence interval

TABLE 7.9. Changes in Percentages of Adults Who Have Ever Looked for Cancer Information Online between 2003 and 2005, Controlling for Age and Sex in the Education-Level Subgroup "College Graduate or More"

Subgroup	Beta Coefficient	Standard Error Beta Coefficient	Odds Ratio	Lower Bound; 95% CI Odds Ratio	Upper Bound; 95% CI Odds Ratio
Intercept	−1.54	0.13	0.21	0.17	0.28
Survey year					
2003	0.00	0.00	1.00	1.00	1.00
2005	0.46	0.09	1.58	1.33	1.88
Age					
18-34	1.24	0.15	3.45	2.56	4.66
35-49	1.12	0.14	3.08	2.33	4.06
50-64	1.13	0.15	3.10	2.32	4.15
65+	0.00	0.00	1.00	1.00	1.00
Gender					
Male	−0.18	0.08	0.84	0.71	0.99
Female	0.00	0.00	1.00	1.00	1.00

CI, confidence interval

GOAL 3: ESTIMATES THAT RELY ON MULTIPLE YEARS OF DATA

With multiple distinct surveys, we can report separate values for each year or one value summarizing the entire time period. If the distinct estimates from the years are quite different, then reporting their average may not be a good idea, as the average may represent distinct values or a single value. In those cases, when the years do not differ substantially, putting the two years together will certainly allow a considerable increase in precision. This may be very useful for population subgroups in which the one-year sample sizes are not large.

An example for which this combining across time periods is done as a matter of course is the National Health and Nutrition Examination Survey (NHANES; www.cdc.gov/nhanes). In NHANES, less than 20 geographic primary sampling units (PSUs[1]) are canvassed each year because of the enormous overhead cost in using the mobile examination centers. It is difficult to obtain sufficient precision for many characteristics unless at least two years are combined. In NHANES, the combined sample across two years becomes the two sets of PSUs across years. The analysis must treat this combined PSU sample as a single sample.

The average of two survey years may be estimated in either of two ways: (a) using two separate data files, and (b) using the combined data file. In the first approach, we use the mean value [(mean1 + mean2)/2] as the parameter of interest. The variance is the sum of the variances divided by 4. The second method estimates the mean of the years using the combined data with the new weights described previously. The mean over the two years (2003 and 2005) using these weights implicitly estimates the weighted parameter $\theta_w = (N_0\theta_0 + N_2\theta_2) / (N_0 + N_2)$, where N_0 and N_2 are the population sizes in the two surveys. When the population sizes in the two surveys are constant, the weighted mean reduces to the unweighted mean. Over a short period of time, the population size of most groups would change very little. However, there may be subgroups increasing or decreasing in size rapidly by immigration. Therefore, one advantage of using the combined data set with the new weights is that it takes into account change in population size.

Table 7.10 presents results for estimating θ_w: the weighted parameter. These calculations use the combined data set with the full set of replicate weights, using SAS/SUDAAN or STATA. The HINTS user's guide contains examples of SAS/SUDAAN and STATA code to carry out these calculations.[2]

---

[1]PSUs are counties or groups of counties that are selected as a first stage of sampling.
[2]Note that these confidence intervals are asymmetric, as the end points are reverse logistic transformations of symmetric confidence intervals on the logit scale. The STATA code provides similar results with a slightly different degree of freedom. Note that the STATA software provides a number of commands for confidence interval formation. For example, for dichotomous response variables, if one uses the svy: mean or svy: proportion command then the confidence interval will be symmetric. If one uses the svy: tabulate command the confidence interval will be asymmetric (it uses the logit transform).

TABLE 7.10. Combined (2003 and 2005) Percentages of Adults Who Have Ever Looked for Cancer Information Online

Subgroup	Weighted 2003 Estimate (%)	Standard Error (%)	Weighted 2005 Estimate (%)	Standard Error (%)	2003 to 2005 θ_w Estimate (%)	Lower Bound; 95% CI (%)	Upper Bound; 95% CI (%)
All	19.7	0.6	28.3	0.7	24.0	23.1	25.0
Age							
18-34	23.5	1.3	32.6	1.5	28.1	26.2	30.1
35-49	23.3	1.2	32.5	1.6	27.9	26.0	29.9
50-64	20.6	1.2	30.0	1.4	25.5	23.7	27.4
65+	4.2	0.5	9.6	0.8	7.0	6.1	7.9
Education level							
Less than high school	6.5	1.4	6.4	1.1	6.4	4.9	8.4
High school graduate	12.0	0.9	19.9	1.6	15.9	14.2	17.8
Some college	23.9	1.3	34.7	1.9	29.9	27.5	32.3
College grad or more	36.0	1.3	46.5	1.6	41.2	39.2	43.2
Race							
Non-Hispanic White	23.1	0.8	33.3	1.1	28.2	26.9	29.5
Non-Hispanic Black	13.6	1.7	23.3	3.4	18.4	15.0	22.4
Hispanic	7.2	1.0	11.2	2.0	9.3	7.2	11.9
Non-Hispanic Other	22.1	2.4	28.2	3.7	25.5	21.2	30.3
Gender							
Male	16.7	0.8	25.3	1.4	21.1	19.5	22.8
Female	22.4	0.9	31.0	0.9	26.8	25.6	28.0
Annual income							
Less than $25,000	10.1	0.9	18.0	1.5	13.7	12.1	15.6
$25,000-$50,000	16.6	1.2	25.6	1.9	20.5	18.5	22.7
$50,000-$75,000	27.3	1.6	30.4	2.0	29.0	26.5	31.6
More than $75,000	36.3	1.8	44.6	2.1	40.8	38.1	43.6

SUMMARY AND OTHER APPLICATIONS

This chapter is an invitation to users to utilize cross-sectional repeated health surveys to estimate change and to increase precision. In brief, our illustration from HINTS showed that there was a significant increase in the percentage of people who have ever accessed the internet to look for cancer information between 2003 and 2005, and that this increase was found among most sociodemographic groups, with important exceptions. We also demonstrated how to control for a set of covariates when implementing a statistical model, and how to test for differential effects of a covariate by year, by including an interaction term. The simplest way to do these analyses is to combine the data sets by generating a set of amalgamated replicate weights. In general, for HINTS, the number of replicate weights for each survey is presently 50, so two years of combined data would produce 100 replicate weights, three years of data would involve 150 replicate weights, and so on. The same principles apply to surveys such as CHIS, which incorporates 80 replicate weights for each survey. The replicate weights generated using the methodology given previously will provide variance estimators that are the sums of the appropriate variances for each individual year, correctly reflecting the independent sampling across years (although note that there is some disagreement on whether the default degrees of freedom used by programs such as SUDAAN and STATA are correct; see the appendix for a suggestion on an improved procedure for computing degrees of freedom using a Satterthwaite method). In SUDAAN, the denominator degrees of freedom (when not specified) is equal to the number of replicate weights, or equivalent to the difference (#PSUs − #STRATA), depending on the specified design. In STATA, the design degrees of freedom is equal to #replicates − 1, or #PSUs − #STRATA, depending on the specified design. These degrees of freedom are correct for working within one survey year, but it is not strictly correct to add the degrees of freedom in analyses comparing two years. Hopefully future versions of these software applications may allow the user more flexibility in assigning degrees of freedom.

A wide variety of analyses can be done with the combined data sets using these and other software packages. This includes linear regression and a wide variety of generalized linear models such as simple dichotomous logistic regression and ordinal logistic regression. Time becomes a predictor variable (e.g., the first year is time = 0, the third year time = 2, etc.), so that parameter coefficients for time can be interpreted as yearly rates of change. With two or three surveys combined, a linear model is appropriate: for a larger number of surveys linearity can be relaxed (variable yearly rates of change). The effect of time (i.e., survey year) can be viewed as a simple intercept effect, or can interact with other independent variables such as age, education level, race, sex, and income level.

This methodology can be adopted to any sequence of independent annual surveys. The CHIS is a good example (see Lee et al., 2007, at www.chis.ucla.edu). Another example is the Behavioral Risk Factors Surveillance Survey (BRFSS; see www.cdc.org/brfss). BRFSS surveys are independent annual random-digit dial surveys, and BRFSS is different from HINTS and CHIS in that standard errors are not estimated using replicate weights. This methodology can also be used for surveys such as the NHIS, which have independent surveys that can be compared. It is important to note that survey years within one full cycle of NHIS (such as 1995-2005) will not be independent, as the PSUs are maintained across years within one cycle. However, in comparing NHIS 2006 to any earlier year, independence can be assumed, as 2006 is the beginning of a new independent cycle for NHIS. NHIS does not provide replicate weights, so linearization rather than replicate-based techniques need to be used. When combining independent years, the new STRATA variables must be recoded so that the alternate survey years have different values for these cluster variables. For example, see http://www.cdc.gov/nchs/data/nhis/2006var.pdf. The degrees of freedom for one NHIS year are the number of PSUs minus the number of strata. Using SUDAAN or STATA for hypothesis testing or computing confidence intervals, the degrees of freedom assumed will be the sum of the two years' degrees of freedom, which is too large a value. Again, a Satterthwaite approximation should in theory be used, to obtain the correct degrees of freedom, although current versions of these software packages does not allow that option in this circumstance.

For comparing or combining years between NHIS cycles (e.g., 1995-2005), the methodology for combining across years is entirely different than that described here for HINTS. In this case the PSUs, which are shared across the years, are viewed as the "sample," and the mean values across years for the PSUs are viewed as differing observations for the single sample unit, constituting a longitudinal sample design at the PSU level (multiple observations across time for single sample units). For such analysis of NHIS, the reader is referred to http://www.cdc.gov/nchs/data/nhis/2006var.pdf. The degrees of freedom here are the same as for the single-year survey (as the PSU set remains the same).

APPENDIX. COMPUTING DEGREES OF FREEDOM

This technical appendix discusses the computing of appropriate degrees of freedom for general estimators of the form $L'\theta$, where $\theta = [\theta_1, \theta_2, \ldots, \theta_T]'$ and L is a vector of length T. It can be assumed as an approximation that the T samples are simple random samples of size n_t (corresponding to the [n]t replicates for each survey: Each replicate provides a "pseudo sample unit") from a normal distribution.[3] We have independent estimates $\hat{\theta}_t$ with variances $Var(\hat{\theta}_t)$. The estimator of $L'\theta$ is $L'\hat{\theta}$ with estimator of variance $v(L'\hat{\theta}) = \sum_{t-1} l_t'v (\hat{\theta}_t)$. Each $v(\hat{\theta}_t)$ has n_t-1 degrees of freedom respectively.[4] The estimating equation referred to the t-distribution in this case is $(L'\hat{\theta} - L'\theta)/\sqrt{(\sum_{t-1}^{T} l_t'v(\theta_t))}$. An approximate degrees of freedom can be obtained from the Satterthwaite approximation (see, e.g., Kotz & Johnson 1988, pp. 261-262). This approximate degrees of freedom is

$$df = \frac{\left(\sum_{t-1}^{T} l_t'v(\hat{\theta}_t)\right)^2}{\sum_{t-1}^{T} \frac{l_t'\{v(\hat{\theta}_t)\}^2}{n_t-1}}$$

A lower bound for this is $df_{lb} = \min\{n_t-1\}$. An upper bound is $df_{ub} = \sum_{t-1}^{T}\{n_t-1\}$. For example, in the simple case of a difference between two years $\hat{\Delta} = \hat{\theta}_2 - \hat{\theta}_1$ (so that $T=2$; $l_2 = +1$ and $l_1 = -1$), the Satterthwaite approximation reduces to the Welch approximation (see, e.g., Bickel & Doksum, 1977, Section 6.4) which computes as the degrees of freedom k for the estimating equation $(\hat{\Delta} - \Delta)/\sqrt{(v(\hat{\theta}_1) + v(\hat{\theta}_2))}$

$$k = \left[\frac{c^2}{n_1-1} + \frac{(1-c)^2}{n_2-1}\right]^{-1} \quad \text{where } c = \frac{v(\hat{\theta}_1)}{v(\hat{\theta}_1) + v(\hat{\theta}_2)}.$$

It should be noted that subgroups may not have the same numbers of degrees of freedom as a national estimate (with [n]t the number of degrees of freedom). For example, if the degrees of freedom are based on PSUs, and the subgroup is only present in particular PSUs, then the appropriate degrees of freedom are based on the number of PSUs which actually cover the subgroup. For the random-digit dial surveys (e.g., HINTS, CHIS, BRFSS), most subgroups will be represented in each replicate, so that assuming [n]t as the degrees of freedom will generally be valid.

---

[3]The pseudo-values may not necessarily have a normal distribution: It is good practice to check this assumption and make sure there is not kurtosis that may reduce the effective degrees of freedom.

[4]It actually may be smaller if for a particular statistic many of the replicates are effectively equal to the full-sample estimator. [n]t is actually the maximum in general.

REFERENCES

Bickel, P., and Doksum, K. A. (1977). *Mathematical statistics.* Oakland, CA: Holden-Day.

Cochran, W. G. (1977). *Sampling techniques,* (3rd ed.). New York: Wiley.

Fitzmaurice, G. M., Laird, N. M., & Ware, J. H. (2004). *Applied longitudinal analysis.* New York: Wiley.

Korn, E. L., & Graubard, B. (1999). *Analysis of health surveys.* New York: Wiley.

Kotz, S., & Johnson, N. L. (1988). *Encyclopedia of statistical sciences* (Vol. 8). New York: Wiley.

Lee, S., Davis, W. W., Nguyen, H. A., McNeel, T. S., Brick, J. M., & Flores-Cervantes, I. (2006). *Examining trends and averages using combined cross-sectional survey data from multiple years.* California Health Interview Survey 2005 Methodology paper, Los Angeles, CA, UCLA Center for Health Policy Research.

Research Triangle Institute. (2004). *SUDAAN Language Manual: Release 9.0.* Research Triangle Park, NC: Author.

StataCorp. (2007). *Stata Statistical Software: Release 10.* College Station, TX: StataCorp LP.

II

EXTENDING REACH
IN HEALTH COMMUNICATION

8

EXPANDING THE IMPACT OF HEALTH COMMUNICATION

Section Overview

Erik M. Augustson
National Cancer Institute

Recent advances in technology have broadened medical treatment, diagnostics, and our ability to disseminate health information through various communication channels. For example, in the field of cancer treatment and prevention, there are now a number of effective screening tools available for early detection, and, perhaps more importantly, a great deal is known regarding the primary prevention of many of the most common forms of cancer in the United States (Hiatt & Rimer, 1999; Stein & Colditz, 2004). This wealth of information, coupled with increased access to health information via electronic sources, such as the Internet, holds great promise in reducing morbidity and mortality associated with cancer. Capitalizing on this promise requires the effective dissemination of health information, which in turn points to the important role of health communication science in reducing population cancer burden. It is ironic then that such advances in technology and resultant access to quality health information are not shared equally across the population and may have the unintended consequence of potentially widening gaps in health-related knowledge. Knowledge gaps may, in turn, lead to further disparities in access to and practice of effective primary and secondary preventive health behaviors between mainstream and at-risk populations (Hiatt & Rimer, 1999; Viswanath et al., 2006).

A large body of literature has highlighted marked disparities in the burden associated with diseases such as cancer among a variety of populations
(ACS, 2006, 2007a, 2007b; Office of Minority Health, 2005). Within the
United States and similar countries, these disparities appear to be fundamentally, but not exclusively, associated with a cluster of individual-level factors
that are markers of socioeconomic status (SES) including education, income,
and occupation (Kawachi & Kroenke, 2006; Singh, Miller, Hankey, &
Edwards, 2003, Ward et al., 2004). For example, national estimates from the
Surveillance, Epidemiology, and End Results (SEER) data indicate that the
lung cancer incidence rate for men in high-poverty counties was at least 12%
greater than for men in low-poverty counties from 1975 to 1999 (Singh et al.,
2003). Trends in lung cancer in women indicate that the incidence rates in
high-poverty counties were 11% greater than the rates for women in counties with poverty levels between 10% and 20% (Singh et al., 2003).
Compared with men in low-poverty counties, the lung cancer mortality for
U.S. men in high-poverty counties was 7% greater in 1975 and 25% greater
in 1999 (Singh et al., 2003). Trends from 1975 to 1999 indicate that men in
high-poverty areas experienced at least 18% higher lung cancer mortality
than men in low-poverty areas (Singh et al., 2003).

Consistent with the SEER findings on incidence and mortality, in 2006
smoking prevalence was higher among adults living below the poverty level
and among those with low educational attainment (CDC, 2007). Individuals
who work in service or blue-collar positions are also at significant risk
(Barbeau, Krieger, & Soobader, 2004). Barbeau and colleagues found that
35% of U.S. blue-collar workers and 31% of U.S. service workers were
smokers, whereas only 20% of white-collar workers smoked (Barbeau et al.,
2004). Quitting success is also impacted by income level and is lowest among
persons with characteristics associated with low income (Barbeau et al., 2004).

Such disparities are evident in use of available cancer screening, adherence to screening recommendations, and in a wide range of secondary preventive health behaviors (Hewitt, Devesa, & Breen, 2004; Rakowski et al.,
2004). Although there have been significant increases in screening rates for
cancer, screening uptake and adherence has been inconsistent across various
racial and ethnic groups. Compared with White and Black women, Hispanic
and Asian women have demonstrated lower rates of screening, even for cancers that have well-established screening protocols such as breast or cervical
cancers (James, Lillie-Blanton, & Garfield, 2006). Although uptake and
maintenance of screening for colorectal cancer is lower than recommended
for both men and women in most racial and ethnic groups within the United
States, some groups lag even further behind in adopting regular colon cancer screening. For example, Hispanics are less likely to adhere to screening
guidelines for colorectal cancer (James et al., 2006).

Although the association between factors such as SES and health-related outcomes is well established in diseases such as cancer, the underlying

causes of these disparities is not well understood and is likely related to a myriad of individual- and system-level factors (Kawachi & Kroenke, 2006). Among these factors, it has been suggested that a key component may be differential access to information about various aspects of cancer care and prevention, which creates "knowledge gaps" that subsequently impact health (Hiatt & Rimer, 1999; Viswanath, 2005; Viswanath et al., 2006). Indeed, it has been clear for more than two decades that there is an inequity between high SES and low SES groups with regard to health information and knowledge (Tichenor, Donohue, & Olien, 1970; Viswanath & Finnegan, 1996). This gap appears to be widening over time and tends to be most pronounced with the development of new information dissemination technologies (Tichenor et al., 1970; Viswanath & Finnegan, 1996; Viswanath et al., 1993). Thus, as the ability to disseminate health information improves, there is often a widening of the existing knowledge gaps.

An explicit set of goals for the National Cancer Institute's Behavioral Research Program is to identify means to extend the reach, improve the effectiveness, and optimize the efficiency of health communication efforts nationwide. This section of the volume focuses on the first of those goals: extending the reach of health communication across vulnerable and underserved populations. The authors in this section explore various aspects of the existing knowledge gaps regarding cancer prevention and screening and the utility of using national surveys to assist in developing evidentiary profiles of diverse audience needs. The overarching question that this section seeks to address is: *How can survey data resources be used to document, diagnose, and address the root causes of health disparities in cancer communication?*

Thompson and Cavazos-Rehg (Chap. 9) open the analytic chapters in this section with a discussion of fundamental issues associated with health communication and health disparities. They then present the results of several analyses aimed at better understanding the nature of the health disparities in the United States, especially as they relate to health communication gaps using Health Information National Trends Survey (HINTS) data and other data sources. Results also are presented from interventions studies, including the highly innovative use of computer kiosks, targeted at reaching populations that have historically been missed by many traditional public health information campaigns. The findings highlight the potential for such inventive approaches as a means to bridge some of the major obstacles associated with the critical information gaps. The material presented in this chapter also points to the utility surveys like HINTS can play in identifying information needs and potential interventions to address those needs.

In their chapter on variation in communication channel preferences by class and race, Blake, Flynt-Wallington, and Viswanath (Chap. 10) attempt to understand how group-level preferences are related to health communication. In particular, these authors discuss how class, race, and urbanicity are related to choices in communication channels, and how the Structural

Influence Model (SIM) can serve as a useful means to understand emerging communication inequalities. Results from their analyses point to strategies to improve health communication efforts to reach various populations in a more consistent and empirically driven fashion.

Hay, Zaid-Muhammad, Ford, and Coups (Chap. 11) present results from a series of analyses using HINTS data to identify cancer knowledge gaps associated with the screening and prevention of colon cancer. Although knowledge gaps were found among some groups, Hay and colleagues also found that the overall level of awareness in the population continues to be poor. Thus, even though colon cancer has been the focus of a number of broadly promoted campaigns and media events in recent years, adequate knowledge regarding this highly detectable cancer remains low. Their analysis provides clear evidence of the need for additional dissemination efforts and identifies barriers that have likely impeded previous attempts to improve colon cancer awareness and knowledge.

Smith, Crammer, and Stefanek, in Chapter 12, discuss key issues in cancer survivorship. Although HINTS has methodological limitations for exploring issues associated with cancer survivorships, the authors demonstrate how databases such as HINTS can expand our understanding of the impact of significant health outcomes on a variety of subsequent health behaviors. Analyses are presented of health beliefs, screening adherence, and other health behaviors such as diet, physical activity, and smoking from cancer survivors and individuals with a family history of cancer. The implications of these findings are discussed in the context of cancer survivorship and the importance of understanding survivor health behavior given the elevated risk of a wide variety of negative health outcomes that survivors can experience. Despite the limits of available data from surveys such as HINTS from cancer survivors and their families, the authors note that information from these data sources effectively expands the understanding of the relationship among health beliefs, health behaviors, and cancer.

In the final chapter of this section, Miller and Kreps (Chap. 13) present the concept of biological literacy and the concern that low basic biology and science literacy levels in the U.S. population present a significant challenge to effective health communication. Their review of research in this area reveals that higher levels of bioliteracy are clearly associated with at least some college education in the sciences. Given that most vulnerable populations have lower levels of education, bioliteracy is in many ways fundamental to communication-related health disparities. As health-related technology becomes increasingly complex and sophisticated, there is considerable risk that those populations most vulnerable to health inequalities and most likely to experience excessive health burden will fall further behind.

Although knowledge gaps and health disparities have long existed, the emergence and rapid expansion of information technologies have presented the field of public health with a number of new challenges. Perhaps one of the most insidious is that the very technologies that hold such potential for diminishing knowledge gaps may serve as agents in widening them. Therefore, a crucial challenge for health communication is to better understand the nature of these gaps, how they contribute to disparities in health behaviors and disease burden, and to identify means to reduce this often overlooked problem that undoubtedly impacts the health of many of our most vulnerable populations. The information provided in this section aims to contribute to the evidence base for addressing these needs.

REFERENCES

ACS. (2006). *Cancer Facts and Figures for Hispanics/Latinos 2006-2008. Statistics for 2007*. Atlanta: Author.

ACS. (2007a). *Cancer Facts and Figures. Statistics for 2007*. Atlanta: Author.

ACS. (2007a). *Cancer Facts and Figures for African Americans. Statistics for 2007*. Atlanta: Author.

Barbeau, E. M., Krieger, N., & Soobader, M. J. (2004). Working class matters: Socioeconomic disadvantage, race/ethnicity, gender, and smoking in NHIS 2000. *American Journal Public Health, 94*(2), 269-278.

Centers for Disease Control and Prevention (CDC). (2007). Cigarette smoking among adults—United States, 2006. *MMWR, 56*(44), 1157-1161.

Hewitt, M., Devesa, S. S., & Breen, N. (2004). Cervical cancer screening among U.S. women: Analyses of the 2000 National Health Interview Survey. *Preventative Medicine, 39*(2), 270-278.

Hiatt, R. A., & Rimer, B. K. (1999). A new strategy for cancer control research. *Cancer Epidemiology Biomarkers Prevention, 8*(11), 957-964.

James, C., Thomas, M., Lillie-Blanton, M., & Garfield, R. (2006). *Key facts race, ethnicity & medical care*. Menlo Park, CA: The Henry J. Kaiser Family Foundation.

Kawachi, I., & Kroenke, C. (2006). Socioeconomic disparities in cancer incidence and mortality. In D. Schottenfeld & J.F.J. Fraumeni (Eds.), *Cancer epidemiology and prevention* (3rd ed., pp. 174-188). Oxford: Oxford University Press.

Office of Minority Health. (2005, October 19). *Eliminating racial & ethnic disparities*. Retrieved June 10, 2007, from http://www.cdc.gov/omhd/About/disparities.htm.

Rakowski, W., Breen, N., Meissner H., Rimer B. K., Vernon S. W., Clark M. A., & Freedman A. N. (2004). Prevalence and correlates of repeat mammography among women aged 55-79 in the year 2000 National Health Interview Survey. *Preventive Medicine, 39*(1), 1-10.

Singh, G. K., Miller, B. A., Hankey, B. F., & Ewards, B. K. (2003). Area socioeconomic variations in U.S. cancer incidence, mortality, stage, treatment, and survival, 1975-1999. In *NCI Cancer Surveillance Monograph Series*, National Cancer Institute. NIH Publication No. 03-5417, Bethesda, MD.

Stein, C. J., & Colditz, G. A. (2004). Modifiable risk factors for cancer. *British Journal of Cancer, 90*(2), 299-303.

Tichenor, P. J., Donohue , G. A., & Olien, C. N. (1970). Mass media flow and differential growth in knowledge. *The Public Opinion Quarterly, 34.*

Viswanath, K. (2005). The communications revolution and cancer control. *Nature Reviews Cancer, 5*(10), 828-835.

Viswanath, K., Breen, N., Meissner, H., Moser, R. P., Hesse, B., Steele, W. R. et al. (2006). Cancer knowledge and disparities in the information age. *Journal of Health Communication, 11*(Suppl 1), 1-17.

Viswanath, K., & Finnegan, J. R., Jr. (1996). *The knowledge gap hypothesis: Twenty-five years later.* Thousand Oaks, CA: Sage.

Viswanath, K., Kahn, E., Finnegan, J. R., Hertog, J., & Potter, J. (1993). Motivation and the knowledge gap: Effects of a campaign to reduce diet-related cancer risk. *Communication Research, 20*(4), 546-563.

Ward, E., Jemal, A., Cokkinides, V., Singh, G. K., Cardinez, C., Ghafoor, A., & Thun, M. (2004). Cancer disparities by race/ethnicity and socioeconomic status. *CA: A Cancer Journal for Clinicians, 54*(2), 78-93.

9

HEALTH INFORMATION NATIONAL TRENDS SURVEY

Implications for Addressing Cancer Health Disparities Through Public Health Surveillance

Vetta L. Sanders Thompson
Washington University in St. Louis

Patricia Cavazos-Rehg
Washington University in St. Louis

The United States continues to increase in diversity (OMHD, 2007). The current health discourse suggests that researchers and practitioners understand that this diversity has developed in a context without equity in the societal structures that shape health outcomes (Budrys, 2003; LaViest, 2005; Williams, Neighbors, Jackson et al., 2003). This increased awareness has led to scrutiny of the health, safety, and well-being of diverse segments of the population. When health outcomes are examined, the differences that exist among populations are obvious, striking, and persistent (Williams et al., 2003). These differences are especially pronounced among the most disadvantaged; those with low income, limited education, lower occupational status and wealth, and ethnic and racial minorities have poorer health outcomes than those with higher incomes, occupational status and wealth, more education, and majority group members (LaViest, 2005; Williams et al., 2003).

HEALTH DISPARITY

The term *health disparity* has gained favor in discussions of differences in health outcomes (Budrys, 2003; Carter-Pokras & Baquet, 2002). There are a number of meanings to the term; in this chapter *health disparity* is discussed as the differences in incidence, morbidity, and mortality for disease; rates of health and preventive behaviors; and quality of life that are likely the result of injustice and inequity in society (Budrys, 2003). Health disparity can also be referred to as health inequality and health inequity (Carter-Pokras & Baquet, 2002). The use of the term *health inequity* is probably more appropriate, although it is not widely used in the United States. Some researchers have argued for its use, because it highlights the issues of social justice that are subtexts of many of our discussions of disparity (Carter-Pokras & Baquet, 2002).

Differences in health outcomes in the United States are well documented (National Center for Health Statistics [NCHS], 2002; Office of Minority Health [OMH], 2005). Black, Native American, and Puerto Rican infants have higher mortality rates than White infants. Blacks have higher rates of heart disease (29% higher), stroke (40% higher), and diabetes (two times more likely) (NCHS, 2002). Blacks and Hispanics represented only 26% of the U.S. population in 2001, yet they accounted for 66% of adult AIDS cases (OMH, 2005). Likewise, it is well documented that people with low income and less education have higher rates of morbidity and mortality than those with more education and higher income (House & Williams, 2000).

The disparity statistics related to cancer, the second leading cause of death in the United States, are no different (Heron, 2007). Although racial disparities have decreased from 1997 to 2007, Blacks continue to suffer from cancer at a higher rate relative to other groups (American Cancer Society [ACS], 2007). Blacks also have a higher cancer incidence and mortality (see Fig. 9.1) for all cancer sites combined than any other racial or ethnic group. In 2003, the death rate for all cancers combined remained 35% higher in Black men and 18% higher in Black women compared with White men and women, respectively (ACS, 2007). Hispanics experience higher cancer incidence and mortality rates for stomach, liver, cervix, acute lymphocytic leukemia, and gallbladder (ACS, 2006). However, broad use of Hispanic data may mask differences experienced by persons of Hispanic ethnicity depending on country of origin.

For all cancer sites combined, residents of poorer counties have 13% higher death rates from cancer in men and 3% higher rates in women compared with more affluent counties (Ward et al., 2004). Five-year survival for all cancers combined is 10 percentage points lower among persons who live in poorer than in more affluent census tracts. However, Black, Native American/Alaskan Native, and Asian/Pacific Islander men and Black and Native American/Alaskan Native women have lower 5-year survival than Whites, even when controlling for poverty.

Preventive health and screening behaviors follow a trend that reflects observed differences in incidence and mortality. Although cancer-screening

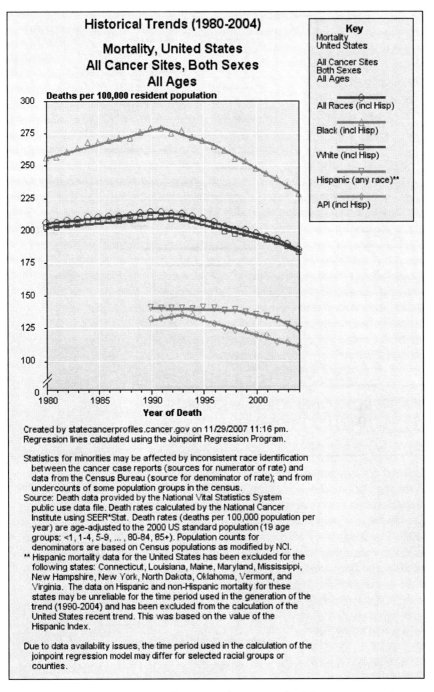

Historical Trends (1980-2004)

**Mortality, United States
All Cancer Sites, Both Sexes
All Ages**

Key
Mortality
United States

All Cancer Sites
Both Sexes
All Ages

All Races (incl Hisp)

Black (incl Hisp)

White (incl Hisp)

Hispanic (any race)**

API (incl Hisp)

Deaths per 100,000 resident population

Year of Death

Created by statecancerprofiles.cancer.gov on 11/29/2007 11:16 pm.
Regression lines calculated using the Joinpoint Regression Program.

Statistics for minorities may be affected by inconsistent race identification
between the cancer case reports (sources for numerator of rate) and
data from the Census Bureau (source for denominator of rate); and from
undercounts of some population groups in the census.
Source: Death data provided by the National Vital Statistics System
public use data file. Death rates calculated by the National Cancer
Institute using SEER*Stat. Death rates (deaths per 100,000 population per
year) are age-adjusted to the 2000 US standard population (19 age
groups: <1, 1-4, 5-9, ... , 80-84, 85+). Population counts for
denominators are based on Census populations as modified by NCI.
** Hispanic mortality data for the United States has been excluded for the
following states: Connecticut, Louisiana, Maine, Maryland, Mississippi,
New Hampshire, New York, North Dakota, Oklahoma, Vermont, and
Virginia. The data on Hispanic and non-Hispanic mortality for these
states may be unreliable for the time period used in the generation of the
trend (1990-2004) and has been excluded from the calculation of the
United States recent trend. This was based on the value of the
Hispanic Index.

Due to data availability issues, the time period used in the calculation of the
joinpoint regression model may differ for selected racial groups or
counties.

FIGURE 9.1. Cancer mortality rates by race/ethnicity (1980-2004).

129

rates have increased over the past two decades, there is substantial variation by race and ethnicity. Hispanic and Asian women are less likely to be screened for breast or cervical cancers than are White or Black women (James, Thomas, Lillie-Blanton, & Garfield, 2006). Hispanic and Asian women also are less likely to have had a pap smear in the past three years than were White, Black, or Native American/Alaska Native women. Men and women from all racial or ethnic groups are less likely to undergo colorectal cancer screening than other cancer-screening tests. However, Hispanics are the least likely to report having been screened for colorectal cancer within the past 2 years. Despite comparable screening rates, as with breast and cervical cancers, mortality rates from colorectal cancer are higher among Blacks than Whites (James et al., 2006).

This chapter examines the role of health communication in the reduction of disparities in cancer outcomes and preventive health behaviors. Specifically, it explores the role that analyses of the Health Information National Trends Survey (HINTS) data may play in suggesting important health communication research questions and innovative intervention strategies targeted toward disadvantaged populations. We attempt to encourage more in-depth analyses of these data sets to inform more culturally sensitive and appropriate cancer communication.

HEALTH COMMUNICATION AND INFORMATION IN THE ELIMINATION OF DISPARITIES

Researchers concerned with health disparities are now moving beyond documenting the populations affected and the relative magnitude of the differences noted in health outcomes, and are increasingly focused on the strategies that will assist in the reduction of such disparities (Angeles & Somers, 2007). The Institute of Medicine (IOM, 2002) has recognized the importance of health communication and literacy in addressing health disparities. Great strides have been made in the use of technology, such as the Internet and wireless communication, bolstering the potential to advance the public's health. Yet, it is likely that technological advances in health care will only exacerbate existing disparities, unless disadvantaged groups make substantial gains in the ability to use, access, and understand relevant health information (Viswanath et al., 2006).

Information-seeking is composed of several behaviors that include actively or passively scanning for and gathering information to clarify or confirm knowledge about a particular topic, in this case health (Janis, 1984). Health educators and communication researchers are concerned about health information-seeking and literacy because well-informed patients are more apt to maintain a sense of control regarding their illness than those individuals with limited information (Janis, 1984; Lerman, Daly, Walsh, Resch, Seay, & Barsevick, 1993; Viney & Westbrook, 1984) and are better able to cope with illness outcomes and treatment consequences (Evans & Clarke, 1983; Mollem, Krabbendam, Annyas, Koops, Sleijfer, & Vermey, 1984). Correspondingly, there is documented evidence that having inadequate health information can have detrimental heath consequences (Denberg, Wong, & Beattie, 2005; Lerman et al., 1993). Importantly, cancer communication has been shown to play a role in reductions of cancer burden (Viswanath, 2005). Cancer communications provide the knowledge and skills that facilitate behavior change (Hornik, 2002); for example, communication campaigns have successfully increased rates of cancer screening (Viswanath, 2005).

Limitations in access to health information and related knowledge have been linked to problems with using preventive care, delayed diagnoses, and difficulty understanding one's medical condition (Wolf, Davis, & Parker, 2007). According to the Agency for Health Care Policy and Research (1997), the inability to access, understand and use health information (the IOM, 2002, definition of health literacy) likely plays a significant role in health disparities. The first national assessment of U.S. adult ability to access, understand, and use health information found that a disproportionate number of ethnic/racial minorities and low-income individuals had low health literacy (Wolf, Davis, & Parker, 2007). Specifically, more than half of Blacks, adults without health insurance, and the elderly had basic or below basic health literacy skills.

Although biological literacy is not discussed as often as health literacy, it has particular relevance as advances in the understanding of cancer biology, genetics, and treatment increase (Miller, 2007). Biological literacy exists along a continuum and varies by sex, education, and other types of literacy such as scientific literacy. Literacy in biology includes the recognition of key terms and concepts belonging to the domain; an accurate understanding and the ability to apply these and understand their place in the human experience; and finally the ability to examine and debate issues that involve the impact of biology on society, such as stem cell research and genetically based medicines (Uno & Bybee, 1994). Miller estimated that in 2005 only approximately 16% of adult Americans were biologically literate (Miller, 2007). Without biological literacy, citizens are ill-prepared to understand the development of genomic technologies that may result in more precise estimates of cancer risk, and new therapies for cancer that are being projected or developed.

Racial and ethnic differences in English proficiency, educational attainment, and general literacy can contribute to communication difficulties that limit health and biological literacy, and access to and processing of health information. Research suggests that approximately 20% of Spanish-speaking Latinos say they do not seek medical advice because of language barriers (IOM, 2002). A survey of 6,722 adults found that minority populations are more likely to have difficulties communicating with their health care providers compared with Whites (Collins, Hughes, Doty, Ives, Edwards, & Tenney, 2002). Specifically, minority populations were more likely than Whites to cite problems not fully understanding their doctor, with their doctor not listening to everything they said, and having questions during the visit but not asking them.

Dervin (2005) discussed the necessity of accommodating the information needs and preferences of individuals in any population. To achieve this goal it is important to understand involvement, situational circumstances, and sense-making needs. Involvement can include whether the message recipient is or has previously considered or been concerned about a topic and the creation of involvement through skill-building or empowerment activities. In the context of information-seeking, situational circumstances refer to lived experiences, such as interactions with health care professionals and systems, family history, and prior experiences with chronic disease. These situational circumstances affect the sense-making needs of information-seekers. Sense-making refers to the strategies used to decide when, what, and how to seek and use health information. These issues can be quite complex. At various times, there may be the need or desire for facts or information from authorities, and/or information provided by peers or supportive others.

According to the IOM (2002), appropriate strategies for addressing health literacy and information needs involve matching the needs of individuals to the information and services provided by health care systems. However, too often there is a mismatch between an individual's skills, needs, preferences, and expectations and the information and services that are available (Dervin, 2005). It is in this context that cultural competence in the development of health communications, interventions, and education becomes relevant.

Although a growing body of research outlines obstacles to the engagement in health preventative behaviors among minority, economically, and socially disadvantaged segments of the population (House & Williams, 2000; Huff & Kline, 1999; Shavers & Brown, 2002), relatively less is known about the barriers that adversely impact these individuals' involvement in health information-seeking, an equally relevant health behavior. The data derived from the HINTS, if properly used, can assist in identifying the gaps between what individuals and groups with adequate health literacy and information concerns need, prefer, access, and can use and what is currently available. This knowledge permits us to design, promote, and disseminate interventions and materials that inform efforts to reduce health disparities.

HINTS

HINTS provides health communications researchers and practitioners with a source of surveillance data related to variables that influence the access to and use of health information and communication (HINTS, 2007). Using a random-digit dialing telephone survey method, data were collected from October 2002 through April 2003 for HINTS 2003 and February 2005 to August 2005 for HINTS 2005. Although there are limitations of the data collected, such as its cross-sectional nature, lower response rates in 2005, and larger confidence intervals around population estimates due to sample size, its examination of issues relevant to health communication and cancer prevention and control make it a valuable resource.

For example, the HINTS survey queries respondents on several broad questions related to their cancer information search; including media exposure, Internet usage for health, sources of cancer information, use, preferences, awareness, trust, and ratings of experience with sources during searches. In 2003 and 2005, survey participants indicated the extent to which "It took a lot of effort," they "Felt frustrated during your search," and "Information was hard to understand" during their search. The data shifts from 2003 to 2005 suggest improvements in the cancer information environment. Participants were less likely to report that it look a lot of effort to find cancer information (2003, 48.4% strongly agreed or somewhat agreed compared with 37.3% in 2005), they felt frustrated during their search for information (2003, 41.9% strongly agreed or somewhat agreed compared with 26.7% in 2005), and found the information too hard to understand (2003, 37.7% strongly agreed or somewhat agreed compared with 23.7% in 2005). Although this trend toward greater ease in obtaining and improved understanding of cancer information was true across racial/ethnic groups, the data also indicates that ethnic/racial minorities, and those with less education and less income, continued to report more difficulties in obtaining and understanding information (see HINTS, 2007, Table 13, p. 52).

The trend identified by HINTS data, suggesting disparities in obtaining and understanding information for disadvantaged individuals, mirrors the literature on cancer burden and disparities (ACS, 2006, 2007); however, as is the case with health and cancer outcomes, we must move beyond merely documenting disparities to answering questions that will reduce the impact of disparities in health information and literacy. What makes information-seeking more effortful for these populations? Is it low literacy, low health literacy, or the result of linguistic barriers? Can HINTS help us gain a better understanding of where minority populations are looking and what *they* are looking for compared with the current channels used to disseminate health information and what current communications provide? Are some sources more frustrating than others? Do seeking experiences vary by population age, education, sex, and income? What makes data hard to understand? Are there styles of presenting data that are more user-friendly and how does data presentation affect perceptions of data quality?

EXTENDING COMMUNICATION REACH
AND EFFECTIVENESS

HINTS data have and can be used to guide exploration of issues that will increase our ability to reach ethnic minority and disadvantaged populations (Nguyen & Bellamy, 2006; Ramirez, 2007; Viswanath et al., 2006). Culturally appropriate communications may assist in reducing the impact of disparities in health information and literacy (Brach & Fraser, 2000; Pornpitakpan, 2004). Every cultural group has a system of attitudes, beliefs, and practices that are comprised of its general worldview (Kavanaugh & Kennedy, 1992). This worldview provides a set of guidelines that outlines socially acceptable activities, behaviors and beliefs, and enables each group to form their own coherent picture of the world (Spector, 1996). The views of the world that develop result in a number of concepts from which individuals can determine ways to maintain, protect, and restore their health.

As with other aspects of culture, beliefs, attitudes, and practices concerning health and well-being are subject to change across time and circumstances. One plausible precipitant of change is exposure to advances in health-related knowledge and expertise within the culture and/or outside of the culture. Media provide a major example of outside influences that may affect health beliefs and attitudes. Media influences may have a more persuasive effect if the appropriate inputs are used, as described by McGuire (1989) in his theory of persuasive communication. Two studies that used HINTS data suggest the need to consider source and channel selection, and highlight the role that English-language facility may play in patterns of information-seeking among ethnic populations (Nguyen & Bellamy, 2006; Ramirez, 2007).

Nguyen and Bellamy's use of HINTS data provide an example of one strategy to derive the information required to develop culturally appropriate communication. The authors examined the information needs and seeking behaviors of Asian Americans using HINTS 2003 data. Asian Americans were less knowledgeable about the benefits of not smoking or quitting smoking and were also less knowledgeable about the benefits of colon cancer screening than Whites. Although Asians Americans and Whites had similar rates of media use and preferences for cancer information from various sources, Asian Americans reported a significantly stronger preference for print materials.

Ramirez (2007) explored U.S. Latino/Hispanic health information behavior compared with non-Latino/Hispanic Whites and as a function of acculturation, using HINTS 2005 data. Latinos/Hispanics who preferred to complete the survey in Spanish were less likely to report: (a) seeking health or cancer information from any source, (b) that anyone had sought health information for them, (c) use of the Internet (20% Spanish-speaking compared with 60% English-speaking Latinos/Hispanics and 68% non-Latino/Hispanic Whites), and (d) reported a different media use pattern compared with English-speaking Latinos/Hispanics and non-Latino/Hispanic Whites.

HINTS data indicate that members of ethnic minority and economically and socially disadvantaged groups also reported greater concerns about the quality of the cancer information they obtained (43.8% of Whites, 61% of Blacks, and 59.2% of Latinos/Hispanics; see HINTS, 2007, p. 53, Table 13). Concerns for quality may relate to mistrust of source or it may reflect an affective or cognitive response to how and why the data are presented. This highlights the need for health communicators to explore the role of data presentation in cultural appropriateness and its influence on emotional and cognitive responses to health and cancer communications.

Health communication researchers (Kreuter, Lukwago, Bucholtz, Clark, & Thompson Sanders, 2003; Rogler, Malgady, Costantino, & Blumenthal, 1987) have described five basic approaches currently used to achieve cultural appropriateness in health communications: constituent-involving, peripheral, linguistic, sociocultural, and evidential. *Constituent-involving* strategies include members of the community in intervention activities as advisory board members or intervention staff, whether they are trained as paraprofessionals or act as natural helpers. *Peripheral* approaches enhance effectiveness of communication by packaging content in colors, fonts, images, photographs or declarative titles likely to appeal to a given group. Rogler et al. (1987) described *linguistic* strategies as those that make materials accessible by providing them in the native or dominant language of a group. These materials may be produced for a specific health-promotion activity or translations of existing materials. *Sociocultural* approaches discuss disease in the context of specific social and/or cultural characteristics of the group.

Evidential approaches (Kreuter et al., 2003) provide and discuss data specific to a group. While most evidence used in health promotion is statistical, it need not be. Testimonials and statements related to personal, family, or group experience can also be used as a form of evidence. Evidential statements seek to raise awareness, concern, and/or perceived personal vulnerability to a health concern by showing that it affects others similar to members of the target audience. Research has suggested that the perception that a problem affects others "like you" can increase thinking about the problem, the decision to engage in prevention, and planning to do so (Weinstein & Sandman, 1992). Previous research (Lipkus, Crawford, Fenn, Biradavolu, Binder, & Marcus, 1999) has confirmed the importance of presenting risk-factor information when informing men and women of their risks of cancer. Presenting risk information increased perceived risk without increasing worry, fear, or anxiety. Additional research (Royak-Schaler, Blocker, Yali, Bynoe, Briant, & Smith, 2004) has explored the presentation of evidence in cancer communications targeting Black and Hispanic women. The data seemed to suggest a preference for information about family history and personal risk, provided in graphic and quantitative forms and the need to explore other elements of data presentation.

The news media are a major source of health and cancer information for the American public (Viswanath, 2005). The majority of news stories about race and risk are comparative and highlight differences between racial groups (Singer & Endreny, 1993), with most of racially comparative stories emphasizing Blacks' poorer outcomes when compared with favorable outcomes of Whites and other groups (Gandy, 1996). Although these communications are developed and published with good intentions (Lambeth, Meyer, & Thorson, 1998), it is unclear whether the goal of motivating positive changes in health behaviors is achieved among Blacks exposed to the information.

The Precaution Adoption Process Model (Weinstein & Sandman, 1992) suggests that the decision whether to take action to prevent a problem is influenced by a person's belief that the problem is likely to occur in his or her community or among similar others. Exposure to racially specific cancer information is believed to produce this effect. However, exposure to racially comparative information might have the opposite effect. Hearing that one's group is worse off could lead to active avoidance, devaluation, or rejection of the information because people tend not to believe information that threatens their self-concept or favorable image of their referent group (Crocker, Voelker, Testa, & Major, 1991; Dunning, Leuenberger, & Sherman, 1995). This may be especially likely among African-Americans given their greater mistrust of the health care system (LaViest, 2005).

To determine whether racially comparative cancer information might have unintended negative consequences, a double-blind randomized study (Nicholson, Kreuter, Lapka, Wellborn, Clark, Thompson Sanders et al., 2008) was conducted. The study compared reactions to four versions of the same colon cancer information presented to a community-based sample of Black men and women. The participants read one of four articles that varied in their framing and interpretation of race-specific colorectal cancer mortality data. The articles either emphasized *impact* (colorectal cancer is an important problem for Blacks), two dimensions of *disparity* (Blacks are doing worse than Whites and Blacks are improving, but less than Whites), or *progress* (Blacks are improving over time).

Participants exposed to disparity articles reported more negative emotional reactions to the information and less intention to be screened for colorectal cancer than those in other groups. In contrast, progress articles elicited more positive emotional reactions and greater intention to be screened. Thus, the data suggest that the widespread practice of focusing on disparities in cancer communication to Black populations may undermine prevention and control efforts. HINTS data analyses that examine satisfaction with cancer information might suggest other data-presentation issues for various populations.

INTERSECTIONAL ANALYSES

To date, researchers' attempts to address cultural appropriateness and social determinants of health and health outcomes have been too simplistic (Mullings & Schulz, 2006). Often, research has failed to address the complex and dynamic structures of the communities most affected by disparity, as well as the intersecting nature of the characteristics associated with disparity. The intersectionality framework begins to focus on these issues. This framework acknowledges that disparities are not unique to health, and are observed in education, income, wealth, and occupational status. The theory, like several health-disparity researchers (LaViest, 2005; Williams, Yu, Jackson, & Anderson, 1997), acknowledges the historical existence of socioeconomic status (SES) inequity in society and how these factors structure the interactions and relationships that play a role in maintaining today's health-disparity dilemma (Mullings & Schulz, 2006). Intersectionality theory emphasizes "the simultaneous production of race, class, and gender inequality, such that in any given situation, the unique contribution of one factor might be difficult to measure" (p. 5). It attempts to explore how health disparity is produced as a function of complex social relationships rather than in and by individuals and groups.

Initial analyses of HINTS 2003 data support the relevance of the intersectionality framework. Simple race × gender analyses (Figs. 9.2 and 9.3) demonstrate the importance of intersectional analyses. Although both Hispanic males (42.2%) and females (45%) reported frustration in their information search, White females (41.2%) and Black males (40.4 %) were the next groups to express frustration. When exploring difficulty understanding cancer information, Hispanic women (46.1%) and Black men (40.5%) reported the greatest difficulty followed by Hispanic men (39.4%) and Black women (37.2%). A similar analysis, focused on race/ethnicity and income, illustrates the information difficulties of those with the least income (Fig. 9.4). However, the racial/ethnic groups most affected varied. Although

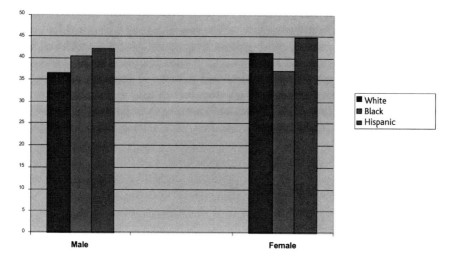

FIGURE 9.2. Percent reporting frustration during a health information search by race/ethnicity and gender.

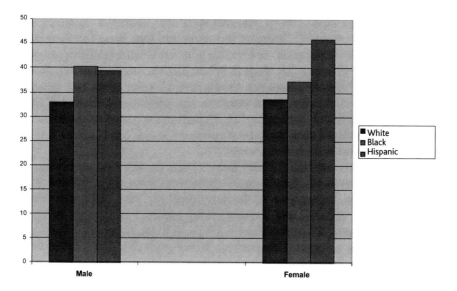

FIGURE 9.3. Percent reporting health information as difficult to understand by race/ethnicity and gender.

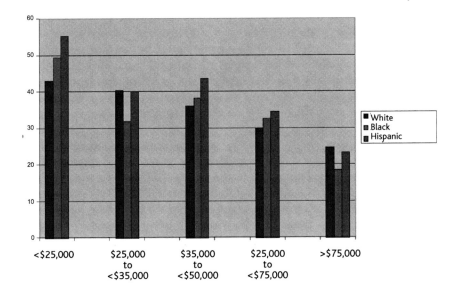

FIGURE 9.4. Percent reporting health information as difficult to understand by race/ethnicity and income.

in most income categories, Hispanics reported the greatest difficulty understanding cancer information, in other income categories, Whites reported greater difficulty. These data clearly suggest the importance of identifying the needs of population segments through simultaneous examination of more than a single category of disadvantage. Such analyses may support the development of more appropriate and targeted interventions.

Analyses by Viswanath et al. (2006) highlight the importance of the simultaneous analysis called for using the intersectionality framework. Using HINTS 2003 data, these researchers sought to understand the role of differential rates of information acquisition on risk behaviors and health disparities between SES groups. The researchers expected to find that SES was related to knowing about the relationship between cancer risk and smoking or sun exposure, but expected this relationship to be affected by the level of media coverage. An important finding of this study was that those with limited income and education also had less knowledge of the link between sun exposure and cancer risk information, regardless of media coverage. They also noted the importance of examining education and income within race, despite the traditional practice of treating racial/ethnic groups as homogenous. More educated Whites had greater awareness of the sun exposure and cancer link than less-educated Whites. This suggests the need to consider income, education, and sex differences within different racial and ethnic groups.

This overview of the use of HINTS data to better understand the health information-seeking patterns, preferences, and needs of vulnerable populations underscores the need to examine a number of factors that may affect information acquisition and use among ethnic/racial minorities and other economically and socially disadvantaged groups, including the identification of source and media channels (newspapers, magazines, Internet, television, etc.) that are the most effective for disseminating health messages to such groups.

In the next section, we describe two dissemination strategies that attempt to address ongoing disparities in access to cancer information. The work undertaken at the National Cancer Institute (NCI)-designated Center of Excellence in Cancer Communication Research (CECCR) at Washington University in Saint Louis provides examples of how research on health and cancer communication trends can be used to overcome barriers to access that make cancer-information seeking difficult and frustrating. The dissemination strategies described focus on identifying trusted media channels and overcoming barriers to the use of new communication technologies.

EFFECTIVE DISSEMINATION

Ozioma

There are more than 200 Black newspapers with a combined audience of 6 to 15 million readers (Muhammad, 2003; National Newspaper Publishers Association, 2008). Black newspapers are read, trusted, and valued by Blacks (Pickle, Quinn, & Brown, 2002). Their coverage is especially attentive to issues that affect local Black communities, and provides information and perspectives that are largely missing from general media (Vercellotti & Brewer, 2006). These characteristics make Blacks newspapers an ideal source for health information aimed at reducing health disparities in the Black community. Despite the cancer burden of the Black community (ACS, 2006, 2007), the mailing lists at most media relations and press offices in national health organizations do not include Black newspapers (Kreuter, 2008).

The Saint Louis CECCR aims to help eliminate cancer disparities by increasing the reach and effectiveness of cancer information in Black communities. As part of this effort, the Ozioma News Service was launched in December 2005 in collaboration with the nationally recognized School of Journalism at the University of Missouri. The Ozioma News Service provides community- and race-specific cancer news releases to Black newspapers. The word "Ozioma" is an Igbo/Nigerian word meaning "good news," which reflects the philosophy of the news service. Rather than focus on cancer disparities that would repeatedly show that Blacks are doing worse than other Americans, Ozioma news releases emphasize progress and opportunity in cancer prevention and control

In a national randomized study in 24 U.S. cities, the Ozioma News Service significantly increased cancer coverage in Black newspapers, and has sustained those changes for nearly 2 years (Cohen, Caburnay, Luke, Cameron, & Kreuter, in press). The study identified and content-analyzed all health and cancer coverage in the Black newspapers of the 24 cities beginning in April 2004. Black newspapers in 12 cities received Ozioma news releases and 12 served as control newspapers. Analyses indicated that intervention papers (receiving Ozioma News Service releases) provided significantly more cancer coverage. Annual surveys were also conducted with a panel of Black newspaper readers from the same 24 cities. Preliminary results suggest that use of Ozioma News Service releases was also associated with an increased likelihood of readers discussing cancer with family and friends, searching for cancer information on the Internet, eating healthier, and making a serious effort to reduce or quit smoking (Cohen et al., in press).

These findings suggest the influential role that Black newspapers can play in cancer communication. It also provides one potential strategy for increasing the use of this media channel to communicate about cancer. An analysis of HINTS media-use data might suggest other populations that would benefit from the use of ethnic-specific media. For example, HINTS analyses indicate that Latino/Hispanic participants are more likely than non-Latino/Hispanic Whites to report frustration during their search for cancer information and find the information obtained hard to understand. A news service directed toward increasing cancer coverage in Spanish-language newspapers and other Spanish-language media might decrease barriers, such as language, that could affect frustration and understanding.

New computer technologies provide an opportunity to provide convenient and rapid access to cancer information. The challenge in the use of the technology is its application in low-income and ethnic-minority populations, whose access to these technologies may be more limited (Lenhart, Horrigan, Rainie, Allen, Madden, & O'Grady, 2003). The next section discusses an example of an effort to use a commercial adaptation of computer technology, the computer kiosk, to provide health information to vulnerable populations.

KIOSKS TO EXTEND REACH

Viswanath (2005) noted that new communication technologies provide opportunities to create interventions that can influence the direction and impact of cancer prevention and control activities. However, interventions using technology have the potential to compound disparities unless the unique position and needs of disadvantaged communities are addressed.

Gaps in Internet use among advantaged and disadvantaged populations are closing and the Pew Internet & American Life Project reported that among nonusers of the Internet, Blacks and Hispanics are more likely than Whites to express a strong interest in gaining access (Lenhart et al., 2003). The report concluded that these groups are not held back by a lack of desire but rather "barriers of circumstance" (Lenhart et al., 2003, p. 34). To reduce gaps in access, the report recommends making more public computers available in accessible places. Public access computing through computer kiosks placed in community settings may help bridge the information divide created by differential access to personal computing technology.

Computer kiosks provide mobile, stand-alone, interactive computer programs that can deliver a variety of communications in easily accessed, user-friendly formats in high-traffic public spaces. Unlike other computer technologies, many kiosk-like devices such as bank ATMs, grocery store self-checkout lanes, museum exhibits, and air travel check-in are familiar to individuals from a wide range of socioeconomic backgrounds. This combination of user familiarity and public access makes computer kiosks attractive as a channel for disseminating evidence-based health education programs in community settings. However, the populations likely to have access to the kiosk must be a concern in selecting community placements (Kreuter, Alcaraz, Pfeiffer, & Kristopher, 2008).

Reach and *specificity* are commonly used to determine the selection of marketing channels (Schooler, Chaffee, Flora, & Roser, 1998). Although reach is defined as the number and type of individuals who participate in a program, specificity refers to a channel's ability to reach a particular, or specific, priority population. These criteria suggest that the optimal channels for disseminating cancer control programs are those that are easily and widely accessible to the target population, provide easy opportunity for participation or use, can be appropriately altered to deliver cancer information, and have wide reach to specific target audiences (Kreuter et al., 2008). The argument can be made that innovative, technological intervention strategies should be evaluated using these criteria to determine the extent to which they will diminish or exacerbate disparities in access to cancer information.

Washington University in Saint Louis CECCR has created computer kiosks designed to create tailored magazines about breast cancer and mammography. Users respond to questions on a touch-screen monitor, and the computer uses this information to generate and print each tailored magazine. All elements of the kiosk program were adapted from a tailored intervention shown in a randomized trial to increase mammography use among Black women (Kreuter, Skinner, Holt, Clark, Haire-Joshu, Fu, 2005). Data were gathered from 10,306 kiosk uses in 92 beauty salons, churches, neighborhood health centers, laundromats, social service agencies, health fairs, and public libraries between June 2003 and March 2007 (Kreuter et al., 2008).

The average number of total users per kiosk day was highest at health fairs, followed by Laundromats and lowest at churches and beauty salons. Among kiosk users aged 40 years and older, those at health fairs were the most likely to report that they knew where to go to get a mammogram and those at laundromats were the least likely to know where to go. Similarly, kiosk users at health fairs were the most likely to report ever having a mammogram and those at laundromats the least likely. Of the seven settings, only laundromats were found to provide both high reach (i.e., frequent kiosk use) and high specificity (i.e., a large proportion of users with no health insurance, unaware of where to get a mammogram, reporting no recent mammogram and barriers to getting one, and having little knowledge about breast cancer and mammography). Given the knowledge gaps established through HINTS analyses, kiosks and similar efforts to present cancer information using technological innovation are necessary. However, these kiosk data suggest the need for careful analysis of the placement of these technologies.

CONCLUSION

This chapter examined the role of HINTS, as a communication surveillance system, in the reduction of disparities in cancer outcomes and preventive health behaviors. Specifically, it explored the role that analyses of HINTS data may play in suggesting important health communication research questions and how these findings might stimulate innovative intervention strategies targeted toward disadvantaged populations. This discussion suggests the need to engage in more complex analyses of HINTS data, including simultaneous consideration of sex, income, and education within racial and ethnic groups. Additionally, the data suggest the utility of examining a variety of issues, including cancer knowledge, attitudes toward screening and preventive behaviors, patterns of information-seeking, and difficulties encountered. These analyses will support efforts to identify information needs that may be addressed through considerations of channel selection, use of technology, and alternative strategies for the presentation of information. Likewise, there should be more in-depth analyses of cultural issues, such as the impact of language preference and use on cancer communication and information.

The intervention strategies described are not exhaustive, and are meant only to suggest that there are numerous options for improving the reach and effectiveness of the work that we do. The intersectional analytic framework highlights the needs of specific subgroups and permits better targeting of interventions. For example, although it is clear that all segments of the

Hispanic community will benefit from more culturally appropriate interventions, the data suggest that among Blacks there is a greater need for programs that target men.

The analyses and studies presented suggest important issues that future HINTS surveys will need to address. Methodological experiments may need to focus on strategies to encourage and improve ethnic minority response in future HINTS surveys. Adequate sampling will affect the ability to conduct analyses of smaller ethnic minority populations, but also the ability to conduct analyses that take into account differences in nationality and culture among Spanish-speaking, Asian, Native American, increasingly people of African descent, and other racial/ethnic groups as well. As we understand the persistence of information disparities among diverse populations, it becomes more important to identify the source of difficulties, frustrations, and concerns with quality. This may require supplemental questions that are periodically administered in order to understand whether these issues are specific to data presented through specific channels, sponsored by particular agencies or organizations, or in particular formats.

ACKNOWLEDGMENTS

This project was supported by grants from the National Cancer Institute's (NCI) Centers of Excellence in Cancer Communication Research program (CA-P50-95815) and Community Networks Program for the Elimination of Cancer Disparities (PECaD) (5-U01-CA114594).

REFERENCES

Agency for Health Care Policy and Research. (1997). Evidence-based practice centers (RFP No. AHCPR-97-001). Washington, DC: HHS.

American Cancer Society (ACS). (2006). *Facts & figures for Hispanics 2006-2008.* Atlanta, GA: Author.

American Cancer Society (ACS). (2007). *Cancer facts & figures for African Americans 2007-2008.* Atlanta, GA: Author.

Angeles, J., & Somers, S. A. (2007). From policy to action: Addressing racial and ethnic disparities at the ground-level. *Center for Health Care Strategies, Inc. Issue Brief.* Retrieved November 28, 2007, from http://www.chcs.org

Brach, C., & Fraser, I. (2000). Can cultural competency reduce racial and ethnic health disparities? A review and conceptual model. *Medical Care Research & Review, 57*(suppl 1), 81-217.

Budrys, G. (2003). *Unequal health: How inequality contributes to health or illness.* Lanham, MD: Rowman & Littlefield.

Carter-Pokras, O., & Baquet, C. (2002). What is a "health disparity"? *Public Health Reports, 117*, 426-433.

Cohen, E., Caburnay, C., Luke, D., Cameron, G., & Kreuter, M. (in press). Cancer coverage in general audience and black newspapers. *Health Communication.*

Collins, K., Hughes, D., Doty, M., Ives, B., Edwards, J., & Tenney, K. (2002). Diverse communities, common concerns: Assessing health care quality for minority Americans. *The Common-wealth Fund 2001 Health Care Quality Survey.* New York: The Commonwealth Fund.

Crocker, J., Voelker, K., Testa, M., Major, B. (1991). Social stigma: The affective consequences of attributional ambiguity. *Journal Personality Social Psychology, 60,* 218-228.

Denberg, T., Wong, S., & Beattie, A. (2005). Women's misconceptions about cancer screening: Implications for informed decision making. *Patient Education & Counseling, 57*(3), 280-285.

Dervin, B. (2005). Libraries reaching out with health information to vulnerable populations: Guidance from research on information seeking and use. *Journal of the Medical Library Association, 93*(suppl), S74-S80.

Dunning, D., Leuenberger, A., & Sherman, D. A. (1995). A new look at motivated inference. Are self-serving theories of success a product of motivated forces? *Journal of Personality and Social Psychology, 69,* 58-68.

Evans, S., & Clarke, P. (1983). When cancer fails to get well: Flaws in health communication. In M. Burgion (Ed.), *Communication yearbook 7, Part 1* (pp. 225-248). New Brunswick, NJ: Transaction Books.

Gandy, O. H. (1996). If it weren't for bad luck: Framing stories of racially comparative risk. In V. Berry & C. Manning-Miller (Eds.), *Mediated messages and African American culture: Contemporary issues* (pp. 55-75). Thousand Oaks: Sage.

Heron, M. (2007) Deaths: Leading causes for 2004. *National Vital Statistics Report, 56*(5), 1-96.

HINTS (2007). *Health Information National Trends Survey (HINTS) Facts.* Retrieved November 26, 2007, from http://hints.cancer.gov

Hornik, R. (2002). *Public health communication: Evidence for behavior change.* Mahwah, NJ: Erlbaum.

House, J., & Williams, D. R. (2000). Understanding and reducing socioeconomic and racial/ethnic disparities in health. In B.D. Smedley & S.L. Syme (Eds.), *Promoting health: Intervention strategies from social and behavioral research* (pp. 81-124), Washington, DC: National Academies Press.

Huff, R., & Kline, M. (Eds.). (1999). *Promoting health in multicultural populations: A handbook for practitioners.* Thousand Oaks, CA: Sage.

Institute of Medicine (IOM). (2002). Committee on Understanding & Eliminating Racial & Ethnic Disparities in Health Care. In B.D. Smedley, A.Y. Stith, & A.R. Nelson (Eds.), *Unequal treatment confronting racial and ethnic disparities in health care.* Washington, DC: National Academies Press.

James, C., Thomas, M., Lillie-Blanton, M., & Garfield, R. (2006). *Key facts race, ethnicity & medical care.* Menlo Park, CA: The Henry J. Kaiser Family Foundation.

Janis, L. (1984). The caller as decision maker. In W. Gentry (Ed.), *Handbook of behavioral medicine* (pp. 326-367). New York: Guilford.

Kavanaugh, K. H., & Kennedy, P. H. (1992). *Promoting cultural diversity: Strategies for health care professionals.* Newbury Park, CA: Sage.

Kreuter, M. (2008). *Research findings and dissemination opportunities from the St. Louis CECCR.* Paper presented at the Centers for Excellence in Cancer Communication Grantees Meeting, Atlanta, GA.

Kreuter, M., Alcaraz, K., Pfeiffer, D., & Kristopher, K. (2008). Using dissemination research to identify optimal community settings for tailored breast cancer information kiosks. *Journal of Public Health Management and Practice, 14*(2), 160-169.

Kreuter, M., Lukwago, S., Bucholtz, D., Clark, E., & Thompson Sanders. V. (2003). Achieving cultural appropriateness in health promotion programs: Targeted and tailored approaches. *Health Education & Behavior, 30,* 133-146.

Kreuter, M., Skinner, C., Holt, C., Clark, E.M., Haire-Joshu, D., Fu, Q. et al. (2005). Cultural tailoring for mammography and fruit and vegetable intake among low-income African American women in urban public health centers. *Preventive Medicine, 41,* 53-62.

Lambeth, E., Meyer, P., & Thorson, E. (Eds.). (1998). *Assessing public journalism.* Columbia: University of Missouri Press.

LaViest, T. A. (2005). *Minority populations and health: An introduction to health disparities in the United States.* San Francisco, CA: Jossey-Bass.

Lenhart, A., Horrigan, J., Rainie, L., Allen, K., Madden, M., & O'Grady, E. (2003). *The ever-shifting internet population: A new look at internet access and the digital divide.* Washington, DC: Pew Internet & American Life Project.

Lerman, C., Daly, M., Walsh, W., Resch, N., Seay, J., & Barsevick, A. (1993). Communication between patients with breast cancer and health care providers. *Cancer, 72*(9), 2612-2620.

Lipkus, I., Crawford, Y., Fenn, K., Biradavolu, M., Binder, R., Marcus, A. et al. (1999). Testing different formats for communicating colorectal cancer risk. *Journal of Health Communication, 4,* 311-324.

McGuire W. (1989). Theoretical foundations of campaigns. In R. Rice & C. Atkin (Eds.), *Public communication campaigns* (2nd ed.). Newbury Park, CA: Sage.

Miller, J. (2007). *Assessing the public's comprehension of biomedical science.* Paper presented at the HINTS Data Users Conference, Pasadena, CA.

Mollem, D., Krabbendam, P., Annyas, A., Koops, H., Sleijfer, D., & Vermey, A. (1984). The significance of the doctor-caller relationship in coping with cancer. *Social Science & Medicine, 18*(6), 475-480.

Muhammad, L. (2003). The black press: Past and present. *Nieman Reports, 57*(3), 13-16.

Mullings, L., & Schulz, A. J. (2006). Intersectionality and health: An introduction. In A. J. Schulz & L Mullings (Eds.). *Gender, race, class and health: Intersectional approaches* (pp. 3-17). San Francisco, CA: Jossey-Bass.

National Center for Health Statistics (NCHS). (2002). *Health, United States, 2002: With chartbook on trends in the health of Americans.* Hyattsville, MD: U.S. Department of Health and Human Services.

National Newspaper Publishers Association. (2008). *NNPA Media Services.* Retrieved January 28, 2008, from http://www.nnpa.org/news/article/article.asp?sID=24

Nguyen, G. T., & Bellamy, S. C. (2006). Cancer information seeking preferences and experiences: Disparities between Asian Americans and whites in the Health Information National Trends Survey (HINTS). *Journal of Health Communication, 11*(suppl 1), 173-180.

Nicholson, R., Kreuter, M., Lapka, C., Wellborn, R., Clark, E. M., Thompson Sanders, V. et al. (2008). Unintended effects of emphasizing disparities in cancer communications to African Americans. *Cancer Epidemiology, Biomarkers and Prevention, 17*(11), 2946-2953.

Office of Minority Health (OMH). (2005, October 19). *Eliminating racial & ethnic disparities.* Retrieved November 17, 2007, from http://www.cdc.gov/omh/AboutUs/disparities.htm.

Office of Minority Health and Health Disparity (OMHD). (2007). *Racial and ethnic populations.* Retrieved December 3, 2007, from http://www.cdc.gov/omhd/Populations/populations.htm (accessed).

Pickle, K., Quinn, S., & Brown, J. (2002). HIV/AIDS coverage in Black newspapers, 1991-1996: Implications for health communication and health education. *Journal of Health Communication, 7*(5), 427-444.

Pornpitakpan, C. (2004). The persuasiveness of source credibility: A critical review of five decades' evidence. *Journal of Applied Social Psychology, 34*, 243-281.

Ramirez, A. S. (2007). Health information media use and cancer information seeking differences between Spanish- and English-speaking Latinos and non-Hispanic Whites. Poster presented at the HINTS Data Users Conference, Pasadena, CA.

Rogler, L. H., Malgady, R. G., Costantino, G., & Blumenthal, R. (1987). What do culturally sensitive mental health services mean? *American Psychologist, 42*, 565-570.

Royak-Schaler, R., Blocker, D., Yali, A., Bynoe, M., Briant, K., & Smith, D. (2004). Breast and colorectal cancer risk communication approaches with low-income African-American and Hispanic women: Implications for healthcare providers. *Journal of the National Medical Association, 96*, 598-608.

Schooler, C., Chaffee, S., Flora, J. A., & Roser, C. (1998). Health campaign channels: Tradeoffs among reach, specificity and impact. *Human Communication Research, 24*(3), 410-432.

Shavers, V. L., & Brown, M. L. (2002). Racial and ethnic disparities in the receipt of cancer treatment. *Journal of the National Cancer Institute, 94*, 334-357.

Singer, E., & Endreny, P. (1993). *Reporting on risk: How the mass media portray accidents, diseases, disasters and other hazards.* New York: Russell Sage.

Spector, R. (1996). *Cultural diversity in health and illness.* Stamford, CT: Appleton & Lange.

Uno, G. E., & Bybee, R. W. (1994). Understanding the dimensions of biological literacy. *Bioscience, 44*(8), 553-557.

Vercellotti, T., & Brewer, P. (2006). "To plead our own cause:" Public opinion toward Black and mainstream news media among African Americans. *Journal of Black Studies, 37*(2), 231-250.

Viney, L., & Westbrook, M. (1984). Coping with chronic illness: Strategy preferences, changes in preferences, and associated emotional reactions. *Journal of Chronic Disease, 37*(6), 489-508.

Viswanath, K. (2005). Science and society: The communications revolution and cancer control. *National Review of Cancer, 5*(10), 828-835.

Viswanath, K., Breen, N., Meissner, H., Moser, R. P., Hesse, B., Steele, W. R., & Rakowski, W. (2006). Cancer knowledge and disparities in the information age. *Journal of Health Communication, 11*(suppl 1), 1-17.

Ward, E., Jemal, A., Cokkinides, V., Singh, G. K., Cardinez, C., Ghafoor, A., & Thun, M. (2004). Cancer disparities by race/ethnicity and socioeconomic status. *CA: A Cancer Journal for Clinicians, 54*, 78-93.

Weinstein, N., & Sandman, P. (1992). A model of the precaution adoption process: Evidence from home radon testing. *Health Psychology, 11*, 170-180.

Williams, D. R., Yu, Y., Jackson, J. S., & Anderson, N. B. (1997). Racial differences in physical and mental health: Socio-economic status, stress, and discrimination. *Journal of Health Psychology, 2*(3), 335-351.

Williams, D. R., Neighbors, H. W., & Jackson, J. S. (2003). Racial/ethnic discrimination and health: Findings from community studies. *American Journal of Public Health, 93*(2), 200-208.

Wolf, M. S., Davis, T. C., & Parker, R. M. (2007). Editorial: The emerging field of health literacy research. *American Journal of Health Behavior, 31*(suppl 1), S3-S5.

10

HEALTH COMMUNICATION CHANNEL PREFERENCES BY CLASS, RACE, AND PLACE

Kelly D. Blake

Sherrie Flynt-Wallington

K. Viswanath

*Harvard School of Public Health
and Dana-Farber Cancer Institute*

Among several factors that influence the effectiveness of health communication, exposure to messages has been offered as one of the more significant determinants (Hornik, 2002). In fact, examining magnitude of exposure has been an important strategy in assessing most communication campaign interventions, and often is cited as an explanation for campaign success or failure (Hornik et al., 2001). Differential exposure and differential use of information channels could potentially influence learning about health from mediated communications. The flow of information on a given topic may lead to differential learning among members of certain groups, delineated by socioeconomic status (SES), race and ethnicity, or geographic area (Viswanath & Finnegan, 1996).

Antecedents to differential exposure and resultant differential learning are explored in this chapter, with an eye toward elucidating the preferred communication channels through which to reach vulnerable populations with health messages. In the world of advertising and marketing, much attention is given to how communication is executed, including the selection of appropriate and effective communication channels, to ensure adequate exposure. Despite the importance of communication channels in ensuring exposure, little attention has been paid to examining channel preferences for health and cancer communications. In general, demographic factors such as age, sex, education, and income are used to understand how people and groups prefer to receive information. And some work has combined demographic factors with psychological factors to develop psychographic profiles. This chapter departs from these conventional approaches in two significant ways. First, we focus on a range of social determinants of health, such as class, race, and place, to understand group-level communication channel preferences as they relate to health and cancer communications. Second, we draw on our recently developed Structural Influence Model (SIM) of health communication, emphasizing the construct of *communication inequality*, to explain how social determinants could be connected to extant health disparities through inequalities in communication access and exposure. We conclude by presenting a multivariable analysis of health communication channel preferences by class, race, and place, with the hope of making both theoretical and practical contributions to efforts aimed at increasing exposure to health promotion and disease prevention messages among audiences beset by health disparities.

HEALTH COMMUNICATION: THE IMPACT OF ACCESS AND EXPOSURE AT MULTIPLE LEVELS

Behavioral Risk Factors

Lifestyle factors and individual behaviors are thought to account for the majority of chronic diseases in the United States (McGinnis & Foege, 1993). As such, major efforts in health promotion and disease prevention have sought to reduce the morbidity and mortality from chronic diseases such as cancer, cardiovascular disease, and diabetes, as well as from infectious diseases such as HIV/AIDS. Communication, in its many forms (including interpersonal communication, mass media, and other types), plays a central role in promoting individual behaviors that are known to prevent disease and poor health, and has the potential to reverse many prevalent chronic illnesses (Institute of Medicine [IOM], 2002).

Indeed, there are several examples of large- and small-scale health communication efforts that have resulted in positive changes in behavior among individuals (Rimer & Glassman, 1999; Snyder & Hamilton, 2002). The "Truth"® campaign, a mass media campaign created to curb adolescent smoking first in Florida and then nationally, proved effective in reducing national smoking rates among adolescents from 25% to 18% between 1999 and 2000 (Farrelly, Davis, Haviland, Messeri, & Healton, 2005; Niederdeppe, Farrelly, & Haviland, 2004). The "Back to Sleep" campaign, aimed at preventing sudden infant death syndrome, affected a significant national decline, from 70% to 17% between 1992 and 1998, in the proportion of infants placed on their backs when put to sleep (Hornik, 2002; Willinger, Ko, Hoffman, Kessler, & Corwin, 2003).

Outside the realm of mass media campaigns, smaller scale communication efforts also have produced improvements in health behaviors at the individual level. The emergence of tailored and targeted communication strategies has been part of a growing approach to customize health information to individuals and groups (Rimer & Kreuter, 2006). There is some evidence that *tailoring*—providing health education messages based on an individual's personal attributes and risk factors such as age and family history—improves adherence to a multitude of health behaviors, including cancer screening, smoking cessation, and diet (Kreuter et al., 2005; Marcus et al., 2005; McBride et al., 2002; Rimer et al., 1999; Rimer et al., 1994). Additionally, *targeting*—developing and disseminating health promotion and disease-specific messages to specific population subgroups (e.g., delineated by race/ethnicity, age, gender, etc.)—also has been a successful health communication and social marketing strategy (Demark-Wahnefried et al., 1998). Early examples of targeted health communication efforts have been well documented (Hornik, 2002), and have included smoking cessation self-help guides for blue-collar and minority smokers (Strecher, Rimer, & Monaco, 1989), Blacks (Robinson, Sutton, James, & Orleans, 1992), pregnant women (Davis, Cummings, Rimer, Sciandra, & Stone, 1992) and women with young children (Keintz, Fleisher, & Rimer, 1994).

Interpersonal communication, such as advice from doctors to patients and information transmitted between and among family members and social networks, is effective in establishing, promoting, and sustaining a variety of behaviors beneficial to health. For example, provider advice delivered in routine practice settings has been shown to have an effect on smoking cessation success rates among both heavy and non-daily smokers (Bao, Duan, & Fox, 2006; Lancaster & Stead, 2004; Tong, Ong, Vittinghoff, & Perez-Stable, 2006). Additionally, provider advice about weight loss is associated with patients eating fewer calories and using exercise to lose weight (Loureiro & Nayga, 2006). Provider recommendation also is an influential determinant of colorectal cancer screening, even among the uninsured (Cairns & Viswanath, 2006). Peer influence, transmitted interpersonally and through social networks, can be either beneficial or detrimental to health. For example, a study examining the effectiveness of a peer-led substance abuse prevention program for adolescents found that programs transmitted through social networks could accelerate the effect of established peer influences. For adolescents with social networks supportive of not using drugs, prevention messages delivered through social networks were effective at reducing drug use; however, for adolescents with social networks that support substance use, programs transmitted through social networks had deleterious effects (Valente et al., 2007).

Yet another form of communication, news media coverage by print and broadcast outlets, is effective at heightening the salience of health issues and framing discussions about health topics in the public arena. There is evidence that health behaviors are responsive to shifts in news media coverage of a topic (Viswanath & Finnegan, 2002). News media play an important role in defining priority health issues and in disseminating new research findings (McCombs & Ghanem, 2001; Reese, Gandy, & Grant, 2001; Schwartz & Woloshin, 2002; Stryker, 2003; Stryker, Emmons, & Viswanath, 2007; Tichenor, Donohue, & Olien, 1980). Through their routine coverage of scientific developments, news media are a critical intermediary in translating research discoveries for the public, patients, practitioners, and policymakers. Some studies suggest that media not only are key sources in defining the importance and relevance of health issues, but also in shaping the public's perceptions of who is responsible for public health problems and their solutions (Caburnay et al., 2003; Shuchman, 2002).

Social Determinants of Health

In addition to individual risk factors, there are several social determinants of health that impact disease outcomes and health-related quality of life either directly (e.g., via environmental exposures) or indirectly (e.g., via opportunity structures that enable or constrain the ability to participate in health-enhancing activities such as buying fresh produce, exercising in safe areas, and getting recommended screening tests for cancer; Berkman & Kawachi, 2000; Emmons et al., 2001). Social determinants of health include, but are not limited to, structural aspects of neighborhoods, poverty, income inequality, racism and discrimination, gender inequality, occupational hazards and job strain, and social cohesion.

Primarily, institutions are responsible for enacting policies to address the larger social determinants of health. As such, communication is a necessary thread in the diffusion of information to those institutions (e.g., business and government), which have the ability to implement changes to improve health at the population level (Hornik, 2002). Policy efforts to modify regulation and taxation in a given area often are referred to as "scaled-up" interventions, where influential policymakers and decision leaders are persuaded that disease prevention and health promotion efforts are most successful when they address multiple levels of influence, and take steps to remedy the socially constructed phenomena that contribute to poor health, especially among disadvantaged populations. The diffusion of scientific knowledge about the dangers of secondhand smoke, for example, illustrates how communication facilitates the process between scientific discovery and the delivery of policy interventions enacted by institutions such as business and government to improve population health, in this case, via

clean indoor air regulations. In many ways, communication efforts intended to affect changes in individual behavior also operate through institutional paths to affect broad changes in the social environment (Hornik &
Yanovitzky, 2003). For example, campaigns designed to deter drunk driving
are thought to have worked more by influencing policy than by directly
changing individual behaviors (Yanovitzky & Bennett, 1999; Yanovitzky &
Stryker, 2001).

Policy-level interventions may impact health directly or indirectly.
Direct effects occur when policies require changes in the exposures that promote or harm health, with little or no agency required on the part of individuals. An often cited example is the mass fluoridation of the water supply
enacted to reduce dental caries in the population. A review of studies on the
effectiveness of water fluoridation conducted in the United States from 1979
to 1989 found that the average reduction in tooth decay among adolescents
was 27% (Newbrun, 1989). Water fluoridation is especially beneficial for
communities of low SES, who have a disproportionate burden of dental
caries and have less access than higher income communities to dental care
services and other sources of fluoride (Riley, Lennon, & Ellwood, 1999).
Additionally, clean indoor air regulations directly reduce individuals' exposure to the harmful effects of secondhand smoke, thereby reducing the overall incidence of tobacco-related illnesses such as lung cancer in adults and
asthma, ear infections, and bronchitis in children (National Cancer Institute
[NCI], 1999). The indirect effects of policy-level interventions are more
subtle, and usually work by changing the structural and social context within which individuals behave, to employ external constraints or incentives on
behavior. For example, policies supportive of investment in the built environment improve neighborhood influences on health by allowing for the
construction of sidewalks, green space, and lighting to enable individuals to
be physically active and engage in social support (Owen, Humpel, Leslie,
Bauman, & Sallis, 2004; Saelens, Sallis, & Frank, 2003).

FUNCTIONS OF HEALTH COMMUNICATION

Communication, and health communication in particular, may serve several
functions including an informational function, an instrumental function, a
social control function, and a communal function (Viswanath, 2006). These
functions are not mutually exclusive; rather, they may operate simultaneously to shape the complex process of health communication.

In public health and medicine, the informational function of communication allows people and patients to acquire knowledge and awareness along
a disease continuum, from prevention to detection, diagnosis, treatment,

survivorship, and end of life. Knowledge acquired from interpersonal interactions such as doctor–patient communication, and from mass communication efforts such as advertising and media campaigns, is considered part of the informational function of health communication.

The instrumental function of communication is best described as the provision of information that enables action. Appointment reminders, information about transportation services to community events, and Internet verification of drug regimens are all examples of how communication can be instrumental at the individual level. At a macro level, the diffusion of scientific evidence to institutions such as the media or advocacy groups can inform elite opinions, which may affect changes in policy (Hornik, 2002).

In performing a function of social control, where social norms are defined and reinforced, communication can create or accelerate secular trends in health. A prominent example comes from tobacco control, where multifaceted efforts, including communication campaigns and heightened media coverage of tobacco control policies, the dangers of tobacco use, and the intentions of the tobacco industry, have influenced the denormalization of smoking in the United States and in other parts of the world (Hammond, Fong, Zanna, Thrasher, & Borland, 2006). Communication techniques also are used in ways that are at odds with public health efforts that aim to change the social norms around tobacco. For example, the tobacco industry frequently uses Hollywood to depict smoking in movies, effectively maintaining the image of tobacco use as part of the social tapestry. A recent review of the effect of viewing smoking portrayal in the movies and subsequent adolescent attitudes and behavior showed that exposure to movie smoking makes viewers' attitudes and beliefs about smoking more favorable, and has a dose–response relationship with adolescent smoking behavior (Charlesworth & Glantz, 2006; Dalton et al., 2003; Sargent et al., 2005).

In its communal function, communication can enhance social support between members of a social network by facilitating norms of reciprocity and access to social capital. In fact, communication is central to the development and maintenance of relationships that could generate social capital (Viswanath, 2008). Disease-specific support groups and online communities of cancer survivors are examples of how health communication can serve a communal function by enabling health-enhancing and supportive interactions among members of a group or community. An assessment of 10 cancer-specific online mailing lists revealed that cancer survivors use Internet lists to offer informational support to other cancer patients, primarily focusing on technical information and explicit advice for how best to communicate with providers; emotional support also is sought and delivered through these online networks (Meier, Lyons, Frydman, Forlenza, & Rimer, 2007). Participation in community groups may also serve as a source of health information (Viswanath, Randolph Steele, & Finnegan, 2006). Certainly, the communal function of communication may not always be beneficial to health. For example, online networks of anorexics and bulimics that use Web sites to communicate and perpetuate eating disorder themes and behaviors can be detrimental to health.

THE KNOWLEDGE GAP AND COMMUNICATION INEQUALITY

The Knowledge Gap Hypothesis

In the 1990s, as disparities in health outcomes and health care by race, ethnicity, sex, and SES (represented by income, education, and occupation; Daly, Duncan, McDonough, & Williams, 2002) received increased attention from U.S. health authorities and public health researchers and practitioners, so too did communication efforts aimed at reducing health disparities among underserved and vulnerable populations (IOM, 2002). Despite the many successes in health communication, for decades investigators have documented differential returns on communication efforts by social group and status. Tichenor et al. (1970) first coined the Knowledge Gap Hypothesis to illustrate how health communication efforts often benefit those of higher SES more than those of low SES, thus widening the already existent gap in health knowledge and contributing another dimension to the notion of health disparities. Several studies have explored the Knowledge Gap Hypothesis, and have confirmed that, indeed, learning remains differential among low SES populations, favoring those of higher SES, despite mass communication efforts and interpersonal communication endeavors that aim to inform equally (Viswanath & Finnegan, 1996).

Differences in knowledge also are pronounced by race and geographic location. For example, despite a plethora of communication efforts aimed at increasing awareness about cancer prevention, early detection, and treatment, one study that assessed popular misconceptions about how cancer spreads revealed interesting differences in knowledge by SES and by race; minorities and people with low levels of education and income consistently demonstrated higher agreement with cancer myths such as, "Surgery can cause cancer to spread" (Gansler et al., 2005). Other studies assessing the sociodemographic correlates of scientifically unsubstantiated beliefs about cancer risk have come to similar conclusions. In assessing agreement with incorrect statements such as, "You cannot get skin cancer from a tanning booth," and "People who smoke low-tar cigarettes have less chance of developing lung cancer than people who smoke regular cigarettes," respondents who were male, older, non-White, less educated, and of lower income were most likely to endorse inaccurate beliefs (Stein, Zhao, Crammer, & Gansler, 2007).

Communication Inequality

Underlying the manifest communication effect of knowledge gaps is a series
of related factors that may contribute to those gaps and to health disparities
generally. Viswanath and colleagues contend that knowledge gaps are one
outcome resultant of communication inequality. *Communication inequality*
is defined as differences among social classes in the generation, manipula-
tion, and distribution of information at the societal level, and differences in
access to and ability to take advantage of information at the individual level
(Viswanath, 2006). Social determinants such as race, class, or geographic area
may work through communication and communication inequality, leading
to health disparities.

Dimensions of Communication Inequality

When considering the dimensions of communication inequality and its
effects, the differences found at the group/societal level are structural influences that facilitate or constrain a group's capacity to act in a manner that is
beneficial to health. Therefore, differences in the way health information is
generated and distributed among groups can create knowledge gaps between
and among groups that do and do not receive adequate exposure to health
information. At the individual level, the dimensions of communication
inequality and its effects include access to and use of information channels
such as television, Internet, radio, and newspapers; attention to health information that is available in the communication environment; recall, knowledge, and comprehension of health information; and personal capacity to act
on information, for example, by having the resources to purchase or obtain
beneficial provisions such as recommended health screenings, healthy foods,
or condoms.

Social epidemiology considers the social contexts within which behavioral risk factors occur (Berkman & Kawachi, 2000; Phelan, Link, Diez-
Roux, Kawachi, & Levin, 2004), and social epidemiologists have asserted the
need for the field to examine the mechanisms that may connect the distal
social determinants of health and with proximal individual risk factors, ultimately to explain known disparities in health (Kaplan, 2004). Communication inequality is among the social determinants of health that may create
and/or exacerbate invidious health disparities, and communication is one
thread that may connect multiple levels of influence on health (Viswanath,
Ramanadhan, & Kontos, 2007).

In 2007, Viswanath and colleagues proposed the SIM of health communication (Viswanath, Ramanadhan, & Kontos, 2007; Fig. 10.1). The model
delineates how communication inequality could help to explain disparities

in health, both as a moderating factor in some cases, and as an independent predictor in others.

According to the SIM, differential communication outcomes (e.g., access, usage, attention, and processing of health communication messages) are influenced by antecedents such as SES and geography, and the effects of those factors may vary by moderating conditions such as age, sex, race/ethnicity, and social networks. All structural antecedents are hypothesized to influence the information environment, thereby leading to differential communication behaviors that may, in turn, affect behavioral outcomes (such as knowledge, beliefs, and adoption of preventive behaviors), and disease outcomes (such as incidence and mortality). Therefore, the model posits that health disparities could potentially be explained by inequalities along the communication continuum, resulting in a cumulative effect on health outcomes. In this chapter, we examine yet another dimension of inequality: differences in preferences for channels to seek health information.

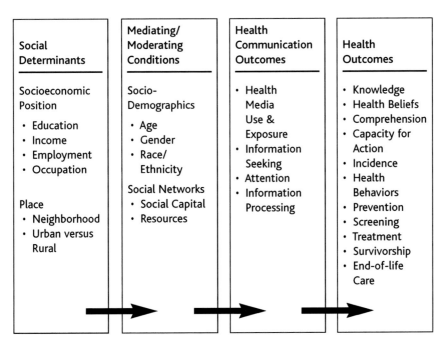

FIGURE 10.1. Structural Influence Model (SIM) of Health Communication (K. Viswanath).

USING SURVEILLANCE TO ADDRESS EXTANT
INEQUALITIES IN COMMUNICATION: EXTENDING REACH
TO VULNERABLE AND UNDERSERVED POPULATIONS

Given the essential role of communication to health as delineated by the SIM, surveillance in health communication is necessary for documenting communication inequalities and developing communication strategies that may guide efforts to reduce health disparities. Earlier work by Viswanath and colleagues, drawing on the communication inequality framework and using NCI's Health Information National Trends Survey (HINTS), reported how a number of social determinants such as SES and race/ethnicity influence communication factors such as access to and use of different media (Viswanath, 2005), attention to health in the media (Viswanath, 2006), information-seeking (Ramanadhan & Viswanath, 2006), and knowledge about smoking and skin cancer (Viswanath et al., 2006).

A 2006 study using HINTS showed that although having a television is universal across income and education strata in the United States, subscription to cable or satellite TV is positively associated with income, education, and employment (Viswanath, 2006). This pattern of association is pronounced for subscription to Internet services as well. Similarly, income and education are associated with daily readership of newspapers. There also are differential patterns of usage of information services by race; Blacks report less time reading newspapers than Whites, and also report less access to cable or satellite TV and the Internet (Viswanath, 2006).

Attention to health information is known to be influenced by SES, but not necessarily by race/ethnicity (Viswanath et al., 2007). For example, there are differences in the degree of attention people from different education and income groups pay to media content. At the same time, data from HINTS has shown that there are no differences among the various racial and ethnic groups in the amount of self-reported attention to health information available in diverse media. This suggests strong interest in health information among all racial and ethnic groups, despite differential access.

Prior work also has shown that certain sociodemographic characteristics are associated with dissatisfaction with attempts to seek and use health information from several media channels. Arora and colleagues (2008) found that people with low levels of education experience difficulty in searching for cancer-related information, and that many express frustration with their searches, say that information-seeking requires a lot of effort, and express concerns about the quality of information found (Arora et al., 2008). Similarly, in a study involving individuals living with HIV/AIDS, those with low levels of education and those living in nonmetropolitan areas reported less preference for using the Internet as a channel to seek health information; the majority of respondents said it is easy to get over-whelmed by information, and one-third said that *not* seeking information can be beneficial (Hogan & Palmer, 2005). With regard to clinical decision making, Levinson and colleagues (Levinson, Kao, Kuby, & Thisted, 2005) found that not all people prefer to be engaged in the health care decision-making process, despite IOM recommendations for physicians to facilitate shared interactions (IOM, 2002; Nielsen-Bohlman, Panzer, & Kindig, 2004). Levinson's study found that women, those with higher levels of education, and healthier people are more likely than men, people with lower levels of education, and people who are less healthy to prefer an active role in health care decision making; in addition, Blacks and Hispanics are more likely to prefer that physicians make the decisions (Levinson et al., 2005).

Given the documented differences in access to communication services, attention to health information, and satisfaction with health communication endeavors — and the knowledge gaps that these and other inequalities induce among disadvantaged groups — HINTS has emerged as an invaluable tool not only for communication surveillance, but also for elucidating evidence that may inform health communication practice in an informed and prag-matic way. In the following section, an analysis of HINTS data is discussed in terms of how it can be used to assist public health and communication practitioners in reaching underserved groups by identifying differences and similarities in information channel preferences for health information across population subgroups. This is important, because evidence from the fields of targeting and tailoring suggests that health outcomes are improved when people and groups receive the information they need, when they need it, and in a format that they prefer (IOM, 2002).

Proposing strategies to address structures of social influence and power that dictate information availability and comprehension among majority and minority groups is not within the scope of this chapter; as such, we do not propose to test the SIM explicitly. Instead, the remainder of the chapter builds on the assumptions denoted by the SIM, using it as a guiding theoret-ical framework and focusing on known differences in several aspects of communication at the group level. The chapter proposes strategies to over-come existing communication inequalities by using communication surveil-lance data to guide efforts to reach underserved groups with health informa-tion. Specifically, a multivariable analysis examines communication channel preferences by class (income and education), race/ethnicity, and place (urban and rural residence). As has been illustrated, selecting appropriate and effec-tive communication channels is essential to ensuring adequate exposure to messaging. As such, the analysis and results that follow may enhance out-reach efforts by providing an evidentiary profile of audience groups and their preferred means to receive health information.

COMMUNICATION CHANNEL PREFERENCES
BY RACE, CLASS, AND PLACE

Methods

HINTS 2003 data were analyzed to model U.S. adults' differential preferences for receiving health information from a variety of channels, including
e-mail or Internet; video; computer CD-ROM; tailored print materials;
books, newspapers, magazines, or other publications; and interpersonal
communication with health care providers, either by telephone or in person.
HINTS is a biennial, telephone-based, nationally representative survey of
the adult U.S. population, conducted by NCI, aimed at tracking trends in
the public's cancer-related communication behaviors, knowledge, attitudes,
and health behaviors. The 2003 survey used a complex stratified sampling
design with an oversampling of Black and Hispanic households (Nelson et
al., 2004).

An initial, descriptive analysis of the percent of HINTS respondents in
each sociodemographic category who said "yes" to preferring to receive
health information from each of the given communication channels showed
that all channels are at least generally acceptable whereas certain others were
more popular (Table 10.1). For example, tailored print materials received
high accolades from 80% to 90% of respondents across all sociodemographic categories. However, preferences for technologically sophisticated channels such as e-mail or Internet and CD-ROMs varied by income and education, illustrating a socioeconomic gradient. Bivariate analyses showed that
group-level categorization was associated with preference for several of the
given communication channels, spurring deeper investigation.

Multivariable logistic regressions were conducted to describe the odds
that specific population groups prefer a given information channel compared to identified referent groups, controlling for respondent age and sex,
and the other class, race, and place variables simultaneously included in each
model (Table 10.2). To demonstrate how communication inequality may
manifest into preferences for specific information channels that are available
and usable among those sociodemographic groups that are less well-off in
terms of information access and exposure, as well as health outcomes generally, referent groups were chosen to represent those who have a better
socioeconomic position, are the racial majority, and are not geographically
isolated. That is, information preference comparisons were made to those
Americans who earn $75,000 or more per year, have a bachelor's degree or
higher, are White, and live in urban areas.

It is important to note that although the analysis was conceptually guid-
ed by the notion of structural inequalities in health information access,

usage, comprehension, and capacity to act, variables assessed only individual-level attributes and did not employ a multilevel approach to modeling the contribution of macro determinants to individual health information channel preferences. What the analysis achieves, however, is an indication of how information channel preferences may mirror extant communication inequalities. Until communication inequality and the many social determinants of health are addressed in a comprehensive way at the policy level, analyses like those presented here, using information from a nationally representative sample of American adults, provide real-time, real-world evidence to inform strategies to aid behavioral interventions for groups at highest risk for poor health outcomes. By summarizing differential preferences for receiving health information through a variety of channels, the following information can be used to guide efforts to reach vulnerable and underserved populations, especially when practitioners must make choices about how best to expend valuable resources in an era of limited funding and still growing disparities in information and health outcomes.

Results

E-mail and Internet. The impact of SES on the likelihood of adults preferring e-mail and the Internet as a resource for health information cannot be overemphasized. Even as we are experiencing a revolution in information technology and are living in an "information age," the digital divide persists as an illustration of communication inequality among individuals with low income and low levels of education compared with those with higher SES. Compared with those making $75,000 or more per year and those with a bachelor's degree or more, lower SES adults are significantly less likely to say that e-mail or the Internet are preferred modes for receiving health information. As with many of the results we present in this section, the differences by income are pronounced not only between those at the highest and lowest income levels; there appears to be a gradient in information preferences at every level of income, mirroring what is known as the socioeconomic gradient in health.

Compared with people in urban areas, those in rural areas are significantly less likely to prefer to receive information from e-mail or the Internet. There is one significant difference by ethnicity: Spanish-speaking Hispanics are significantly less likely than Whites to prefer e-mail and the Internet, whereas Blacks and English-speaking Hispanics are equally as likely as Whites to prefer this mode of communication. Although there is evidence of a digital divide across some racial and ethnic groups in information *access*, our findings suggest that inequality in access to health information does not necessarily define health information preferences. Most minority populations are equally as interested in new technologies and communication

TABLE 10.1. Bivariate Associations Between Sociodemographic Categories and Preferences for Health Communication Channels, and Weighted Percentages of Respondents Preferring Each Channel

	E-MAIL OR INTERNET	VIDEO	COMPUTER CD-ROM
	% Yes	% Yes	% Yes
RACE/ETHNICITY	$p < 0.0001$	$p < 0.0001$	$p = 0.0013$
White	59.05	48.86	59.88
Black	55.53	68.07	62.61
English-speaking Hispanic	60.97	59.38	67.89
Spanish-speaking Hispanic	30.56	81.30	36.40
INCOME	$p < 0.0001$	$p < 0.0001$	$p < 0.0001$
⩾$75K	74.65	40.05	71.92
$50K-<$75K	66.16	53.30	69.36
$35K-<$50K	60.11	53.17	64.28
$25K-<$35K	52.50	57.21	56.87
$25K	42.13	63.40	44.08
EDUCATION	$p < 0.0001$	$p < 0.0001$	$p < 0.0001$
Bachelor's degree or higher	69.24	47.21	68.70
High school diploma or less	44.96	60.09	49.01
PLACE	$p < 0.0001$	$p = 0.0246$	$p = 0.0234$
Urban	59.11	52.64	59.78
Rural	49.48	56.75	54.54
AGE	$p < 0.0001$	$p < 0.0073$	$p < 0.0001$
18-34	68.60	50.67	72.37
35-39	66.75	60.50	68.57
40-44	63.62	54.68	65.16
45+	46.46	53.45	46.29
SEX	$p = 0.0120$	$p = 0.3699$	$p = 0.0090$
Male	59.63	54.20	60.96
Female	55.35	52.71	59.81

Cell values reflect weighted percents of HINTS respondents within each sociodemographic category, who said "yes" to specified channels.

Group-level significance values reflect χ^2 tests with (# categories–1) degrees of freedom for each sociodemographic variable.

Note: Health Information National Trends Survey 2003

TAILORED MATERIALS	READING BOOK, MAGAZINE, OR PUBLICATION	CALL FROM HEALTH CARE PROVIDER	MEETING WITH HEALTH CARE PROVIDER
% Yes	% Yes	% Yes	% Yes
$p = 0.1923$	$p = 0.6129$	$p < 0.0001$	$p = 0.2761$
86.25	78.10	60.60	79.21
88.77	80.01	67.94	81.56
85.88	78.46	59.99	78.06
83.84	79.50	79.92	83.46
$p = 0.0007$	$p = 0.0007$	$p = 0.0316$	$p < 0.0001$
90.37	81.83	60.34	84.70
88.35	82.37	60.76	82.85
87.96	77.70	63.28	74.98
85.18	76.59	63.00	78.31
82.45	74.83	66.27	74.24
$p < 0.0001$	$p < 0.0001$	$p = 0.0937$	$p < 0.0001$
88.92	81.99	60.06	81.63
83.10	74.14	63.87	76.34
$p = 0.1783$	$p = 0.0009$	$p = 0.6983$	$p = 0.3382$
86.28	79.36	62.37	79.36
84.26	72.77	61.66	77.68
$p < 0.0001$	$p < 0.0001$	$p = 0.0292$	$p < 0.0001$
89.88	81.27	62.97	81.73
90.47	82.59	66.83	84.62
90.16	80.01	66.09	84.17
81.36	74.67	59.92	74.94
$p < 0.0001$	$p < 0.0001$	$p = 0.0027$	$p = 0.3332$
81.69	71.95	59.69	78.39
89.78	83.77	64.59	79.65

TABLE 10.2. Multivariable Logistic Regressions: Health Communication Channel Preferences by Class, Race, and Place

	E-MAIL OR INTERNET	VIDEO	COMPUTER CD-ROM
	N = 5,235	N = 5,214	N = 5,206
	OR (95% CI)	OR (95% CI)	OR (95% CI)
CLASS			
Income: <$25K	0.39*** (0.31, 0.48)	1.82*** (1.45, 2.27)	0.42*** (0.32, 0.55)
Income: $25K-<$35K	0.50*** (0.39, 0.64)	1.64** (1.28, 2.10)	0.59** (0.44, 0.80)
Income: $35K-<$50K	0.63*** (0.51, 0.78)	1.53** (1.21, 1.95)	0.82 (0.62, 1.08)
Income: $50K-<$75K	0.74** (0.58, 0.94)	1.62*** (1.33, 1.99)	0.94 (0.73, 1.20)
Education: ≤ High School Diploma	0.55*** (0.47, 0.65)	1.24** (1.06, 1.46)	0.61*** (0.52, 0.72)
RACE/ETHNICITY			
Spanish-speaking Hispanic	0.40*** (0.28, 0.59)	3.49*** (2.36, 5.15)	0.42*** (0.29, 0.62)
English-speaking Hispanic	0.97 (0.71, 1.31)	1.50** (1.15, 1.96)	1.30 (0.93, 1.83)
Black	0.951 (0.74, 1.23)	2.01*** (1.58, 2.56)	1.26 (0.97, 1.64)
PLACE			
Rural	0.82* (0.69, 0.98)	1.20* (1.01, 1.43)	1.04 (0.85, 1.26)

Key: *$p < 0.05$, **$p < 0.01$, ***$p < 0.0001$
Referent Categories: *Class*: Income>$75K, Bachelor's degree or higher; *Race/Ethnicity*: White; *Place*: Urban
Health Information National Trends Survey 2003
Odds ratios (OR) and 95% confidence intervals (CI) for fitted logistic regression models that describe the odds of saying that a given communication channel is a preferred source for cancer information, controlling simultaneously for each sociodemographic characteristic and respondent age and sex.

TAILORED MATERIALS N = 5,218	READING BOOK, MAGAZINE, OR PUBLICATION N = 5,230	CALL FROM HEALTH CARE PROVIDER N = 5,206	MEETING WITH HEALTH CARE PROVIDER N = 5,222
OR (95% CI)	OR (95% CI)	OR (95% CI)	OR (95% CI)
0.66* (0.46, 0.94)	0.71* (0.54, 0.95)	1.09 (0.86, 1.38)	0.52*** (0.40, 0.68)
0.84 (0.56, 1.25)	0.77 (0.55, 1.08)	0.99 (0.76, 1.28)	0.63* (0.42, 0.94)
1.03 (0.70, 1.51)	0.85 (0.66, 1.10)	1.07 (0.85, 1.35)	0.67** (0.49, 0.91)
1.28 (0.86, 1.92)	1.11 (0.85, 1.44)	1.00 (0.84, 1.20)	0.88 (0.61, 1.26)
0.74* (0.58, 0.94)	0.75** (0.60, 0.93)	1.04 (0.87, 1.22)	0.88 (0.73, 1.07)
1.04 (0.69, 1.55)	1.39 (0.91, 2.14)	2.54*** (1.63, 3.96)	1.61* (1.09, 2.37)
0.85 (0.59, 1.23)	0.99 (0.70, 1.40)	0.97 (0.73, 1.28)	0.90 (0.65, 1.24)
1.40 (0.89, 2.20)	1.24 (0.94, 1.64)	1.33** (1.06, 1.66)	1.22 (0.93, 1.59)
1.02 (0.74, 1.40)	0.81 (0.64, 1.01)	0.96 (0.79, 1.15)	1.11 (0.85, 1.45)

channels as Whites. This finding adds to previous research that showed that although there are differences in the degree of attention people from different education and income groups pay to media content, there is no evidence of differences among the various racial and ethnic groups in the amount of self-reported attention to health information available in diverse media, suggesting strong interest in health information among all racial and ethnic groups, despite differential access (Viswanath et al., 2007).

Video. Non-White, rural, and low SES Americans are significantly more likely to say that they would like to receive health information on video than are White, urban, and high SES Americans. The preference for video is most striking among Spanish-speaking Hispanics, who are 3.5 times more likely than Whites to say that health information by video would be effective. Blacks are about two times more likely than Whites to prefer videos, and English-speaking Hispanics also are significantly more likely than Whites to say that videos would be effective. Among all the communication channels examined, video was universally preferred among disadvantaged populations, signifying its usefulness as a format for communicating complex health information.

Computer CD-ROM. Americans with a high school education or less are significantly less likely than those with a bachelor's degree or more to say they would like to receive a health-related CD-ROM, and those in the lowest income categories (<$25,000 and $25,000-$35,000 per year) were significantly less likely than those who make $75,000 or more to say that a CD-ROM would be effective. There were no significant differences between those in middle-income groups and the highest income group, indicating that those groups are equally likely to say that CD-ROMs are a preferred channel for health information. Urban versus rural residence does not seem to be differentially associated with preference for CD-ROMs.

Tailored Print Materials. As was foreshadowed in our bivariate analyses, there was almost no variance in preference by sociodemographic groups for tailored print materials; this channel for communicating health information is highly regarded across groups. However, controlling for race/ethnicity, levels of SES, urbanity, age, and sex, we found a few striking differences in preference for tailored materials at the lowest levels of SES. Those in the lowest income group (<$25,000 per year) and those with lower levels of education (high school diploma or less) are significantly less likely than those in the highest income group ($75,000 or more) and those with a bachelor's degree or more to say they would like to receive print materials tailored on information such as their age and family history. It is unclear why these groups may be less receptive to tailored materials than higher SES groups, although we posit that this finding could represent a lack of health literacy among low SES populations, such that even print materials containing tailored information may be burdensome.

Books, Magazines, Newspapers, and Other Publications. There are no significant differences in preferring to read about health information in books, magazines, newspapers, or other publications between middle and upper income groups ($25,000-$35,000, $35,000-$50,000, or $50,000-$74,999) compared with those Americans with the highest income levels ($75,000 or more). However, differences are pronounced between the lowest income group and others, with those making less than $25,000 per year being significantly less likely to say they would like to receive health information this way. Individuals with lower levels of education also are less likely than individuals with a bachelor's degree or more to say that books, magazines, newspapers, and other publications are an effective mode for communicating about health. There appear to be no significant differences by geographic area or race/ethnicity.

Call from a Health Care Provider. Individuals from all socioeconomic groups and both urban and rural areas are equally likely to say that they would like to receive a telephone call from a health care provider as a way of acquiring information about health. The only pronounced differences are by race/ethnicity, with Spanish-speaking Hispanics being more than twice as likely as Whites to say they would like to receive a telephone call. Blacks also are significantly more likely than Whites to say that receiving a telephone call from a health care provider would be effective.

Meeting in Person with a Health Care Provider. HINTS has shown us that Americans most trust health care providers as a source of health information (Hesse et al., 2005). Despite this, our analysis shows that low SES populations are significantly less likely than high SES populations to say that visiting a health care provider in person is a preferred means of receiving information about health. In fact, those Americans who make less than $50,000 per year are significantly less likely than those who make $75,000 or more to prefer to receive information by visiting with a health care provider. There is again a pronounced socioeconomic gradient, with those who make less than $25,000 per year being the least likely to say that in-person meetings with health care providers are a preferred mode of communication. We posit that this could reflect the known disparities in access to health care, as well as levels of comfort with navigating the health care system.

Holding constant the effects of income, there remains one ethnic difference in preferences for meeting in person with a health care provider. Spanish-speaking Hispanics are significantly more likely than Whites to say that they would like to receive information about health by meeting in person with a provider. This is similar to our finding that Spanish-speaking Hispanics are more likely than Whites to prefer telephone calls with providers, signaling what could be a cultural preference for interpersonal communication. There were no significant differences between Blacks or English-speaking Hispanics and Whites, or rural versus urban residents.

SUMMARY AND IMPLICATIONS

Our analysis of differential preferences for health and cancer communication channels revealed interesting insights that may be used in developing strategies to reach vulnerable and underserved populations with health information. Our multivariable analyses adjusted simultaneously for several social determinants of health and communication inequality, and found some real, remaining differences in channel preferences among groups delineated by race/ethnicity, geographic location, and levels of SES. Our referent group selections allow for group comparisons that correspond to other examinations of social inequalities in health, thus enhancing our ability to inform decisions about executing health communication strategies to increase message exposure among populations that bear the largest burden of many diseases and disease risk factors.

Our analysis suggests that new media channels generally are more preferred by higher income and more highly educated groups compared to low SES groups, and therefore may not be the most effective means of reaching the most vulnerable and underserved populations defined by SES. Importantly, racial and ethnic minority populations are equally as likely as Whites to embrace new technologies and communication channels for health information. Although there are few differences in preferences for traditional media across sociodemographic groups, health communication and public health practitioners should pay special attention to messages delivered via tailored print materials and books, magazines, newspapers, or other publications, as those in the lowest income groups and those with a high school education or less still are less likely than higher SES groups to say they would like to receive health information from tailored and traditional print media channels. Across all disadvantaged populations, there were strong differential preferences for receiving health information on video, indicating that video may be an appropriate and effective communication channel to reach certain underserved groups.

Interpersonal communication channels are more preferred by Spanish-speaking Hispanics and Blacks than by Whites, suggesting the usefulness of patient–provider communication as a means of reaching those racial and ethnic groups with health information, especially by telephone. Despite these strong preferences for interpersonal communication, particularly among Spanish-speaking Hispanics, low SES populations are significantly less likely to prefer meeting in person with health care providers, signaling a need to be sensitive to low SES groups' time constraints, access issues, and comfort level with navigating the health care system.

CONCLUSION

Health communication efforts can be most effective when audiences are heavily exposed to information they need, in a format they can use. In this chapter, we presented an abbreviated overview of the individual and social determinants of health, and the ways in which communication can influence individual level health behavior and societal level change. Our focus has been on the notion of *communication inequality*, and how knowledge gaps resultant of communication efforts can contribute to health disparities. Just as other studies have documented inequalities in communication usage, access, information-seeking, and attention to health messages (Viswanath, 2006; Viswanath et al., 2006), our analysis adds another dimension, to demonstrate differences in communication channel preferences by several sociodemographic factors. Findings from our analysis reinforce and refine the SIM and the communication inequality thesis, especially with regard to the influence of SES on communication outcomes. Our findings further add a cultural dimension, by demonstrating differential preferences for health communication channels among Whites, Blacks, and English- and Spanish-speaking Hispanics. Perhaps paramount in our consideration of differential channel preferences by racial and ethnic group is our finding that Hispanics are heterogeneous when it comes to channel preferences, with English-speaking Hispanics having similar preferences as Whites, but Spanish-speaking Hispanics showing marked differences.

Our findings may help to explain why reliance on conventional media such as mass media and the Internet may exacerbate knowledge gaps and health disparities. We hope that readers take away an appreciation of the potential health effects of communication inequality, and realize that a "one-size-fits-all" approach is untenable in this period of increasing social inequalities in health. It was our intention to provide an evidentiary profile of specific sociodemographic groups' differential information channel preferences, in order to facilitate effective communication outreach to address health disparities across the cancer care continuum.

REFERENCES

Arora, N. K., Hesse, B. W., Rimer, B. K., Viswanath, K., Clayman, M. L., & Croyle, R. T. (2008). Frustrated and confused: The American public rates its cancer-related information-seeking experiences. *Journal of General Internal Medicine, 23*(2), 223-228.

Bao, Y., Duan, N., & Fox, S. A. (2006). Is some provider advice on smoking cessation better than no advice? An instrumental variable analysis of the 2001 National Health Interview Survey. *Health Services Research, 41*(6), 2114-2135.

Berkman, L. F., & Kawachi, I. (Eds.). (2000). *Social epidemiology.* New York: Oxford University Press.

Caburnay, C. A., Kreuter, M. W., Luke, D. A., Logan, R. A., Jacobsen, H. A., Reddy, V. C. et al. (2003). The news on health behavior: Coverage of diet, activity, and tobacco in local newspapers. *Health, Education & Behavior, 30*(6), 709-722.

Cairns, C., & Viswanath, K. (2006). Colorectal cancer screening among the uninsured: Data from the Health Information National Trends Survey. *Cancer Causes and Control, 17*(9), 1115-1125.

Charlesworth, A., & Glantz, S. A. (2006). Tobacco and the movie industry. *Clinics in Occupational and Environmental Medicine, 5*(1), ix, 73-84.

Dalton, M. A., Sargent, J. D., Beach, M. L., Titus-Ernstoff, L., Gibson, J. J., Ahrens, M. B. et al. (2003). Effect of viewing smoking in movies on adolescent smoking initiation: A cohort study. *Lancet, 362*(9380), 281-285.

Daly, M. C., Duncan, G. J., McDonough, P., & Williams, D. R. (2002). Optimal indicators of socioeconomic status for health research. *American Journal of Public Health, 92*(7), 1151-1157.

Davis, S. W., Cummings, K. M., Rimer, B. K., Sciandra, R., & Stone, J. C. (1992). The impact of tailored self-help smoking cessation guides on young mothers. *Health Education Quarterly, 19*, 495-504.

Demark-Wahnefried, W., McClelland, J., Campbell, M. K., Hoben, K., Lashley, J., Graves, C. et al. (1998). Awareness of cancer-related programs and services among rural African Americans. *Journal of the National Medical Association, 90*(4), 197-202.

Emmons, K. M., Wong, M., Hammond, S. K., Velicer, W. F., Fava, J. L., Monroe, A. D. et al. (2001). Intervention and policy issues related to children's exposure to environmental tobacco smoke. *Preventive Medicine, 32*(4), 321-331.

Farrelly, M. C., Davis, K. C., Haviland, M. L., Messeri, P., & Healton, C. G. (2005). Evidence of a dose-response relationship between "truth" antismoking ads and youth smoking prevalence. *American Journal of Public Health, 95*(3), 425-431.

Gansler, T., Henley, S. J., Stein, K., Nehl, E. J., Smigal, C., & Slaughter, E. (2005). Sociodemographic determinants of cancer treatment health literacy. *Cancer, 104*(3), 653-660.

Hammond, D., Fong, G. T., Zanna, M. P., Thrasher, J. F., & Borland, R. (2006). Tobacco denormalization and industry beliefs among smokers from four countries. *American Journal of Preventive Medicine, 31*(3), 225-232.

Hesse, B. W., Nelson, D. E., Kreps, G. L., Croyle, R. T., Arora, N. K., Rimer, B. K. et al. (2005). Trust and sources of health information: The impact of the Internet and its implications for health care providers: Findings from the first Health

Information National Trends Survey. *Archives of Internal Medicine, 165*(22), 2618-2624.

Hogan, T. P., & Palmer, C. L. (2005). Information preferences and practices among people living with HIV/AIDS: Results from a nationwide survey. *Journal of the Medical Library Association, 93*(4), 431-439.

Hornik, R. (Ed.). (2002). *Public health communication: Evidence for behavior change.* Mahwah, NJ: Erlbaum.

Hornik, R., Maklan, D. M., Judkins, D., Cadell, D., Yanovitzky, I., Zador, P. et al. (2001). *Evaluation of the National Youth Anti-Drug Media Campaign: Second semiannual report of findings.* Washington, DC: National Institute on Drug Abuse.

Hornik, R., & Yanovitzky, I. (2003). Using theory to design evaluations of communication campaigns: The case of the National Youth Anti-Drug Media Campaign. *Communication Theory, 13*(2), 204-224.

Institute of Medicine (IOM). (2002). *Speaking of health: Assessing health communication strategies for diverse populations.* Washington, DC: National Academies Press.

Kaplan, G. A. (2004). What's wrong with social epidemiology, and how can we make it better? *Epidemiologic Reviews, 26,* 124-135.

Keintz, M. K., Fleisher, L., & Rimer, B. K. (1994). Reaching mothers of pre-school aged children with a targeted quit smoking intervention. *Journal of Community Health, 19*(1), 25-40.

Kreuter, M. W., Sugg-Skinner, C., Holt, C. L., Clark, E. M., Haire-Joshu, D., Fu, Q. et al. (2005). Cultural tailoring for mammography and fruit and vegetable intake among low-income African-American women in urban public health centers. *Preventive Medicine, 41*(1), 53-62.

Lancaster, T., & Stead, L. (2004). Physician advice for smoking cessation. *Cochrane Database of Systematic Reviews, 4,* CD000165.

Levinson, W., Kao, A., Kuby, A., & Thisted, R. A. (2005). Not all patients want to participate in decision making. A national study of public preferences. *Journal of General Internal Medicine, 20*(6), 531-535.

Loureiro, M. L., & Nayga, R. M., Jr. (2006). Obesity, weight loss, and physician's advice. *Social Science and Medicine, 62*(10), 2458-2468.

Marcus, A. C., Mason, M., Wolfe, P., Rimer, B. K., Lipkus, I., Strecher, V. et al. (2005). The efficacy of tailored print materials in promoting colorectal cancer screening: Results from a randomized trial involving callers to the National Cancer Institute's Cancer Information Service. *Journal of Health Communication, 10*(suppl 1), 83-104.

McBride, C. M., Bastian, L. A., Halabi, S., Fish, L., Lipkus, I. M., Bosworth, H. B. et al. (2002). A tailored intervention to aid decision-making about hormone replacement therapy. *American Journal of Public Health, 92*(7), 1112-1114.

McCombs, M. E., & Ghanem, S. I. (2001). The convergence of agenda setting and framing. In S. D. Reese, O. H. Gandy, & A. E. Grant (Eds.), *Framing public life: Perspectives on media and our understanding of the social world.* Mahwah NJ: Erlbaum.

McGinnis, J. M., & Foege, W. H. (1993). Actual causes of death in the United States. *Journal of the American Medical Association, 270*(18), 2207-2212.

Meier, A., Lyons, E. J., Frydman, G., Forlenza, M., & Rimer, B. K. (2007). How can-
    cer survivors provide support on cancer-related Internet mailing lists. *Journal of
    Medical Internet Research, 9*(2), e12.
National Cancer Institute (NCI). (1999). *Smoking and tobacco control monograph
    10: Health effects of exposure to environmental tobacco smoke.* Bethesda, MD.
Nelson, D. E., Kreps, G. L., Hesse, B. W., Croyle, R. T., Willis, G., Arora, N. K. et
    al. (2004). The Health Information National Trends Survey (HINTS):
    Development, design, and dissemination. *Journal of Health Communication,
    9*(5), 443-460.
Newbrun, E. (1989). Effectiveness of water fluoridation. *Journal of Public Health
    Dentistry, 49*, 279-289.
Niederdeppe, J., Farrelly, M. C., & Haviland, M. L. (2004). Confirming "truth":
    More evidence of a successful tobacco countermarketing campaign in Florida.
    American Journal of Public Health, 94(2), 255-257.
Nielsen-Bohlman, L., Panzer, A. M., & Kindig, D. A. (Eds.). (2004). *Health literacy:
    A prescription to end confusion.* Washington, DC: Institute of Medicine,
    National Research Council, The National Academies Press.
Owen, N., Humpel, N., Leslie, E., Bauman, A., & Sallis, J. F. (2004). Understanding
    environmental influences on walking; Review and research agenda. *American
    Journal of Preventive Medicine, 27*(1), 67-76.
Phelan, J. C., Link, B. G., Diez-Roux, A., Kawachi, I., & Levin, B. (2004).
    "Fundamental causes" of social inequalities in mortality: A test of the theory.
    Journal of Health and Social Behavior, 45(3), 265-285.
Ramanadhan, S., & Viswanath, K. (2006). Health and the information non-seekers:
    A profile. *Health Communication, 20*(2), 131-139.
Reese, S. D., Gandy, O. H., & Grant, A. E. (Eds.). (2001). *Framing public life:
    Perspectives on media and our understanding of the social world.* Mahwah, NJ:
    Erlbaum.
Riley, J., Lennon, M., & Ellwood, R. (1999). The effect of water fluoridation and
    social inequalities on dental caries in 5-year-old children. *International Journal
    of Epidemiology, 28*, 300-305.
Rimer, B. K., Conaway, M., Lyna, P., Glassman, B., Yarnall, K. S., Lipkus, I. et al.
    (1999). The impact of tailored interventions on a community health center pop-
    ulation. *Patient Education and Counseling, 37*(2), 125-140.
Rimer, B. K., & Glassman, B. (1999). Is there a use for tailored print communications
    in cancer risk communication? *Journal of the National Cancer Institute
    Monographs, 25*, 140-148.
Rimer, B. K., & Kreuter, M. (2006). Advancing tailored health communication: A
    persuasion and message effects perspective. *Journal of Communication,
    56*(suppl), S184-S201.
Rimer, B. K., Orleans, C. T., Fleisher, L., Cristinzio, S., Resch, N., & Telepchak, J.
    (1994). Does tailoring matter? The impact of a tailored guide on ratings and
    short-term smoking-related outcomes for older smokers. *Health Education
    Research: Theory & Practice, 9*(1), 69-84.
Robinson, R. G., Sutton, C. D., James, D. A., & Orleans, C. T. (1992). *Pathways to
    freedom: Winning the fight against tobacco.* Philadelphia: Fox Chase Cancer
    Center.

Saelens, B. E., Sallis, J. F., & Frank, L. D. (2003). Environmental correlates of walking and cycling: Findings from the transportation, urban design, and planning literatures. *Annals of Behavioral Medicine, 25*(2), 80-91.

Sargent, J. D., Beach, M. L., Adachi-Mejia, A. M., Gibson, J. J., Titus-Ernstoff, L. T., Carusi, C. P. et al. (2005). Exposure to movie smoking: Its relation to smoking initiation among US adolescents. *Pediatrics, 116*(5), 1183-1191.

Schwartz, L. M., & Woloshin, S. (2002). News media coverage of screening mammography for women in their 40s and tamoxifen for primary prevention of breast cancer. *Journal of the American Medical Association, 287*(23), 3136-3142.

Shuchman, M. (2002). Journalists as change agents in medicine and health care. *Journal of the American Medical Association, 287*(6), 776.

Snyder, L. B., & Hamilton, M. A. (2002). A meta-analysis of U.S. health campaign effects on behavior: Emphasize enforcement, exposure, and new information, and beware of secular trend. In R. Hornik (Ed.), *Public health communication: Evidence for behavior change* (pp. 357-383). Mahwah, NJ: Erlbaum.

Stein, K., Zhao, L., Crammer, C., & Gansler, T. (2007). Prevalence and sociodemographic correlates of beliefs regarding cancer risks. *Cancer, 110*(5), 1139-1148.

Strecher, V. J., Rimer, B. K., & Monaco, K. D. (1989). Development of a new self-help guide: Freedom from smoking for you and your family. *Health Education Quarterly, 16*(1), 101-112.

Stryker, J. E. (2003). Media and marijuana: A longitudinal analysis of news media effects on adolescents' marijuana use and related outcomes, 1977-1999. *Journal of Health Communication, 8*(4), 305-328.

Stryker, J. E., Emmons, K. M., & Viswanath, K. (2007). Uncovering differences across the cancer control continuum: A comparison of ethnic and mainstream cancer newspaper stories. *Preventive Medicine, 44*(1), 20-25.

Tichenor, P. J., Donohue, G. A., & Olien, C. N. (1980). *Community conflict and the press.* Newbury Park, CA: Sage.

Tong, E. K., Ong, M. K., Vittinghoff, E., & Perez-Stable, E. J. (2006). Nondaily smokers should be asked and advised to quit. *American Journal of Preventive Medicine, 30*(1), 23-30.

Valente, T. W., Ritt-Olson, A., Stacy, A., Unger, J. B., Okamoto, J., & Sussman, S. (2007). Peer acceleration: Effects of a social network tailored substance abuse prevention program among high-risk adolescents. *Addiction, 102*(11), 1804-1815.

Viswanath, K. (2005). The communications revolution and cancer control. *Nature Reviews of Cancer, 5*(10), 828-835.

Viswanath, K. (2006). Public communications and its role in reducing and eliminating health disparities. In G. E. Thomson, F. Mitchell, & M. B. Williams (Eds.), *Examining the health disparities research plan of the National Institutes of Health: Unfinished business* (pp. 215-253). Washington, DC: Institute of Medicine.

Viswanath, K. (2008). Social capital and health communications. In I. Kawachi, S. V. Subramanian & D. Kim (Eds.), *Social capital and health.* New York: Springer.

Viswanath, K., Breen, N., Meissner, H., Moser, R. P., Hesse, B., Steele, W. R., et al. (2006). Cancer knowledge and disparities in the information age. *Journal of Health Communication, 11*(suppl 1), 1-17.

Viswanath, K., & Finnegan, J. R. (1996). The knowledge gap hypothesis: Twenty five years later. In B. Burleson (Ed.), *Communication yearbook 19* (pp. 187-227). Thousand Oaks: Sage.

Viswanath, K., & Finnegan, J. R. (2002). Community health campaigns and secular trends: Insights from the Minnesota Heart Health Program and Community Trials in Heart Disease Prevention. In R. Hornik (Ed.), *Public health communication: Evidence for behavior change* (pp. 289-312). Mahwah, NJ: Erlbaum.

Viswanath, K., Ramanadhan, S., & Kontos, E. (2007). Mass media. In S. Galea (Ed.), *Macrosocial determinants of population health* (pp. 275-294). New York: Springer.

Viswanath, K., Randolph Steele, W., & Finnegan, J. (2006). Social capital and health: Civic engagement, community size, and recall of health messages. *American Journal of Public Health, 96*(8), 1456-1461.

Willinger, M., Ko, C. W., Hoffman, H. J., Kessler, R. C., & Corwin, M. J. (2003). Trends in infant bed sharing in the United States, 1993-2000: The National Infant Sleep Position study. *Archives of Pediatric and Adolescent Medicine, 157*(1), 43-49.

Yanovitzky, I., & Bennett, C. (1999). Media attention, institutional response, and health behavior change: The case of drunk driving, 1978-1996. *Communication Research, 26,* 429-453.

Yanovitzky, I., & Stryker, J. (2001). Mass media, social norms, and health promotion efforts: A longitudinal study of media effects on youth binge drinking. *Communication Research, 28,* 208-239.

11

USING THE HEALTH INFORMATION NATIONAL TRENDS SURVEY TO IDENTIFY CANCER KNOWLEDGE DEFICITS

Jennifer Hay
Memorial Sloan-Kettering Cancer Center

Soye Zaid-Muhammad
Pace University

Jennifer S. Ford
Memorial Sloan-Kettering Cancer Center

Elliot J. Coups
Fox Chase Cancer Center

In the United States, the burden of cancer disproportionately affects underserved populations. According to the National Cancer Institute's (NCI) Center to Reduce Cancer Health Disparities, disparities are defined as differential rates of cancer incidence, prevalence, or mortality for one subgroup of people (Harper & Lynch, 2005). Individuals at the lower end of the socioeconomic continuum, with less formal education and lower income, and those drawn from racial/ethnic minority groups tend to experience the burdens associated with cancer at higher rates than those individuals drawn from higher socioeconomic status (SES) groups and Whites (ACS, 2007a, 2007b, 2007c). Disparities operate throughout the cancer continuum, from prevention and early detection to treatment, end-of-life care, mortality, and survivorship. For example, non-Hispanic Blacks, and other minorities are less likely to be adherent to colorectal cancer (CRC) screening than Whites (ACS, 2007b, 2007c; Ananthakrishnan, Schellhase, Sparapani, Laud, & Neuner, 2007; Lloyd, Harvey, Hebert, Daguise, Williams, & Scott, 2007). Black men diagnosed with CRC are more likely to be diagnosed at a later stage than Whites (Polite, Dignam, & Olopade, 2005). Additionally, mortality rates from CRC are higher for Black men as compared with stage-matched White men (ACS, 2007b; Alexander, Waterbor, Hughes,

Funkhouser, Grizzle, & Manne, 2007; Baquet & Commiskey, 1999; Du, Meyer, & Franzini, 2007). Some disparities are evident in specific geographical locations, for example rural, underserved women in Appalachia have one of the highest rates of cervical cancer in the United States (Brandt, Modayil, Hurley, Pirisi-Creek, Johnson, Davis et al., 2006; Drake, Keane, Mosley, Adams, Elder, Modayil et al., 2006; Fouad et al., 2004, 2006; Powell, 2006; Yabroff, Lawrence, King, Mangan, Washington, Yi et al., 2005). Similar disparities operate within other ethnicities (ACS, 2006, 2007a) and across other common cancers, such as cancers of the prostate (Chu, Tarone, & Freeman, 2003; Reddy, Shapiro, Morton, & Brawley, 2003; Vijayakumar, Winter, Sause, Gallagher, Michalski, Roach et al., 1998), lung (Abidoye, Ferguson, & Salgia, 2007; Alberg, Horner, Daguise, Carpenter, Mosley, Vincent et al., 2006; Berger, Lund, & Brawley, 2007; Flenaugh & Henriques-Forsythe, 2006), and breast (Adams, Hebert, Bolick-Aldrich, Daguise, Mosley, Modayil et al., 2006; Bowen, Alfano, McGregor, Kuniyuki, Bernstein, Meeske et al., 2007; Du & Gor, 2007; Hirschman, Whitman, & Ansell, 2007; Lantz, Mujahid, Schwartz, Janz, Fagerlin, Salem et al., 2006; Sassi, Luft, & Guadagnoli, 2006; Tammemagi, 2007).

Although cancer disparities have a complex etiology, differential access to information about cancer prevention, early detection, and treatment options has been proposed as an important factor underlying these disparities (Hiah & Rimer, 1999). Information disseminated by mass media is acquired by those at higher SES at a faster rate than their lower SES counterparts, so that gaps in knowledge acquisition tend to increase over time, and are particularly dramatic in the context of new innovations (Tichenor, Donohue, & Olien, 1970; Viswanath & Finnegan, 1996; Viswanath, Kahn, Finnegan, Hertog et al., 1993). This knowledge gap hypothesis is highly relevant in the context of cancer prevention and control for those at increased risk as well as in the general population, where rapidly burgeoning knowledge of cancer risk factors, prevention strategies, early detection recommendations, and treatment options require concomitant knowledge transfer through multiple communication channels. Accordingly, the detection of cancer knowledge gaps represents an important step in pinpointing useful opportunities to help close these gaps in cancer knowledge and important health outcomes in the United States. In this chapter we review the work we have conducted over the past few years to identify cancer prevention and control knowledge gaps in the United States using the NCI-sponsored Health Information National Trends Surveys (HINTS 2003, 2005; Hesse, Moser, Rutten, & Kreps, 2006; Nelson, Kreps, Hesse, Croyle, Willis, Arora et al., 2004; NCI, 2004, 2005; Yach, 2004). We then advance a set of research priorities that illustrate the value of our HINTS findings in providing the groundwork for further work to close knowledge gaps in cancer prevention and control, and to close disparities in important cancer outcomes.

Much of the work we have conducted using HINTS data has focused on knowledge gaps relevant to CRC. There are a number of reasons for this. First, according to the U.S. Preventive Services Task Force (2002), screening for CRC is proven efficacious. CRC screening is also recommended for a large proportion of society (the general population for those individuals aged 50 and older) for both men and women, and includes multiple strategies for screening that have been developed over recent years (ACS, 2007a; NCI, 2006; USPSTF, 2002). This presents an opportunity to examine age and sex differences in knowledge gaps. Despite evidence for efficacy, only 50% of the general population is adherent with guidelines for CRC screening (Cokkinides, Chao, Smith, Vernon, & Thun, 2003), This adherence rate lags significantly behind the 2010 U.S. Department of Health and Human Services (2007) goal for 80% of the population to be adherent to recommendations for CRC screening. Current guidelines for CRC screening include one of the following strategies: fecal occult blood testing (FOBT) annually; flexible sigmoidoscopy or double contrast barium enema every 5 years; or colonoscopy every 10 years (Jonas, Russell, Sandler, Chou, & Pignone, 2007; NCI, 2006). Of note, these current recommendations have only been in place for 11 years (Winawer, Fletcher, Miller, Godlee, Stolar, Mulrow et al., 1997) and Medicare has provided reimbursement for screening colonoscopy since then (Cooper & Kou, 2008; Jonas et al., 2007; Schenck, Klabunde, Warren, Peacock, Davis, Hawley et al., 2007; Sonnenberg, Amorosi, Lacey, & Lieberman, 2008; USDHHS, 2007), making it a newer innovation than mammography screening. Additionally, there is growing consensus that lifestyle factors play an important role in the development and prevention of CRC, so this knowledge is critical to state-of-the-art prevention guidelines for this malignancy. For example, engaging in regular physical activity, maintaining a healthy body weight, limiting intake of red meat, avoiding high alcohol consumption, and refraining from smoking have each been linked with a reduced risk for CRC (Calle, Rodriguez, Walker-Thurmond, & Thun, 2003; Chao, Thun, Connell, McCullough, Jacobs, Flanders et al., 2005; Giovannucci, 2001; Slattery, 2007; Cho, Smith-Warner, Ritz, van den Brandt, Colditz, Folsom et al., 2004; James, Jackson-Leach, Mhurchu, Kalamara, Shayeghi, Rigby et al., 2004; Samad, Taylor, Marshall, & Chapman, 2005). We have examined CRC prevention and early detection knowledge deficits as well as demographic differences in perceived risk for CRC in our studies utilizing multiple HINTS datasets. We also review an additional study examining gaps in cancer information-seeking among cancer survivors that provides perspective on the determinants of cancer knowledge gaps in the United States. The findings from our studies are summarized in Table 11.1.

TABLE 11.1. Summary of HINTS Knowledge Gap Findings

Primary Outcome	Sample	Multivariate Predictors of Reduced Knowledge	Primary Source

Knowledge of colorectal cancer screening	3,131 HINTS 2003 participants	Age
		Education
		Race
		Married/partnered
		No. of health care
		  provider visits in last year
		Ever done FOBT
		Ever looked for cancer
		  information
			Ford, Coups, & Hay (2006)

Colorectal cancer prevention awareness	1,932 HINTS 2005 participants	Age Knowing colorectal cancer symptoms	Coups, Hay, & Ford (2008)
Knowledge of colorectal cancer risks	2,949 HINTS 2003 (at least 45 years) no personal history of colon cancer	*Predictors of comparative perceived risks* Age Interview language General anxiety Colon cancer worry Information overload *Predictors of absolute perceived risks* Overall health Personal history of cancer Family history of cancer Colon cancer worry Afraid of finding colon cancer if checked	Hay, Coups, & Ford (2006)
Information-seeking behaviors	711 HINTS 2005 cancer survivors	Education Age Income Race	Ford, Coups, & Hay (2009)

FOBT, fecal occult blood testing

KNOWLEDGE OF COLORECTAL CANCER SCREENING GUIDELINES

Using HINTS 2003, we examined the prevalence and patterns of CRC screening knowledge among a subsample of 3,131 HINTS respondents (Ford, Coups, & Hay, 2006). Although the screening strategies examined are sensitive to finding cancers in the rectum as well as the colon, given that more than 70% of CRC originates in the colon, and the fact that the question phrasing adopted in HINTS includes the colon only, we limit our findings to screening regarding cancers of the colon only. We excluded participants who were under the age of 45, because we believed that recommendations for colon cancer screening would legitimately lack salience to younger members of the general population and that knowledge of colon cancer screening would be most relevant to adults who were at or near the age of recommended screening. Also excluded were individuals who had a history of colon cancer, those who were missing age and colon cancer history data, and those who were missing data on the screening knowledge criterion variable.

In this study, we had the unique opportunity to examine knowledge of three elements of colon screening across multiple screening modalities, including being able to name a screening procedure for colon cancer screening, the age at which screening should begin, and knowledge of the recommended screening interval for different types of screening. Participants in the study were denoted as having "complete knowledge" of a test if they conjointly identified a colon cancer screening test, knew the start age for that test, and correctly identified its recommended screening frequency. For example, a participant with "complete knowledge" of FOBT would have recalled that this test must be initiated by age 50 years, and should be conducted every year. Participants were denoted as having knowledge of colon cancer screening if they gave the correct responses reflecting knowledge of either FOBT or sigmoidoscopy/colonoscopy. In this way, we examined the joint information necessary to maintain at least one colon screening modality through recommended screening intervals.

Overall, knowledge of colon cancer screening was low, with only 21% of participants having "complete knowledge" of at least one screening modality. Only 15% had FOBT screening knowledge, and 7% had sigmoidoscopy/colonoscopy screening knowledge. Based on multivariate findings, knowledge was particularly poor among participants who were aged 45 to 49 years or over age 70, with 14% and 15% from these groups, respectively, having knowledge of at least one screening modality. Rates were significantly reduced for those with less than a high school education and among unmarried individuals, with only 8% and 14%, respectively, having adequate screening knowledge. Black participants had lower levels of screening knowledge (10%) than other racial/ethnic groups, as did those who had not visited a health care provider in the past year (10%). Of those who had never undergone an FOBT, only 16% had screening knowledge. Among those individuals who had never looked for cancer information, only 16% had adequate screening knowledge.

It is important to highlight that adequate overall knowledge of CRC screening was low among all participants, with 80% of the entire sample evidencing knowledge deficits around CRC screening. Even among the most "advantaged" individuals in our sample we found significant knowledge deficits. For example, only 30% of those at highest education levels had adequate knowledge of CRC screening. This study was the first to examine the combined knowledge of cancer screening tests, age at initiation, and recommended interval for completion, that we believe is critical to follow through with adherence to screening guidelines. Our findings reveal the presence of knowledge gaps for colon cancer screening in the United States wherein knowledge deficits are most pronounced among those with lower educational attainment, non-Hispanic Blacks, older adults, those who have never had FOBT, and those who have not looked for cancer information. These findings justify the development of targeted interventions for those segments of the population with the greatest knowledge deficits. Such interventions could usefully engage with communication channels at multiple levels of public policies and health, including the mass media, managed care, and face-to-face exchanges between patients and physicians (Street, 2003). However, the development of interventions for specific subpopulations should not neglect general population strategies to raise level of awareness for colon cancer screening. The study also points out that communications regarding colon cancer recommendations should stress multiple aspects of the test, which may allow individuals to initiate screening, and then to retain the information required to continue screening at recommended intervals for many years.

COLON CANCER PREVENTION AWARENESS

We also recently examined knowledge gaps regarding awareness of the role of physical activity in the prevention of colon cancer in the 2005 HINTS sample (Coups, Hay, & Ford, 2008). This study was conducted in a sample of 1,932 HINTS participants. In order to measure their awareness of the role of physical activity in cancer prevention, participants responded to the following open-ended question: "What are some things that people can do to reduce their chances of getting colon cancer?" Participants who listed exercise or physical activity in their responses were denoted as being aware of the role of physical activity in colon cancer prevention. As with CRC screening knowledge, awareness of the role of physical activity in reducing the risk of colon cancer was low among the overall sample. Indeed, only 15% of participants indicated that physical activity reduces the risk for colon cancer. Based on our multivariate findings, knowledge was significantly less for older age groups; only 9.5% of those aged 70 and older reporting awareness of the role of physical activity in preventing colon cancer. Additionally, among participants with high school education attainment or less or who reported being sedentary, fewer than 1 in 10 individuals indicated that physical activity plays a role in preventing colon cancer. Those who had lower levels of knowledge reported lower levels of information-seeking and knowledge about cancer prevention recommendations. For instance, individuals who agreed that physical activity recommendations are confusing, those reporting not being exposed to any information about physical activity and cancer in the past year, those who have never looked for cancer information, and individuals not knowing any symptoms of colon cancer were more likely to lack knowledge of the role of physical activity in preventing colon cancer. Knowledge did not differ significantly across gender or racial/ethnic subgroups.

The results of this national probability survey of U.S. adults revealed that fewer than one in six study participants (15%) was aware that physical activity plays a role in reducing risk for colon cancer. This low level of awareness suggests that public heath communication efforts regarding the strong protective effective of physical activity against colon cancer are lacking and/or ineffective. Although we found no specific knowledge deficits among racial/ethnic groups, those who are older and less educated could be singled out for targeted interventions. As knowledge increases on a population level, it may be necessary to monitor and counteract potential differential gains in knowledge across vulnerable and underserved populations. Furthermore, the study results suggest that individuals' lack of awareness of the role of physical activity in colon cancer prevention may be one component of a broader lack of information exposure and low information-seeking about cancer prevention. This study also illustrates how individuals who engage in less information-seeking are less knowledgeable, pointing out potential opportunities to improve the clarity and user-friendly nature of health information across multiple delivery channels.

KNOWLEDGE OF COLON CANCER RISKS

In a third study (Hay, Coups, & Ford, 2006), we examined individuals' perception of their colon cancer risks. Although knowledge and cancer risk perceptions are distinct constructs, knowledge gaps are likely to perpetuate inaccuracies in cancer risk perceptions in the general population and could represent one route through which knowledge gaps lead to optimistic biases about risk. In this study we utilized a subsample of 2,949 HINTS 2003 (NCI, 2004, 2005; Nelson et al., 2004; Yach, 2004) participants who were at least 45 years of age with no personal history of colon cancer. Perceived risk for colon cancer was measured in two ways, including absolute perceived risk for developing colon cancer (responses ranged from *very low* to *very high*) and comparative perceived colon cancer risk (responses ranged from *much less likely* to *much more likely* than individuals of the same age and gender).

As has been shown in many prior studies, our study confirms the existence of optimistic biases in perceptions of risk across the sample as a whole. Of the sample, 48% reported that their risk for colon cancer was less than that for others their age and gender, and 62% reported that their absolute risk for colon cancer was either somewhat or very low. Multivariate examination of the uniquely important predictors of comparative risk perceptions found that psychosocial factors (cancer worry, fear of finding colon cancer), family cancer history, poor/fair subjective health status, and the perception of information overload about cancer were related to increased perceptions of being at risk for colon cancer. Of all the sociodemographic factors examined, only age and Spanish-language preference for the HINTS interview were related to increased perceptions of being at risk for colon cancer. Although it is difficult to formulate firm conclusions regarding language preference given that only about 3% of participants overall fell into this category, these effects indicated that those aged 65 and older were more likely to perceive that they were at *reduced* risk compared with individuals of the same age and gender than were younger participants; those who completed the interview in Spanish felt they were at *increased* risk for colon cancer than were those who completed the interview in English. Nonsignificant predictors included most socioeconomic factors, including gender, education, and race, and lifestyle factors (cigarette smoking, fruit and vegetable consumption, and body mass index). Significant multivariate predictors of higher absolute perceived risk were even more limited, and included only poor/fair health status, personal and family history of colon cancer, cancer worry and fear of finding a cancer. The findings reported here highlight, again, that knowledge deficits may be critical in older adults, who may come to see themselves at less risk for developing colon cancer in part based on their lack of information about early detection and prevention for colon cancer. It is also valuable to note that there is much inconsistency across sociodemographic groups regarding perceived colon cancer risk, making it difficult to draw generalizations regarding which groups are most deficient in their knowledge, and why. These results are important because perceived risk for CRC is likely an important precursor to uptake of screening and risk reduction strategies for CRC. There is evidence that perceived risk for CRC prospectively increases CRC screening intentions and utilization (McCrae, Hill, St. John, Ambikapathy, Garner, & the Ballarat General Practitioner

Research Group, 1984; Vernon, Myers, Tilley, & Li 2001; Watts, Vernon, Myers, & Tilley, 2003).

INFORMATION SEEKING BEHAVIORS

In one final study (Ford, Coups, & Hay, 2009), we examined the cancer information-seeking experiences of a sample of cancer survivors using HINTS 2005. Specifically, we were interested in the prevalence of, and barriers to, health information-seeking that could be related to knowledge gaps among cancer survivors or subpopulations of cancer survivors. We examined 711 cancer survivors, excluding those with nonmelanoma skin cancers who participated in HINTS 2005. The survivors were mostly female (65.5%), non-Hispanic White (82.3%), over the age of 60 (66.7%), and had graduated from high school (84.3%). The most common cancer diagnoses reported were breast (21%), prostate (15.4%), melanoma (14.3%), cervical (10.9%), and colon (8%). Most were long-term survivors and had been diagnosed more than 5 years prior to the telephone interview (62.8%).

Overall, 63.6% of the survivors reported having looked for cancer information. Consistent with the knowledge gap hypothesis, our findings reveal SES, race/ethnicity, and age discrepancies in cancer information-seeking among these cancer survivors. For instance, only 52% of those who were non-Hispanic Blacks, 27% of those with less than a high school education, 50% of those with annual incomes of less than $25,000, and 48% of those over age 70 years reported ever having looked for information about cancer from any source. Overall, survivors were confident that they could get advice or information about cancer if they needed it (61.5% were very to completely confident), although many reported that it took a lot of effort to get the information they needed. More than one-fourth (25.8%) felt frustrated during their search for information. Based on their most recent search for information about cancer, 47.6% of survivors were concerned about the quality of information they obtained. Additionally, 26.4% felt that the information they found was too difficult to understand and that it took a lot of effort to get the information they needed (33.5%). Accordingly, cancer information-seeking is lower among those who are disadvantaged in terms of education and income, as well as among older adults and non-Hispanic Blacks. This highlights a question regarding whether some individuals avoid information-seeking because of their concerns about the quality of the information they are finding.

Given what survivors reported in the HINTS 2005 about cancer information-seeking, it is possible that many survivors are not receiving the information they are interested in and/or are receiving incorrect cancer information. Additionally, they are having difficulty understanding the information and are not confident in the quality of information they are receiving. These implications point to many useful areas of future inquiry and intervention.

DISCUSSION

There are some important overarching themes to our findings reported across four studies. First, despite our focus on gaps in knowledge for colon cancer, we found universally low levels of knowledge *across all groups*. Given that only 21% had adequate knowledge of colon cancer screening, and only 15% had knowledge of the role of physical activity in preventing colon cancer, strategies to improve dissemination of CRC prevention and control information would be useful and seem necessary at the population level. We also found that most participants (62%) saw themselves as being at very or somewhat low risk for colon cancer; 48% thought that their risk was less than for others their age and sex. Knowledge gaps in the United States regarding screening and prevention strategies for cancer were noted in the 1992 National Health Interview Survey Cancer Control Supplement (Breslow, Sorkin, Frey, & Kessler, 1997); CRC-specific knowledge gaps have been confirmed recently as well, in a large survey study conducted across 21 European countries (Keighley, O'Morain, Giacosa, Ashorn, Burroughs, Crespi et al., 2004). Knowledge about the risks associated with colon cancer are likely important predictors of risk perceptions for the disease (Robb, Miles, & Wardle, 2004), so knowledge gaps may set the stage for this unrealistic optimism concerning colorectal cancer risk. Inadequate knowledge about what factors contribute to risk for various cancers has been confirmed in recent studies in the general population (Breslow et al., 1997; Keighley et al., 2004). Some of this may be explained by the fact that people are aware that dietary factors and adequate exercise contribute to good health overall, but do not necessarily relate these factors to the prevention of specific cancers (Goldman, Barbeau, Hunt, Acevedo-Garcia, Emmons, Gagne et al., 2008). Unfortunately, efforts to increase awareness of cancer risk factors could compound the problem; a recent population-based national survey reported that 50% of those surveyed believe that there are so many recommendations for cancer risk reduction that it is difficult to know what to believe (Hesse et al., 2006; Hornik, Bettinghaus, Gurmankin, Kimmel, Kelly, Shim et al., 2005; NCI, 2004, 2005; Nelson et al., 2004; Yach, 2004). Perhaps a team effort to develop unified media messages linking prevention and early detection information for many cancers, or cancer and heart disease, could limit overload and frustration.

In terms of race and ethnicity, our results were mixed, showing that it is not the only, or the most important, factor in determining the knowledge gaps we examined. We found some evidence for knowledge gaps among non-Hispanic Black participants as well as those who completed their interview in Spanish. Recently, Shokar, Vernon, and Weller (2005) conducted qualitative individual interviews with non-Hispanic Black, Hispanic, and non-Hispanic White participants, and found knowledge deficits among the non-White populations; however, they did not observe expected fatalistic attitudes about cancer, pointing the way for possibly high levels of receptivity for early detection messages in diverse populations. Although race/ethnicity may be an important factor to consider when addressing cancer knowledge disparities, it is not the only one to take into account. Therefore, we need to think about our efforts in targeted and tailored interventions. Alternatively, older individuals show consistent deficits in colon cancer knowledge based on our HINTS findings; these deficits may be exacerbated among less educated, non-White older adult populations and across other cancer sites (Donovan & Tucker, 2000; Hislop, Teh, Lai, Ralston, Shu, & Taylor, 2004; Jones, Thompson, Oster, Samadi, Davis, Mayberry et al., 2003; Loehrer, Greger, Weinberger, Musick, Miller, Nichols et al., 1991; Ralston, Taylor, Yasui, Kuniyuki, Jackson, Tu et al., 2003; Viswanath, Breen, Meissner, Moser, Hesse, Steele et al., 2006). For instance, Jones and colleagues (2003) noted the increased need for mammography and clinical breast examination education in older Black women. Furthermore, true population-based samples may be even less knowledgeable than those who are self-referred for survey research (Henrikson, Harris, & Bowen, 2007). Research is certainly warranted to examine the multiple sources of knowledge deficits in older adults. This research represents a valuable priority given the heightened cancer risk faced by older adults that dictates a need for them to maintain cancer screening strategies, in particular, over the age of 65 (Sheinfeld Gorin, Gauthier, Hay, Miles, & Wardle, 2008). Finally, further research regarding the predictors of cancer information-seeking is an important priority, as reduced information-seeking is consistently related to knowledge gaps. In the case of cancer survivors, participants reported that they have trouble trusting the quality of the information, and/or may not understand the information they have obtained. Clinicians and health behavior interventionists need to develop strategies to assist people throughout the information-seeking process starting from the point of eliciting unmet informational needs and directing people to the most reliable sources.

Prior literature has shown deficits in knowledge regarding cancer risk among non-Hispanic Blacks (Breslow et al., 1997; Donovan & Tucker, 2000) and Hispanics (Breslow et al., 1997), as well as those with lower education and income levels, and among older adults (Breslow et al., 1997; Donovan & Tucker, 2000; Hislop et al., 2004, Viswanath et al., 2006). For example, Breslow et al. (1997) assessed the knowledge of cancer-related risks and survival among 12,035 participants in the National Health Interview Survey, and found that the identification of multiple sex partners as a risk factor for cervical cancer was lowest among women who had the lowest income and education levels. Additionally, the identification of high-fat diet with multiple cancers, family history of breast and colon cancer, low-fiber diet with colon cancer, and smoking with cervical cancer were lowest among participants who were Hispanic or Black and had the lowest education and income levels. Similarly, in Chinese women, knowledge of cervical cancer risks and pap screening practices has been shown to be higher in those women with higher education and income levels (Hislop et al., 2004).

Knowledge gaps regarding cancer screening have been established for other malignancies, as well. For example, lack of basic cancer knowledge and a poor understanding of cancer screening has been shown to be higher for Non-Hispanic Blacks and Hispanics as compared with non-Hispanic Whites (Shokar, Vernon, & Weller, 2005). Age effects are important as well; Jones and colleagues (2003) compared Black women from three different age cohorts (65–74, 75–84, and >85 years), and found that women from the youngest group were more likely than the women from the middle and oldest groups to correctly assume that women aged 65 or older should undergo annual mammography screenings. Additionally, 94% of women from the two younger cohorts, as compared with 80.5% from the older cohort, knew that early diagnosis and treatment of breast cancer can prevent death.

In summary, collective research from HINTS as well as other sources indicates that cancer knowledge deficits in the general population and knowledge gaps between certain subgroups continue to exist. In our studies we focused primarily on knowledge and risk perceptions regarding colon cancer, and we found that these gaps were most consistently problematic in older adults, the less educated, and among those who do not look for cancer information. Although with somewhat less consistency, individuals from certain racial/ethnic subgroups demonstrate knowledge deficits as well. Importantly, our results indicate that knowledge of available colon cancer screening modalities and physical activity as a prevention strategy for colon cancer is generally low in the population. Findings from HINTS will provide an evidence base to guide intervention development and mechanistic research. These efforts will serve to advance initiatives to address and surmount cancer knowledge gaps in the United States.

ACKNOWLEDGMENTS

We acknowledge the support of NIH CA098106 (Jennifer Hay), the ACS MRSG-07-165-01-CPPB (Jennifer Ford), and NIH 5R25CA057708 and CA006927 (Elliot Coups).

REFERENCES

Abidoye, O., Ferguson, M.K., & Salgia, R. (2007). Lung carcinoma in African Americans. *Nature Clinical Practice Oncology, 4*(2), 118-129.

ACS, Cancer Facts and Figures for Hispanics/Latinos 2006-2008. (2006). *Statistics for 2007.* Atlanta: American Cancer Society.

ACS, Cancer Facts and Figures. (2007a). *Statistics for 2007.* Atlanta: American Cancer Society.

ACS, Cancer Facts and Figures for African Americans. (2007b). *Statistics for 2007.* Atlanta: American Cancer Society.

ACS, Global Cancer Facts & Figures (2007c). *Statistics for 2007.* Atlanta: American Cancer Society.

Adams, S.A., Hebert, J.R., Bolick-Aldrich, S., Daguise, V.G., Mosley, C.M., Modayil, M.V. et al. (2006). Breast cancer disparities in South Carolina: Early detection, special programs, and descriptive epidemiology. *Journal of the South Carolina Medical Association, 102,* 231-239.

Alberg, A.J., Horner, M.J., Daguise, V.G., Carpenter, M.J., Mosley, C.M., Vincent, B. et al. (2006). Lung and bronchus cancer disparities in South Carolina: Epidemiology and strategies for prevention. *Journal of the South Carolina Medical Association, 102*(7), 183-191.

Alexander, D.D., Waterbor, J., Hughes, T., Funkhouser, E., Grizzle, W., & Manne, U. (2007). African-American and caucasian disparities in colorectal cancer mortality and survival by data source: An epidemiologic review. *Cancer Biomark, 3*(6), 301-313.

Ananthakrishnan, A.N., Schellhase, K.G., Sparapani, R.A., Laud, P.W., & Neuner, J.M. (2007). Disparities in colon cancer screening in the Medicare population. *Archives of Internal Medicine, 167,* 258-64.

Baquet, C.R., & Commiskey, P. (1999). Colorectal cancer epidemiology in minorities: A review. *Journal of the Association for Academic Minority Physicians, 10*(3), 51-58.

Berger, M., Lund, M.J., & Brawley, O.W. (2007). Racial disparities in lung cancer. *Current Problems in Cancer, 31*(3), 202-210.

Bowen, D.J., Alfano, C.M., McGregor, B.A., Kuniyuki, A., Bernstein, L., Meeske, K. et al. (2007). Possible socioeconomic and ethnic disparities in quality of life in a cohort of breast cancer survivors. *Breast Cancer Research and Treatment, 106*(1), 85-95.

Brandt, H.M., Modayil, M.V., Hurley, D., Pirisi-Creek, L.A., Johnson, M.G., Davis, J. et al. (2006). Cervical cancer disparities in South Carolina: An update of early detection, special programs, descriptive epidemiology, and emerging directions. *Journal of the South Carolina Medical Association, 102*(7), 223-230.

Breslow, R.A., Sorkin, J.D., Frey, C.M., & Kessler, L.G. (1997). Americans' knowledge of cancer risk and survival. *Preventive Medicine, 126*(2), 170-177.

Calle, E.E., Rodriguez, C., Walker-Thurmond, K., & Thun, M.J. (2003). Overweight, obesity, and mortality from cancer in a prospectively studied cohort of U.S. adults. *New England Journal of Medicine, 348*(17), 625-638.

Chao, A., Thun, M.J., Connell, C.J., McCullough, M.L., Jacobs, E.J., Flanders, W.D. et al. (2005). Meat consumption and risk of colorectal cancer. *Journal of the American Medical Association, 293*(2), 172-182.

Cho, E., Smith-Warner, S.A., Ritz, J., van den Brandt, P.A., Colditz, G.A., Folsom, A.R. et al. (2004). Alcohol intake and colorectal cancer: A pooled analysis of 8 cohort studies. *Annals of Internal Medicine, 140*(8), 603-613.

Chu, K.C., Tarone, R.E., & Freeman, H.P. (2003). Trends in prostate cancer mortality among black men and white men in the United States. *Cancer, 97*(6), 1507-1516.

Cokkinides, V.E., Chao, A., Smith, R.A., Vernon, S.W., & Thun, M.J. (2003). Correlates of underutilization of colorectal cancer screening among U.S. adults, age 50 years and older. *Preventive Medicine, 36*(1), 85-91.

Cooper, G.S., & Doug Kou, T. (2008). Underuse of colorectal cancer screening in a cohort of medicare beneficiaries. *Cancer, 112*(2), 293-299.

Coups, E.J., Hay, J., & Ford, J.S. (in press). Awareness of the role of physical activity in colon cancer prevention. *Patient Education.*

Donovan, K.A., & Tucker, D.C. (2000). Knowledge about genetic risk for breast cancer and perceptions of genetic testing in a sociodemographically diverse sample. *Journal of Behavioral Medicine, 23*(1), 15-36.

Drake, B.E., Keane, T.E., Mosley, C.M., Adams, S.A., Elder, K.T., Modayil, M.V. et al. (2006). Prostate cancer disparities in South Carolina: Early detection, special programs, and descriptive epidemiology. *Journal of the South Carolina Medical Association, 102*(7), 241-249.

Du, X.L., Meyer, T.E., & Franzini, L. (2007). Meta-analysis of racial disparities in survival in association with socioeconomic status among men and women with colon cancer. *Cancer, 109*, 2161-2170.

Du X.L., & Gor, B.J. (2007). Racial disparities and trends in radiation therapy after breast-conserving surgery for early-stage breast cancer in women, 1992 to 2002. *Ethnicity and Disease, 17*(1), 122-128.

Flenaugh, E.L., & Henriques-Forsythe, M.N. (2006). Lung cancer disparities in African Americans: Health versus health care. *Clinics in Chest Medicine, 27*(3), 431-439, vi.

Ford, J.S., Coups, E.J., & Hay, J.L. (2006). Knowledge of colon cancer screening in a national probability sample in the United States. *Journal of Health Communication, 11*(Suppl1), 19-35.

Ford, J.S., Coups, E.J., & Hay, J.L. (2009) *Health information seeking of cancer survivors.* Manuscript in preparation.

Fouad, M.N., Nagy, M.C., Johnson, R.E., Wynn, T.A., Partridge, E.E., & Dignan, M. (2004). The development of a community action plan to reduce breast and cervical cancer disparities between African-American and White women. *Ethnicity and Disease, 14*(3 Suppl 1), S53-560.

Fouad, M.N., Partridge, E., Dignan, M., Holt, C., Johnson, R., Nagy, C. et al. (2006). A community-driven action plan to eliminate breast and cervical cancer disparity: Successes and limitations. *Journal of Cancer Education, 21*(1 Suppl), S91-100.

Giovannucci, E. (2001). An updated review of the epidemiological evidence that cigarette smoking increases risk of colorectal cancer. *Cancer Epidemiology, Biomarkers & Prevention, 10*(7), 725-731.

Goldman, R.E., Barbeau, E., Hunt, M.K., Acevedo-Garcia, D., Emmons, K.M., Gagne, J. et al. (2008). Perceptions of health promotion and cancer prevention among adults in working-class occupations and neighborhoods. *Health Education & Behavior.*

Harper, S., & Lynch, J. (2005). Methods for measuring cancer disparities: Using data relevant to healthy people 2010 cancer-related objectives. *NCI Cancer Surveillance Monograph Series* (Number 6). Bethesda, MD: National Cancer Institute.

Hay, J., Coups, E.J., & Ford, J.S. (2006). Predictors of perceived risk for colon cancer in a national probability sample in the United States. *Journal of Health Communication, 11*(Suppl 1), 71-92.

Henrikson, N.B., Harris, J.N., & Bowen, D.J. (2007). Predictors of self-referral into a cancer genetics registry. *Cancer Epidemiology, Biomarkers & Prevention, 16*(7), 1387-1392.

Hesse, B.W., Moser, R.P., Rutten, L.J., & Kreps, G.L. (2006). The health information national trends survey: Research from the baseline. *Journal of Health Communication, 11*(Suppl 1), vii-xvi.

Hiatt, R.A., & Rimer, B.K. (1999). A new strategy for cancer control research. *Cancer Epidemiology, Biomarkers & Prevention, 8*(11), 957-964.

Hirschman, J., Whitman, S., & Ansell, D. (2007). The black:white disparity in breast cancer mortality: The example of Chicago. *Cancer Causes & Control, 18*(3), 323-333.

Hislop, T.G., Teh, C., Lai, A., Ralston, J.D., Shu, J. & Taylor, V.M. (2004). Pap screening and knowledge of risk factors for cervical cancer in Chinese women in British Columbia, Canada. *Ethnicity & Health, 9*(3), 267-281.

Hornik, R., Bettinghaus, E., Gurmankin, A.D., Kimmel, L.G., Kelly, B., Shim, M. et al. (2005). Health communication/media. *Health Information National Trends Survey Data Users Conference*, St. Pte Beach, FL.

James, W.P.T., Jackson-Leach, R., Mhurchu, C.N., Kalamara, E., Shayehgi, M., Rigby, N.J. et al. (2004). Overweight and obesity (high body mass index). In M. Ezzati (Ed.), *Comparative quantification of health risks: Global and regional burden of disease attributable to selected major risk factors.* Geneva: World Health Organizations.

Jonas, D.E., Russell, L.B., Sandler, R.S., Chou, J., & Pignone, M. (2007). Patient time requirements for screening colonoscopy. *American Journal of Gastroenterology, 102*(11), 2401-2410.

Jones, A.R., Thompson, C.J., Oster, R.A., Samadi, A., Davis, M.K., Mayberry, R.M. et al. (2003). Breast cancer knowledge, beliefs, and screening behaviors among low-income, elderly black women. *Journal of the National Medical Association, 95*(9), 791-797, 802-805.

Keighley, M.R., O'Morain, C., Giacosa, A., Ashorn, M., Burroughs, A., Crespi, M. et al. (2004). Public awareness of risk factors and screening for colorectal cancer in Europe. *European Journal of Cancer Prevention, 13*(4), 257-262.

Lantz, P.M., Mujahid, M., Schwartz, K., Janz, N.K., Fagerlin, A., Salem, B. et al. (2006). The influence of race, ethnicity, and individual socioeconomic factors on breast cancer stage at diagnosis. *American Journal of Public Health, 96*(12), 2173-2178.

Lloyd, S.C., Harvey, N.R., Hebert, J.R., Daguise, V., Williams, D., & Scott, D.B. (2007). Racial disparities in colon cancer. Primary care endoscopy as a tool to increase screening rates among minority patients. *Cancer, 109*(2 Suppl), 378-385.

Loehrer, P.J., Sr., Greger, H.A., Weinberger, M., Musick, B., Miller, M., Nichols, C. et al. (1991). Knowledge and beliefs about cancer in a socioeconomically disadvantaged population. *Cancer, 68*(7), 1665-1671.

McCrae, F.A., Hill, D.J., St. John, J.B., Ambikapathy, A., Garner, J.F. & the Ballarat General Practitioner Research Group. (1984). Predicting colon cancer screening behavior from health beliefs. *Preventive Medicine, 13*, 115-126.

NCI. (2004). Health Information National Trends Survey (HINTS). Retrieved November 3, 2004, from http://cancercontrol.cancer.gov/hints/instrument.html.

NCI. (2005). Health Information National Trends Survey. Available: http://www.cancercontrol.cancer.gov/hints/.

NCI (2006). *What you need to know about cancer of the colon and rectum.*

Nelson, D.E., Kreps, G.L., Hesse, B.W., Croyle, R.T., Willis, G., Arora, N.K. et al. (2004). The Health Information National Trends Survey (HINTS): Development, design, and dissemination. *Journal of Health Communication, 9*(5), 443-460; discussion 81-84.

Polite, B.N., Dignam, J.J., & Olopade, O.I. (2005). Colorectal cancer and race: Understanding the differences in outcomes between African Americans and whites. *Medical Clinics of North America, 89*(4), 771-793.

Powell, T.R. (2006). Breast and cervical cancer disparities in SC: African-American perspective. *Journal of the South Carolina Medical Association, 102*(7), 240.

Ralston, J.D., Taylor, V.M., Yasui, Y., Kuniyuki, A., Jackson, J.C., & Tu, S.P. (2003). Knowledge of cervical cancer risk factors among Chinese immigrants in Seattle. *Journal of Community Health, 28*(1), 41-57.

Reddy, S., Shapiro, M., Morton, R., Jr., & Brawley, O.W. (2003). Prostate cancer in black and white Americans. *Cancer Metastasis Review, 22*(1), 83-86.

Robb, K.A., Miles, A., & Wardle, J. (2004). Demographic and psychosocial factors associated with perceived risk for colorectal cancer. *Cancer Epidemiology, Biomarkers & Prevention, 13*(3), 366-372.

Samad, A.K., Taylor, R.S., Marshall, T., & Chapman, M.A. (2005). A meta-analysis of the association of physical activity with reduced risk of colorectal cancer. *International Journal of Colorectal Disease, 7*(3), 204-213.

Sassi, F., Luft, H.S., & Guadagnoli, E. (2006). Reducing racial/ethnic disparities in female breast cancer: Screening rates and stage at diagnosis. *American Journal of Public Health, 96*(12), 2165-2172.

Schenck, A.P., Klabunde, C.N., Warren, J.L., Peacock, S., Davis, W.W., Hawley, S.T. et al. (2007). Data sources for measuring colorectal endoscopy use among Medicare enrollees. *Cancer Epidemiology, Biomarkers & Prevention, 16*(10), 2118-2127.

Sheinfeld Gorin, S., Gauthier, J., Hay, J., Miles, A. & Wardle, J. (2008). Cancer screening and aging: Research barriers and opportunities. *Cancer, 113*, 3493-504.

Shokar, N.K., Vernon, S.W., & Weller, S.C. (2005). Cancer and colorectal cancer: Knowledge, beliefs, and screening preferences of a diverse patient population. *Family Medicine, 37*(5), 341-347.

Slattery, M.L. (2007). Physical activity and colorectal cancer. In M. Feuerstein (Ed.), *Handbook of cancer survivorship* (pp. 75-90). New York: Springer.

Sonnenberg, A., Amorosi, S.L., Lacey, M.J., & Lieberman, D.A. (2008). Patterns of endoscopy in the United States: Analysis of data from the Centers for Medicare and Medicaid Services and the National Endoscopic Database. *Gastrointestinal Endoscopy.*

Street, R.L. (2003). Communications in medical encounters: An ecological perspective. In T. L. Thompson et al. (Eds.), *Handbook of health communication* (pp. 63-89). Mahwah, NJ: Erlbaum.

Tammemagi, C.M. (2007). Racial/ethnic disparities in breast and gynecologic cancer treatment and outcomes. *Current Opinion in Obstetrics and Gynecology, 19*(1), 31-36.

Tichenor, P.J., Donohue, G.A., & Olien, C.N. (1970). Mass media flow and differential growth in knowledge. *The Public Opinion Quarterly, 34.*

USDHHS. (2007). *Healthy People 2010: Understanding and improving health.* Available: http://www.healthypeople.gov/Document/tableofcontents.htm# under.

USPSTF. (2002). *Screening for colorectal cancer: Recommendations and rationale.* Rockville, MD: Agency for Healthcare Research and Quality. Available: http://www.ahrq.gov/clinic/3rduspstf/colorectal/colorr.htm.

Vernon, S.W., Myers, R.E., Tilley, B.C., & Li, S. (2001). Factors associated with perceived risk in automotive employees at increased risk of colorectal cancer. *Cancer Epidemiology, Biomarkers & Prevention, 10*(1), 35-43.

Vijayakumar, S., Winter, K., Sause, W., Gallagher, M.J., Michalski, J., Roach, M. et al. (1998). Prostate-specific antigen levels are higher in African-American than in white patients in a multicenter registration study: Results of RTOG 94-12. *International Journal of Radiation Oncology, Biology, Physics, 40*(1), 17-25.

Viswanath, K., Breen, N., Meissner, H., Moser, R.P., Hesse, B., Steele, W.R. et al. (2006). Cancer knowledge and disparities in the information age. *Journal of Health Communication, 11*(Suppl 1), 1-17.

Viswanath, K., & Finnegan, J.R., Jr. (1996). *The knowledge gap hypothesis: Twenty-five years later.* Thousand Oaks, CA: Sage.

Viswanath, K., Kahn, E., Finnegan, J.R., Hertog, J. et al. (1993). Motivation and the knowledge gap: Effects of a campaign to reduce diet-related cancer risk. *Communication Research, 20*(4), 546-563.

Watts, B.G., Vernon, S.W., Myers, R.E., & Tilley, B.C. (2003). Intention to be screened over time for colorectal cancer in male automotive workers. *Cancer Epidemiology, Biomarkers & Prevention, 12*(4), 339-349.

Winawer, S.J., Fletcher, R.H., Miller, L., Godlee, F., Stolar, M.H., Mulrow, C.D. et al. (1997). Colorectal cancer screening: Clinical guidelines and rationale. *Gastroenterology, 112*(2), 594-642.

Yabroff, K.R., Lawrence, W.F., King, J.C., Mangan, P., Washington, K.S., Yi, B. et al. (2005). Geographic disparities in cervical cancer mortality: What are the roles of risk factor prevalence, screening, and use of recommended treatment? *Journal of Rural Health, 21*(2), 149-157.

Yach, D. (2004). The Health Information National Trends Survey (HINTS): Development, design, and dissemination. *Journal of Health Communication, 9*(5), 481-482.

12

HEALTH BEHAVIORS AND BELIEFS AMONG CANCER SURVIVORS, FAMILY MEMBERS, AND THE GENERAL POPULATION

The HINTS Perspective

Tenbroeck Smith

Corinne Crammer

Michael Stefanek

Behavioral Research Center
American Cancer Society

A number of national organizations, including the American Cancer Society (ACS), the Institute of Medicine (IOM), and the National Cancer Institute (NCI), have identified cancer survivors as individuals with unique health needs, and cancer survivorship as an area in need of better scientific understanding. Cancer survivors experience the distress of a cancer diagnosis, the physical consequences of the disease, the complexity of treatment decisions, and the side effects of treatment. Furthermore, post-treatment cancer survivors face physical and psychological late effects as well as the social and financial impact of the cancer, all of which can persist for years. Many family members of those diagnosed with cancer also are highly impacted. Although not well studied, research to date suggests that these experiences impact survivor health behavior, including information-seeking.

The Health Information National Trends Survey (HINTS) has contributed to the nascent but growing body of literature investigating survivor health behavior and health beliefs. HINTS brings a number of strengths to the area of survivorship research, including population-based methods, a sufficient number of cancer survivors for many analyses, a built-in comparison group recruited via identical methods, and, most uniquely, a concentration on health communications, behaviors, and beliefs. The first four sections of this chapter provide a brief overview of cancer survivor and family caregiver issues as background. Limitations of HINTS and potential improvements also are discussed. Later sections describe the contribution of HINTS-based studies on survivorship research, making select comparisons to other studies in the literature to place them in context.

THE TERM *CANCER SURVIVOR*

The term *cancer survivor* is widely used, yet no consensus definition exists, and the meaning attributed to it varies by context and user. Thus, any discussion of cancer survivorship must first deal with this ambiguity. Traditional definitions included those still disease-free at 5 years or more from diagnosis. Currently, the most commonly used definition is the one established by the National Coalition for Cancer Survivorship (NCCS) in 1986: An individual is considered a cancer survivor from the time of cancer diagnosis through the balance of his or her life. NCCS credits Fitzhugh Mullan (1985) with the concept of calling individuals diagnosed with cancer *survivors*, rather than cancer victims or patients. Mullan based his use of the term on his own experience, which led him to believe that "survival, in fact, begins at the point of diagnosis because that is the time when cancer patients are forced to confront their own mortality" (p. 270). This definition may be useful for advocates who wish to cast their net widely in order to gather a sufficient advocate community to promote legislation and policies that address the needs of survivors and their families.

This definition of the term *cancer survivor* is not, however, universally accepted. Some individuals undergoing treatment for cancer may feel that the term is inappropriate until they are found to be cancer-free. One study of patients with breast and prostate cancers undergoing curative treatment found that the majority disliked being referred to as a "survivor"; most liked being referred to as a "patient" (Deber, Kraetschmer, Urowitz, & Sharpe, 2005). Those who are post-treatment may want to distance themselves from the cancer (Twombly, 2006). A study of survivors of prostate cancer 1 to 8 years from diagnosis showed that 57% identified themselves as "someone who has had prostate cancer," and only 26% self-identified as "survivors" (Bellizzi & Blank, 2007). The design of clinical and communications interventions and study recruitment materials should take into consideration the evidence that many individuals undergoing cancer treatment dislike the term *survivor*, and many of those with a history identify more closely with other terms.

One recent trend is to include all those who have been touched by cancer—family, friends, and informal caregivers—under the umbrella of survivorship. In recognition that cancer strongly affects family and close friends of the person diagnosed with the disease, several major organizations have expanded the meaning of survivor to include them (CDC, n.d.; NCCS, n.d.). For example, the NCI's Office of Cancer Survivorship definition of survivor includes more than the person with cancer: "An individual is considered a cancer survivor from the time of diagnosis, through the balance of his or her life. Family members, friends, and caregivers are also impacted by the survivorship experience and are therefore included in this definition."

Given the variety of existing definitions for the term *cancer survivor*, it is important for researchers and authors to provide precise definitions of the survivor populations to which they refer. In this chapter, the term *cancer survivor* refers to those who have been diagnosed with cancer, regardless of stage, prognosis, or treatment status. Because HINTS identifies not only survivors but also those with a family history of cancer, who are known to be affected by the diagnosis of a loved one, these persons are referred to separately as those with a family history of cancer (FHC).

THE DEMOGRAPHICS OF CANCER AND RELEVANT HINTS VARIABLES

As a result of advances in cancer treatment and early detection, cancer survival rates have been steadily increasing. This, combined with the general growth of the population of the United States and the growing number of older Americans as the baby-boom generation ages, has resulted in increasing numbers of cancer survivors (see Fig. 12.1). Estimates suggest that the

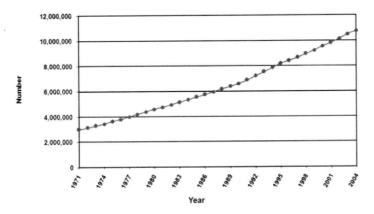

FIGURE 12.1. Number of cancer survivors in the United States from 1971 to 2004 (from NCI, 2007).

proportion of the U.S. population that had a history of cancer grew from 1.5% in 1971 to 3.7% in 2004, with more than 11.4 million people with a history of cancer living in the United States as of January 2007 (Horner, Ries, Krapcho, Neyman, Aminou, Howlader et al., 2009). The numbers of cancer survivors can be expected to continue to rise (Edwards, Howe, Ries, Thun, Rosenberg, Yancik et al., 2002; Hewit, Greenfield, & Stovall, 2006) for several reasons, including increasing incidence rates associated with the aging of the U.S. population and increasing survival rates (Jemal et al., 2004).

SEER data provides the demographic characteristics of cancer survivors (Ries, Melbert, Krapcho, Stinchcomb et al., 2008). Because cancer is a disease of aging, cancer survivors are older than the general population, with a majority (60%) 65 or older (see Fig. 12.2). In 1997, an estimated 16% of those aged 65 or older were cancer survivors (Hewitt, Rowland, & Yancik, 2003). There are more female than male survivors. As to race, survivors are less diverse than the general population: 88.5% are White and 7.8% are Black. More than half were initially diagnosed with breast (23%), prostate (19%), or colorectal cancer (10%, see Fig. 12.3). The majority of cancer survivors are less than 10 years past diagnosis. The majority of those with a history of cancer are post-treatment, disease-free survivors because only a small fraction of survivors were diagnosed within the last year (see Fig. 12.4).

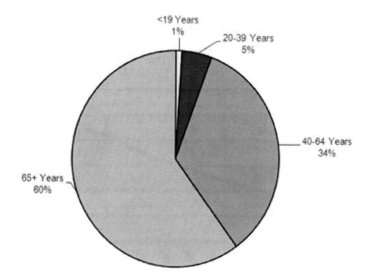

FIGURE 12.2.   Number of cancer survivors in the United States on January 1, 2004 by current age (from NCI, 2007).

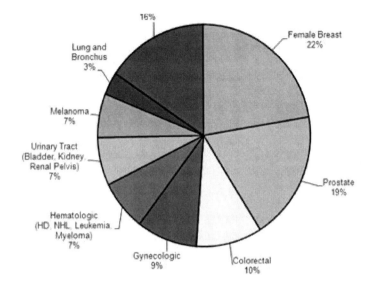

FIGURE 12.3. Number of cancer survivors in the United States on
January 1, 2004 by site (from NCI, 2007).

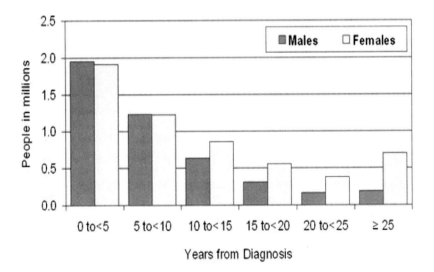

FIGURE 12.4. Number of cancer survivors in the United States on
January 1, 2004 by time from diagnosis and gender (from NCI, 2007).

ISSUES OF CANCER SURVIVORS

The cancer survivorship continuum can be divided into diagnosis, treatment, remission, advanced cancer or recurrence, and end of life. Considerable research has addressed the challenges of cancer diagnosis and treatment. In the past decade, research has turned to the unique issues faced by those post-treatment and disease-free. Because the majority of survivors in the HINTS sample and the general U.S. population fall into this category, this section focuses on the issues of post-treatment, disease-free survivors. Analyses of data from the National Health Interview Survey (NHIS) documented that survivors as a whole experience a range of long-term problems, including poorer general health than matched peers (Hewitt et al., 2003; Yabroff, Lawrence, Clauser, Davis, & Brown, 2004). For many individuals, however, overall health status returns to normal within 1 to 2 years after completion of treatment: This has been observed among survivors of local breast, prostate, or colorectal cancers (Anthony, Jones, Antoine, Sivess-Franks, & Turnage, 2001; Bloom, Stewart, Chang, & Banks, 2004; Ganz et al., 2002; Helgeson, Snyder, & Seltman, 2004; Helgeson & Tomich, 2005; Hoffman et al., 2004; Hurria et al., 2006). This illustrates that survivors as a whole continue to report health deficits years after diagnosis, although the overall functioning of certain subgroups returns to normative levels not long after completion of treatment.

Regardless of their overall health status, many cancer survivors experience physical and psychosocial long-term or late effects of cancer and its treatment (Kattlove & Winn, 2003; Stein, Syrjala, & Andrykowski, 2008). Fatigue, one of the most common symptoms associated with cancer and its treatment (Stasi, Abriani, Beccaglia, Terzoli, & Amadori, 2003), is one of the most prevalent long-term effects, beginning around the time of treatment and sometimes persisting for years afterwards (Ahn et al., 2007; Baker, Denniston, Smith, & West, 2005; Bower, 2005; Bower, Ganz, Aziz, Fahey, & Cole, 2003; Bower et al., 2000; Cella, Davis, Breitbart, & Curt, 2001; Fossa, Dahl, & Loge, 2003; Jereczek-Fossa, Marsiglia, & Orecchia, 2001; Vistad, Fossa, Kristensen, & Dahl, 2007). The debilitating effects of fatigue can impede return to precancer roles and activities, leading to employment limitations and social problems, including isolation and loneliness (Pryce, Munir, & Haslam, 2007; Short, Vasey, & Tunceli, 2005; Stasi et al., 2003).

Late effects are the long-term health changes resulting from cancer and its treatment that are absent immediately after treatment but appear later in a cancer-free survivor. For example, chemotherapeutic agents can result in cardiomyopathy, ischemia, and dysrhythmias, which may occur years after completion of treatment (Carver et al., 2007; Doyle, Neugut, Jacobson, Grann, & Hershman, 2005; Ganz et al., 2008; Steinherz & Yahalom, 2001). Radiotherapy can also lead to cardiovascular late effects (Eriksson et al.,

2000; Harpham, 1998; Prosnitz et al., 2007). The list of potential long-term and late effects is long and includes pulmonary disease (McDonald, Rubin, Philips, & Marks, 1995), chronic pain (Burton, Fanciullo, Beasley, & Fisch, 2007; Robb, Duvivier, & Newham, 2006), lymphedema (Petrek, Senie, Peters, & Rosen, 2001; Velanovich & Szymanski, 1999), chemotherapy-induced peripheral neuropathies (Lyne, Coyne, & Watson, 2002), avascular necrosis and other bone diseases (Cook, Dzik-Jurasz, Padhani, Norman, & Huddart, 2001; Pfeilschifter & Diel, 2000), and infertility (Huddart et al., 2005; Knobf, 2006; Nieman et al., 2006; Wenzel et al., 2005). The risk varies by cancer type and treatment. Long-term effects such as fatigue may negatively affect health behaviors, such as exercise, whereas risk of cardiac late-effect could motivate survivors to improve health behavior.

Cancer survivors may also experience difficulty in adjusting to life after treatment ends (McKinley, 2000; Mullen, 1985). Two of the more common psychological sequelae of cancer are depression and cognitive impairment (Bender et al., 2006; Bower, 2008; Hurria, Somlo, & Ahles, 2007). Estimates of the prevalence of symptoms of depression in survivors vary by study (Massie, 2004); a number of studies show elevated levels of depression in cancer survivors (Deimling, Kahana, Bowman, & Schaefer, 2002; Shinn, Basen-Engquist, Thornton, Spiess, & Pisters, 2007). Long-term survivors of breast, lung, and ovarian cancers, and lymphoma, may have cognitive (Ahles, 2004; Schultz, Beck, Stava, & Vassilopoulou-Sellin, 2003; Tannock, Ahles, Ganz, & van Dam 2004; Tchen et al., 2003; Wefel, Lenzi, Theriault, Davis, & Meyers, 2004) and neurological (Padovan et al., 1998) complications, such as memory loss, caused by systemic chemotherapy. Although only a subgroup of survivors suffer long-term cognitive dysfunction, these deficits can be disabling (Ahles & Saykin, 2001; Ahl et al., 2002). On the other hand, some report that the cancer experience has influenced them in a positive way via improved relationships, changed priorities, a greater appreciation of life, and personal or spiritual growth (Bellizzi et al., 2006; Kinsinger et al., 2006; Lechner et al., 2003). The new priorities and improved social support engendered in these benefits may also influence health behavior.

Perhaps the most important late effect that cancer survivors face is the return of cancer. Survivors not only face the possibility of recurrence of the original cancer, but are also at higher risk than the general populace for developing new or "second" cancers (Ng & Travis, 2008; Mariotto, Rowland, Ries, Scoppa, & Feuer, 2007). These second cancers are medically and biologically distinct from the initial cancer, for example, leukemia developing after treatment for lung cancer. The high rate of second cancers among survivors can be treatment-related (Brown et al., 2005; Hemminki, Lenner, Sundquist, & Bermejo, 2008; Kwong et al., 2008), the result of genetic propensity (Allan, 2008; Andersson et al., 2008; Travis, 2006), or related to the same behaviors that placed the individual at risk for the first cancer diagnosed (Garces et al., 2007). A 2007 study (Mariotto et al., 2007) estimated that 8% of cancer survivors (756,467 people) in the United States have been affected by cancer more than once between 1975 and 2001.

A significant proportion of cancer survivors experience recurrence, but rates vary widely by cancer type, disease characteristics, and treatment. For example, a study of survivors of local lung cancer showed 5-year recurrence rates varied from 27% to 50% depending on the type of surgery (Martini et al., 1995). A study of prostate carcinoma survivors who received radical radiotherapy showed that 10-year recurrence rates varied from 20% for stage T1 cancer to 87% for stage T4 (Duncan et al., 1993). Data on recurrence is not collected by state cancer registries, so national estimates are not available, but clearly much more than 8% of survivors have experienced either recurrence or a second cancer.

The threat of recurrence and increased risk of new cancers are particularly relevant here, as they may be factors that influence survivor health behavior. The possibility of the return of cancer has been described as a Damocles sword hanging over survivors (Muzzin, Andersen, Figueredo, & Gudelis, 1994) and is one of their most common concerns (Baker et al., 2005). Mullan (1985) and others argue that because of the threat of recurrence, in a sense, a person never really "gets over" cancer. A study of older cancer survivors found that one-third worried about cancer recurrence, and one-third worried about developing a second cancer (Deimling, Bowman, Sterns, Wagner, & Kahana, 2006). On the other hand, fear of recurrence has also been shown to be predictive of positive behavior changes like increasing exercise (Stein et al., 2008).

Based on the risk of recurrence, second cancers, and other late effects, it is important for cancer survivors to be followed by health providers who are knowledgeable about these issues. For recurrence, health providers can refer to the post-treatment surveillance guidelines issued by the National Comprehensive Cancer Network (NCCN; Kattlove & Winn, 2003; Sunga, Eberl, Oeffinger, Hudson, & Mahoney, 2005). Evidence-based guidelines are, however, missing for most other aspects of survivor care, including relatively well-studied areas like cardiac and pulmonary late effects (Earle, 2007). Coordination of care also emerges as an issue, with survivors and health providers unclear which responsibilities should fall to the primary care provider and which to the oncologist (Edwards et al., 2002; Hewitt et al., 2006). Lack of definitive guidelines for dealing with late effects and confusion regarding which physician to consult may influence survivor satisfaction with health information and behavior seeking it.

In summary, even after treatment ends, "survivors are never truly done" (McKinley, 2000). Although the overall functioning of many cancer survivors returns to normative levels not long after the completion of curative treatment, the vast majority of survivors are at risk for a number of long-term or late effects, most notably the return of cancer via recurrence or a second cancer. The level of risk, however, depends on the cancer type and the treatments received, leading to a complex landscape of risks that can be difficult for both survivor and health provider to fully understand. Survivors diagnosed and treated years ago may have only limited medical information available. Inadequate information about the cancer diagnosis and the treatments received may further complicate risk assessment, even for the most knowledgeable physicians. The variety of long-term effects and the issues of coordination of care provide the milieu in which the survivors make decisions about health behavior and interact with health information.

ISSUES OF THOSE WITH A FAMILY HISTORY OF CANCER

It has been said that it is not an individual who gets cancer, but a whole family. A family member's cancer diagnosis affects the family system and the individual family members in a number of ways, often for years after the diagnosis (Kim & Given, 2008; Mellon & Northouse, 2001; Rolland, 2005). The impact of cancer in the family is particularly great for family members providing informal care to the person with cancer. Compared with those caring for relatives with dementia or the frail elderly, cancer caregivers often provide greater intensity care over a shorter period (Kim & Schulz, 2008). The burdens experienced by these informal caregivers may include having to take time off work, which may contribute to the financial burden of cancer (Sherwood et al., 2007). These demands can be especially challenging for caregivers with multiple social roles, which results in them reporting more stress and greater negative affect (Kim, Baker, Spillers, & Wellisch, 2006).

The strain of providing this care can impact the family member in a number of ways. Compared with demographically comparable noncaregivers, caregivers have been shown to have poorer physical health, lower immune functioning, and elevated levels of psychological disorders (Hodges, Humphris, & Macfarlane, 2005). Caregivers may have more symptoms of psychological distress than the person cared for (Bambauer et al., 2006). Family caregivers of those with cancers with a poor prognosis or where the cancer has recurred are particularly at risk (Northouse et al., 2002). A study of caregivers for persons with advanced gastrointestinal or lung cancer found that 38.9% of caregivers exhibited symptoms of depression compared with 23% of the individuals with cancer (Braun, Mikulincer, Rydall, Walsh, & Rodin, 2007).

In the context of this chapter, the issues of caregivers are most important with regard to their influence on health behaviors. Relatives of those with cancer may assist the index case with information-seeking and decision making, as reflected by increased rates of cancer information-seeking and scanning among those with an FHC relative to the general public (Shim,

Kelly, & Hornik, 2006). Although having a family member with cancer may lead to an increase in healthy behaviors (Bowman, Rose, & Deimling, 2005), many caregivers neglect their own health, including good nutrition, exercise, and adherence to cancer screening guidelines (Beach, Schulz, Yee, & Jackson, 2000; Burton, Newsom, Schulz, Hirsch, & German, 1997). This is particularly of concern because for a number of cancers, first-degree relatives are at increased risk.

HINTS SURVIVOR/FHC VARIABLES AND LIMITATIONS

The contribution of HINTS to survivorship research relies on a limited number of items that assess how cancer has touched the respondent's life. In HINTS 2005, survivors were identified by the question "Have you ever been told by a doctor that you had cancer?" The survey provides a significant amount of additional information on cancer survivors including cancer type, year of diagnosis, treatment status, and time since treatment was completed. FHC is assessed based on the question "Have any of your family members ever had cancer?" The type of cancer with which the family member was diagnosed is also collected. These variables allow the researcher to target specific survivor or FHC subpopulations in the HINTS sample.

HINTS 2005 contains a large sample (N = 5,586) of the adult U.S. population. The proportion of this sample that report being cancer survivors — 11.4% (N = 873) — is higher than estimates from other sources. According to the 2005 NHIS, 7.4% of the adult U.S. population has a history of cancer. The significantly lower prevalence reported by SEER (3.7%) can be partially attributed to three factors.

1. SEER includes the entire U.S. population, whereas HINTS and NHIS are restricted to those 18 years and older.
2. Unlike HINTS and NHIS, SEER excludes non-melanoma skin cancers.
3. SEER uses cancer registry data, whereas HINTS and NHIS rely on self-report.

Nonetheless, HINTS appears to overreport cancer prevalence. A similar problem emerges in estimates of cancer-screening rates derived from HINTS, which are higher than those from either NHIS or the Behavioral Risk Factor Surveillance System (BRFSS; Mayer et al., 2007b). Both of these overestimates may be due to the HINTS 2005 recruitment procedure, which began by describing the survey as "about health issues related to cancer," and the mention of sponsorship by the NCI. Both statements are likely to lead to higher response rates among those who are particularly concerned about cancer (Groves, Singer, & Corning, 2000), including cancer survivors, those with a FHC, and those who screen at higher rates. Consequently, researchers should acknowledge said limitations around survivor or FHC prevalence rates from HINTS 2005. Furthermore, because survivors and those with a FHC differ from others with regard to health behaviors and beliefs (as described later in this chapter), the overrepresentation of these groups could influence general population results. Therefore, researchers may benefit from controlling for cancer history in nonsurvivor analyses.

Additional HINTS variables on cancer history can be used to create subgroups of survivors. Researchers may find it helpful to filter out the 21.4% of survivors in the HINTS 2005 sample who reported only non-melanoma skin cancer, a cancer that generally has much lower impact than other cancer types because of highly effective and less severe treatments. In contrast, one can select those reporting multiple cancers (19.7%), which likely reflects a mix of new primary cancers and recurrences. Another variable affecting the impact of cancer is time since diagnosis, which is reported for HINTS 2005 in Table 12.1. Cancer treatment variables are also included in HINTS, although they have not been used in published research to date, perhaps because of difficulties in interpretation. For example, although 11.9% of survivors report they are currently on treatment, some portion of these are undoubtedly on maintenance regimes that can last for years after curative treatment. When asked if they underwent treatment for their cancer, 17.3% of HINTS survivors indicate that they did not; an unexpected finding. Given the challenges in interpreting these cancer treatment variables, consideration is being given to the revision of these questions in future versions of HINTS.

Because a FHC influences health behaviors and beliefs, attention should be paid to the nearly 61% of the HINTS 2005 sample that report a positive FHC. The FHC experience, however, varies widely. Compare, for example, the experiences of a wife who provided significant care to her husband who recently died of lung cancer, to those of a grandson whose grandmother was quickly and successfully treated for skin melanoma 10 years ago. This sort

TABLE 12.1. Time Since Diagnosis (HINTS 2005)

Years Since Diagnosis	Frequency	Unweighted %
1 or less	119	13.82
2-5	231	26.83
6-10	160	18.58
11+	351	40.77

of variation could be described by collecting variables such as relationship to index case and years since diagnosis, variables that are arguably more important than the type of cancer of the index case.

CANCER INFORMATION, CANCER SURVIVORS AND FHC

Perhaps the area of survivorship research to which HINTS can make the most unique contribution is increasing the understanding of survivor cancer knowledge, beliefs, and informational behaviors. As a survey intended to describe "access, sources, and trust of cancer-related, information or factors that facilitate or hinder communication on a population-wide basis," HINTS includes data on constructs that have received little attention in the field of survivorship research to date, such as information needs, sources, and use. Even less research has focused on the outcomes associated with information use among survivors. This dearth of research is illustrated by a recent systematic review, which found that few studies assessed the information needs and sources of post-treatment survivors. Instead, most informational studies with survivors retrospectively focused on patients' needs around treatment (Finney Rutten, Nelson, & Meissner, 2004).

The importance of cancer information has been established in the other, nonsurvivor, populations. Knowledge about cancer risk, prevention, and detection is included in most current health behavior theories as a necessary but not sufficient predictor of behavior (Glanz & Rimer, 1997). The informational needs of patients and their family members facing treatment is well established: These groups need information about cancer, its treatment, and side effects (Manfredi, Czaja, Price, Buis, & Janiszewski, 1993). This information can help with decision making, reduce anxiety, increase treatment compliance, and provide realistic expectations among patients and their family members (Eysenbach, 2003). In the case of cancer survivors, information may have a number of uses including influencing health behaviors, forming realistic expectations, and making decisions about their on-going care. The designers of HINTS have long considered the value of maximizing the potential of HINTS to add to the understudied areas of survivors' informational needs, sources of information, and the effects of information on survivors and have considered the possibility of conducting a separate HINTS focused exclusively on the information needs and experiences of patients with cancer.

The few studies focused on the informational needs of post-treatment survivors show that they had fewer cancer-specific but more rehabilitative information needs than those still facing treatment (Finney Rutten, Arora,

Bakosc, Aziz, & Rowland, 2004). A recent population-based study of non-Hodgkin's lymphoma (NHL), leukemia, colorectal, or bladder cancer survivors 2 to 5 years from diagnosis showed that they continued to experience significant informational needs (Beckjord et al., in press). Survivors in this sample indicated they needed information about the following topics: Cancer tests and treatment (70.8%), health promotion to increase health or reduce cancer risk (67.8%), side effects of cancer (63.3%), interpersonal or emotional issues related to cancer (54.4%), insurance (42.1%), and sex and fertility (30.9%). These areas of survivor information needs align with the areas that the IOM proposed survivorship care plans should address (Edwards et al., 2002; Hewitt et al., 2006); the convergence of these two sources suggests that these are areas of importance for long-term survivors.

Publications based on HINTS have already begun to provide descriptions of the informational needs and information-related behaviors of survivors. The majority of survivors in the HINTS sample indicate that they are confident in their ability to find cancer information (Mayer et al., 2007a), yet 44.6% of information-seeking survivors indicate they are concerned about the quality of the information they find (Hesse, Arora, Beckjord, & Finney Rutten, 2008). Hesse et al. used HINTS data to describe a number of survivor information-related behaviors. Survivors were more likely to have ever searched for cancer information (63.1%) than those untouched by cancer (27.6%). Additionally, those with a FHC were also more likely to have ever searched (54.5%). The data also showed that, like the general population, survivors prefer health providers as a source of information. Phase of survivorship plays an important role in information-seeking. Survivors within 1 year of diagnosis almost universally report having searched for information in that same period (97.2%). In contrast, approximately 50% of those further from diagnosis have searched for cancer-related information in the last year, regardless of whether they are 2 to 5, 6 to 10, or 11 years or more from diagnosis, suggesting that longer-term survivors continue to have informational needs. The Internet was the most prevalent first source of cancer-related information reported both by survivors 2 to 10 years from diagnosis and the general public. In contrast, 1-year survivors and those more than 10 years from diagnosis were most likely to report their health care provider as their first source of cancer information.

In an innovative and theoretically provocative use of HINTS data, Shim et al. (2006) investigated cancer information-scanning and -seeking behaviors. Information *scanning* was defined as the amount of attention paid to health topics in the media. Information *seeking* was defined as looking for cancer information in the last year. Although scanning and seeking behaviors were related (e.g., information seekers were more likely to scan than nonseekers), these behaviors also showed a degree of independence, with 30.2% of the sample consisting of scanners who did not seek, and 9.9% of seekers who did not scan. The authors also showed that both behaviors were correlated with cancer knowledge and health behaviors such as diet, exercise, and screening, thus establishing the theoretical importance of informational behaviors.

Shim et al. also explored how experience with cancer affected the likelihood of engaging in scanning and seeking behaviors. Table 12.2 shows odds ratios of scanning or seeking for survivors, FHC, and the top two other predictors based on logistic regression. Relationship to cancer was the strongest predictor of information-seeking when controlling for a variety of other factors. Results for scanning behaviors were quite different: The propensity of survivors to scan was similar to that of those untouched by cancer, whereas those with a FHC showed only mild elevation in the likelihood of scanning. The authors offered no explanation for this unexpected finding, although health belief variables included in HINTS might be used to explore possible theoretical explanations.

Understanding the health information needs and the impact of health information on survivors is critical, because health communications are one of the primary strategies employed by large public health organizations such as the NCI and the ACS. As demonstrated in this review, HINTS has contributed significantly to the understanding of cancer-related informational behaviors and attitudes of survivors. Survivors and their family members are more likely to seek information than the general public. Not surprisingly, survivors' informational needs are greatest around the time of diagnosis and treatment, but continue after the completion of treatment. Other research suggests that the type of information that survivors need broadens from an intense treatment-related focus around the time of treatment. As they move further from diagnosis, other needs emerge, such as maintaining health and the late effects of cancer treatment. Younger, high-income, female survivors with a regular health care provider are the most likely to seek information (Mayer et al., 2007a). HINTS national prevalence data on survivor and FHC information-related behavior provide the foundation for building informational interventions for survivors. Furthermore, HINTS could be used to

TABLE 12.2. Odds of Seeking or Scanning by Select Variables

Odds Ratio: Seeking Information on Cancer	Odds Ratio: Being a "High Scanner"
Survivor (1.80)	Survivor (n.s.)
Family history of cancer (1.81)	Family history of cancer (1.20)
Female (1.79)	Female (1.97)
Hispanic (0.60)	Black (1.98)

Note: Data from Shim et al. (2006)

test and develop theories by exploring the interrelation among a person's history with cancer (e.g., survivor, FHC), beliefs and knowledge about cancer, information-related behavior, and other health behaviors Theories developed in this way could inform interventions not only among survivors, but also in the general population.

HEALTH BEHAVIOR AND BELIEFS AMONG SURVIVORS AND FHC

The journey through cancer diagnosis and treatment generally leaves survivors and their loved ones forever changed. Having faced a life-threatening disease and the existential crisis it engenders leads many survivors to reassess their priorities; this may include placing greater importance on their health. The cancer experience leads survivors to a new perspective on their physical vulnerability. Additionally, survivors are at risk for a number of adverse health outcomes, such as recurrence, second cancers, and other medical conditions (e.g., fatigue, cardiovascular disease, depression). The risk of other diseases among cancer survivors is underscored by a recent Australian study reporting that cancer patients were more likely to die of noncancer causes than the general population (Baade, Fritschi, & Eakin, 2006). Combining the increased health risks faced by cancer survivors with new attitudes resulting from the cancer experience, the time after treatment has been referred to as a teachable moment that may leave survivors more inclined to improve their health behaviors (Ganz, 2005). These health-protective behaviors include primary preventive behaviors, such as exercise and diet, and secondary preventive behaviors, including cancer screening. HINTS provides an excellent vehicle for testing theories that might elucidate the specific mechanisms that make this a teachable moment.

Regarding primary preventive behaviors, estimates suggest that the majority of cancer deaths in the United States are caused by risky health behaviors, such as physical inactivity, poor nutrition, obesity, and smoking (Rueben, 2007). Given the wealth of evidence that healthy behaviors, such as exercise, appropriate diet, and smoking cessation, can reduce the risk of developing cancer, it is not unreasonable to suspect that the same behaviors could protect cancer survivors from recurrence, second cancers, and other diseases. In fact, a small but growing body of research provides evidence that various health behaviors are protective for survivors (Do et al., 2004; Meyerhardt et al., 2006; Meyerhardt et al., 2007). In a study of survivors of stage III colon cancer, Meyerhardt and colleagues (2006) found that post-treatment physical activity was associated with improved recurrence-free survival and overall survival. An analysis of data from the same sample of survivors of colon cancer found that lower intake of foods typically found in the Western diet was associated with a lower risk of recurrence and over-all mortality (Meyerhardt et al., 2007). Survivors of head and neck cancers who continue to smoke after treatment have a higher risk for developing a smoking-related second primary cancer (Do et al., 2004). The degree to which findings from studies on specific cancers can be generalized to sur-vivors of other types of cancer is unclear, but these findings suggest a link between health behavior and both cancer recurrence and the development of second primaries.

Health behaviors have also been shown to benefit survivors' function-ing and quality of life. A correlational study of survivors of several different cancers showed that health behaviors were related to quality of life (Blanchard et al., 2004). Another study showed that survivors who quit smoking after the diagnosis with non-small cell lung cancer had better per-formance status at 6 and 12 months after diagnosis than those who contin-ued to smoke (Baser et al., 2006). Data from a growing number of clinical trials demonstrate the positive effects of improving health behaviors among cancer survivors. For example, Courneya et al. (2003) demonstrated that exercise improved cardiopulmonary function and quality of life among sur-vivors of breast cancer. A number of studies of survivors have demonstrat-ed that exercise is an effective treatment for cancer-related fatigue (see Mustian et al., 2007, for a review). In accord with the growing evidence that primary preventive health behaviors are highly beneficial to survivors, the ACS has developed a guide for physical activity and nutrition during and after cancer treatment (Kushi et al., 2006).

Regarding secondary preventive behaviors, cancer screening is an important technique for decreasing the risk of advanced cancers. Detection of the cancer at an earlier stage, especially before solid tumors have spread to other parts of the body, can lead to more effective treatment, better prog-nosis, longer survival, and higher quality-of-life survival. Scientific support of the importance of cancer screening is provided by evidenced-based guide-lines produced by the ACS and the U.S. Preventive Task Force. In survivors, secondary prevention includes both surveillance for recurrence and screen-ing for new primaries. The NCCN provides surveillance guidelines for sur-vivors of more common cancers.

Survivor Health Behavior

Research on health behavior change after diagnosis in survivors and those with a FHC has shown mixed results. Retrospective studies, in which sur-vivors or those with an FHC are asked to report the degree to which their health behaviors have changed as a result of a cancer diagnosis, generally report positive changes in health behaviors (Bellizzi, Miller, Arora, & Rowland, 2007; Humpel, Magee, & Jones, 2007). The most consistent and compelling evidence of positive health behavior change after a cancer diagnosis involves cancer screening. Comparisons between screening rates of cancer survivors and the general population conducted with NHIS data have provided convincing evidence that survivors screen at higher rates. Bellizzi and colleagues found that female survivors were more likely than controls to adhere to breast and cervical cancer-screening recommendations, and male survivors were more likely to have had a prostate-specific antigen (PSA) test (Bellizzi, Rowland, Jeffery, & McNeel, 2005). In a study addressing a greater number of screening tests, Trask et al. (2005) found that, compared with cancer-free individuals, survivors were more likely to have had a colorectal exam (odds ratio [OR], 2.2), a fecal occult blood test (FOBT; OR, 1.4), or a total body skin exam (OR, 4.0) within the recommended time frame. Female survivors were more likely to have had a screening mammogram (OR, 1.8), a clinical breast exam (OR, 2.2), or a pap smear test (OR, 1.3). Male survivors were more likely to have had a PSA test (OR, 2.5). Notably, a similar pattern was found when survivors diagnosed with the cancer for which a given screening test was designed to detect were excluded from analysis for that screen. This suggests that for survivors as a group, the cancer experience affects their behavior in a broad way, generalizing to adherence to screening for other cancers. Results from HINTS indicate that survivors are more likely to meet guidelines for colorectal cancer than the general public (Mayer et al., 2007b) although breast and prostate cancer-screening rates were similar to general population levels. Mayer et al. (2007b) suggested two explanations for the difference between HINTS and other sources:

1. The HINTS study controlled for access to health care, whereas NHIS analyses did not.
2. Estimates of screening rates derived from HINTS were higher than those from NHIS or BRFSS, which may have lead to a ceiling effect, in which there was little room for survivors to achieve higher rates.

In any event, the evidence suggests that survivors screen at higher rates than the general public, even in cancer other than that for which they were diagnosed.

As to primary prevention behaviors, such as physical activity, diet, and exercise, evidence for survivor behavior change after diagnosis is mixed. In several retrospective studies, survivors reported positive behavior changes (Bellizzi et al., 2007; Humpel et al., 2007). For example, the American Cancer Society's Studies of Cancer Survivors, a population-based study, has shown that survivors are much more likely to report either positive or no change in health behavior since diagnosis than they are to report negative health behavior change (see Table 12.3; Stein et al., 2008). A significant number of survivors, however, indicate decreased exercise, possibly because of physical impairments, such as fatigue, related to the cancer and its treatment. These retrospective designs, however, are subject to recall bias. Combining the results of retrospective studies with the strong evidence that survivors screen at higher rates than the general population, one might expect survivors to engage in a number of other health behaviors at a higher level than the general public.

Results from population-based studies with noncancer comparison groups provide mixed results with regard to primary preventive behaviors. In an analysis of HINTS data, Mayer and colleagues (2007a) found that cancer survivors did not differ from the general population with respect to physical activity, diet, smoking, or maintaining a healthy weight. In fact, both survivors and the general population were deficient in these areas, with only 7.4% of the cancer survivors and 6.4% of the cancer-free comparison group reporting positively on all three health behaviors and weight. Belizzi et al. (2005) found that survivors were more likely to meet physical activity recommendations than controls, but had similar rates of smoking. Their subgroup analyses revealed that younger survivors (aged 18–40 years) were at greater risk for smoking than controls. Although results are not consistent across health behaviors or studies, the evidence does suggest that the experience of cancer does lead to changes in survivor health behavior.

TABLE 12.3. Reported Changes in Behavior since Cancer Diagnosis

Behavior	More (%)	Same (%)	Less (%)	Never or N/A (%)
Getting regular health check-ups	49.1	48.0	1.1	1.7
Taking vitamins and/or supplements	46.3	41.4	1.5	10.8
Eating healthy foods (e.g., fruits and vegetables)	40.4	57.4	1.3	1.0
Using sunscreen	35.7	43.5	2.0	18.8
Trying to lose weight	35.1	43.1	4.2	17.6
Avoiding exposure to the sun	34.3	52.5	8.3	4.9
Wearing sun-protective clothing	30.6	56.1	1.9	11.4
Making efforts to control stress	30.4	59.1	1.8	8.8
Exercising	28.7	51.2	15.5	4.7
Avoiding alcohol	14.6	42.1	1.3	42.1
Avoiding cigarettes	7.5	8.4	1.3	82.8

Note. All proportions are weighted. From Stein et al. (2008).

FHC and Health Behaviors

Researchers have just begun to turn their attention to the effect of a FHC on health behaviors. Those with a FHC have vicariously experienced a life-threatening disease and, depending on their relationship to the person diagnosed, may have engaged in extensive research about cancer, provided care during treatment, or simply witnessed some of the adverse effects of cancer treatment. Additionally, for some cancers, a family history is associated with higher cancer risk (Fuchs et al., 1994). Consequently, the ACS (2008) recommends a different screening protocol for those at high risk for breast, colorectal, and skin cancers, which would include those with a strong family history of these cancers.

Using the NHIS, Shah et al. (2007) found that, when controlling for sociodemographic variables, women with a family history of any cancer were more likely to engage in breast (OR, 1.1) or colorectal (OR, 1.5) cancer screenings than those without such a history, but were not more likely to engage in skin cancer screening. The effect of FHC was stronger when the family member's cancer matched the cancer that the test was designed to detect. Based on a convenience sample and retrospective recall of prediagnosis behavior, Humpel et al. (2007) found that significant numbers of individuals with a family member or friend diagnosed with cancer reported positive health behavior change following diagnosis: 24.3% reported increased physical activity, 36.2% of smokers quit, 59% improved sun-safe behavior, and the majority made positive dietary changes (e.g., 58.5% increased intake of fruit and vegetables). The increased odds of cancer screening among FHC reported by Shah et al. (2007) appear to be somewhat weaker than those reported by Trask et al. (2005) for survivors. It is presently unclear whether the retrospective reports of positive primary preventive behavior change among FHC reported by Humpel et al. will be contradicted by more rigorous, population-based studies, although this is the pattern found with survivors. In any event, the results reported here suggest that the vicarious experience of cancer through a loved one's diagnosis leads to behavior change in some individuals.

Health Beliefs

Most contemporary health behavior theories posit that individuals' knowledge, attitudes, beliefs, and personality traits influence health behavior. Glanz and Rimer (1997) provided three concepts regarding health beliefs that cut across theories:

1. Behavior is mediated by cognitions; that is, what people know and think affects how they act.

2. Knowledge is necessary for, but not sufficient to produce, most behavior changes.
3. Perceptions, motivations, skills, and the social environment are key influences of behavior.

The HINTS survey includes items assessing a number of health beliefs, such as perceived cancer risk, cancer worry, and beliefs about cancer causes and preventability. Research has demonstrated links between these beliefs and various health behaviors.

Taking cancer worry as an example, a number of studies have shown links between various measures of cancer risk or worry and health behavior outcomes. Using data from HINTS, Moser, McCaul, Peters, Nelson, and Marcus (2007) showed that perceived cancer risk and cancer worry were associated with regular mammography screening and having had a screening sigmoidoscopy or colonoscopy but with neither FOBT nor PSA screening. Stein et al. found that cancer survivors' fear of recurrence was one of the strongest predictors of reporting health behavior improvements since diagnosis (Stein et al., 2008). Survivors with higher perceived risk for developing another cancer were more likely to abstain from smoking (Hay, Ostroff, Burkhalter, Li, Quiles, & Moade, 2007). For those with FHC, perceived cancer risk has also been linked to reported improvements in health behavior since diagnosis of the family member's cancer (Humpel et al., 2007). This suggests that perceived risk of cancer may be useful in motivating positive health behavior changes in the general public, cancer survivors, and those with a FHC.

Given the higher risk of cancer among survivors and those with n FHC, one might expect them to display higher levels of perceived cancer risk and worry. Indeed, simple bivariate analyses of data from HINTS 2005 show that survivors and those with a FHC are less likely to indicate their absolute risk of cancer is "very low" (survivor, 34.8%; FHC, 35.4%) than those untouched by cancer (46.7%, X^2-square p = 0.003). Similar results occur with comparative risk: Survivors and FHC were less likely to indicate they were "less likely than others" to get cancer (survivor, 43.1%; FHC, 44.5%) than those untouched by cancer (52.9%, X^2-square p = 0.03). Cancer worry did not significantly differ between these groups, perhaps because the question was asked for specific cancers and not asked of those with that cancer (e.g., colorectal cancer worry was not asked of colorectal survivors). In HINTS 2007, the cancer worry questions will address cancer in general and be asked of all survivors. Given the demonstrated links between perceived cancer risk, cancer worry, and health behavior in general population and survivor studies, these variables may play a role in explaining differences in health behavior rates between survivors, those with a FHC, and the general populace.

A similar, but less complete, picture can be painted for the fatalistic beliefs assessed by the HINTS survey. Niederdeppe and Levy (2007) used HINTS data to explore fatalistic beliefs in the general populace. They found that the public endorsed the various beliefs at different levels: "It seems like almost everything causes cancer" (47.1%), "There's not much people can do to lower their chances of getting cancer" (27%), and "There are so many recommendations about preventing cancer, it's hard to know which ones to follow" (71.5%). Furthermore, those endorsing these beliefs were less likely to exercise weekly, less likely to meet guidelines for daily fruit and vegetable intake, and more likely to smoke cigarettes (Niederdeppe & Levy, 2007). In a separate HINTS-based study, both survivors and those with a FHC were more likely to believe that "everything causes cancer" than those untouched by cancer (Lykins et al., 2008). Given that survivors are more likely to endorse that fatalistic belief, and that fatalism is related to poorer health behavior, perhaps fatalistic beliefs play a role in health behavior change related to either a personal or a family history of cancer.

Given survivors' greater risk of cancer and exposure to the health system, one might expect them to be more aware of various causes of cancer than those with a FHC or the general public, especially for well-established causes such as smoking. Research in this area, however, suggests otherwise. Using HINTS data, Lykins et al. (2008) found that a personal history of cancer was related to only 1 of 15 cancer-causation beliefs thought by the majority of the scientific community to be true, whereas FHC was related to higher endorsement rates of 8 of 15 beliefs. The authors noted that other studies also found that those with a personal history of cancer had weaker causal beliefs about cancer than cancer-free controls. These results demonstrate that the effect of FHC on health beliefs is unique, and not simply a weaker version of the effect of a personal diagnosis of cancer. Furthermore, these causal beliefs may play a role in behavior change after a diagnosis of cancer.

Summary

Given survivors' increased risk for multiple negative health outcomes, a thorough understanding of their health behaviors is important. HINTS is uniquely positioned to provide prevalence benchmarks among survivors for a number of health beliefs not included in other regularly occurring national surveys. Combining results from HINTS with studies from other sources provides a varied picture of postdiagnosis health behavior among survivors and those with a FHC. Some health behaviors appear to change in a positive direction after diagnosis, others are maintained at prediagnosis levels, and one study found that smoking increased among younger survivors (Bellizzi et al., 2005).

Research regarding health beliefs serves two purposes. First, this research can help identify links between specific beliefs and specific health behaviors, such as physical activity, diet, and smoking. Second, these empirically derived links can provide the theoretical framework for designing interventions to improve survivor and FHC health behavior. Results from HINTS-based studies and other sources raise several interesting theoretical questions, with implications for interventions intended to improve survivor and even general population health behavior. Why do survivors show improvements in some behaviors, whereas others remain unchanged or even worsen? Why do survivors report improving behavior but not show better health behavior than the general populace? At what rates do those with a FHC engage in health behaviors?

HINTS-based studies present a complex picture of the interrelationships between an individual's personal or vicarious cancer history, health beliefs, and health behaviors. Perceived cancer risk and cancer worry are associated with increased adherence to cancer-screening guidelines. Survivors and those with FHC experience higher levels of cancer risk and cancer worry than those untouched by cancer. This suggests that cancer worry may increase in survivors after diagnosis, which may lead to better cancer-screening behavior. In contrast, higher levels of the fatalistic belief that "everything causes cancer" among survivors and those with a FHC may act in the opposite direction because this belief is associated with poorer health behaviors. These results suggest that the mediators of the effect of cancer experiences on health behavior work in opposite directions. With the combination of population-based sampling, identification of respondent personal and familial cancer history, and coverage of a wide range of health beliefs, HINTS is well positioned to add to the literature describing the impact of diagnosis on survivor and FHC health behaviors.

CONCLUDING REMARKS

HINTS has contributed considerably to the understanding of cancer information behavior, health behavior, and health beliefs in cancer survivors and those with a FHC (see Table 12.4), areas in need of further investigation. The population-based, national prevalence data on information-related behaviors of survivors and those with a FHC provided by HINTS is essential to those designing informational interventions for survivors. These prevalence numbers can be expected to change over time, as the information landscape changes with advancing technologies; researchers and interventionists will want to use the most recent data whenever possible. As a survey designed to assess the health information needs and practices of the U.S. public on a

TABLE 12.4. HINTS Survivor and FHC Studies

INFORMATION-SEEKING AND SCANNING	
Survivors, even long-term survivors, and FHC are more likely to seek cancer information than the noncancer population.	Hesse et al. (2008)
For both survivors and FHC, health providers are the preferred information source.	
Survivor and FHC status are the strongest predictors of information-seeking.	Shim et al. (2006)
FHC are more likely than the noncancer population to scan for cancer information, but survivors are not.	
Information-seeking and scanning are related to cancer knowledge and health behaviors.	
HEALTH BELIEFS AND HEALTH BEHAVIORS	
Survivors are more likely to adhere to guidelines for colorectal cancer screening than the noncancer population.	Mayer et al. (2007)
Survivors and FHC perceive their absolute and relative risk of cancer as somewhat higher than the noncancer population.	This chapter
Cancer risk and cancer worry are associated with some cancer screening behaviors.	Moser et al. (2007)
Survivors are more likely to correctly endorse 1 of 15 cancer-causation beliefs than the noncancer population, whereas FHC are more likely to endorse eight of these beliefs.	Lykins et al. (2008)
Survivors and FHC are more likely to endorse the fatalistic belief "everything causes cancer" than the noncancer population.	
Fatalistic beliefs are associated with health behaviors.	Niederdeppe and Levy (2007)

periodic basis, HINTS also enables surveillance of trends in these areas among survivors and those with a FHC.

Perhaps more unexpected is the potential of HINTS to develop and test theories exploring the relationship between a person's cancer experience and his or her health beliefs and health behaviors. In many respects, the variety of experiences of cancer that exist in the general population—a personal history, a FHC, or being untouched by cancer—can serve as a natural experiment. As detailed in the previous section, these groups vary in terms of health beliefs and health behaviors, sometimes in unexpected ways. Survivors perceive themselves to be at higher cancer risk, and this is often associated with improved health behavior. On the other hand, as a group, survivors have elevated levels of cancer fatalism, which is associated with worse health behaviors. By containing variables on health behaviors, health beliefs, and cancer history, HINTS provides the tools to begin to elucidate the reasons why some health behaviors change after a cancer diagnosis, whereas others do not. This increased understanding will improve existing health behavior theories and can inform interventions not only among survivors, but also in the general populace.

One limitation of HINTS 2005 is the apparent overreporting of the proportion of survivors in population and cancer-screening rates. This has been addressed through changes in the recruitment protocol for HINTS 2007. A unique strength of HINTS is that it is the only regularly occurring national study that collects FHC. This strength could be built on by adding variables that describe the variability in FHC experiences—relationship to the survivor and years since diagnosis. Variables such as these would not significantly increase respondent burden and could replace less important variables, such as the survivor's cancer type.

REFERENCES

Ahles, T.A. (2004). Do systemic cancer treatments affect cognitive function? *Lancet Oncology, 5*(5), 270-271.

Ahles, T.A., & Saykin, A. (2001). Cognitive effects of standard-dose chemotherapy in patients with cancer. *Cancer Investigation, 19*(8), 812-820.

Ahles, T.A., Saykin, A.J., Furstenberg, C.T., Cole, B., Mott, L.A., Skalla, K. et al. (2002). Neuropsychologic impact of standard-dose systemic chemotherapy in long-term survivors of breast cancer and lymphoma. *Journal of Clinical Oncology, 20*(2), 485-493.

Ahn, S.H., Park, B.W., Noh, D.Y., Nam, S.J., Lee, E.S., Lee, M.K. et al. (2007). Health-related quality of life in disease-free survivors of breast cancer with the general population. *Annals of Oncology, 18*(1), 173-182.

Allan, J.M. The genetics of cancer survivorship. *Hematology/Oncology Clinic of North America, 22*(2), 257-vii.

American Cancer Society. *Cancer Facts and Figures.* (2008). Atlanta, GA: Author.

Andersson, A., Enblad, G., Tavelin, B., Bjorkholm, M., Linderoth, J., Lagerlof, I. et al. (2008). Family history of cancer as a risk factor for second malignancies after Hodgkin's lymphoma. *British Journal of Cancer, 98*(5), 1001-1005.

Anthony, T., Jones, C., Antoine, J., Sivess-Franks, S., & Turnage, R. (2001). The effect of treatment for colorectal cancer on long-term health-related quality of life. *Annals of Surgical Oncology, 8*(1), 44-9.

Baade, P.D., Fritschi, L., & Eakin, E.G. (2006). Non-cancer mortality among people diagnosed with cancer (Australia). *Cancer Causes and Control, 17*(3), 287-297.

Baker, F., Denniston, M., Smith, T., & West, M.M. (2005). Adult cancer survivors: How are they faring? *Cancer, 104*(11 Suppl), 2565-2576.

Bambauer, K.Z., Zhang, B., Maciejewski, P.K., Sahay, N., Pirl, W.F., Block, S.D. et al. (2006). Mutuality and specificity of mental disorders in advanced cancer patients and caregivers. *Social Psychiatry and Psychiatric Epidemiology, 41*(10), 819-824.

Baser, S., Shannon, V.R., Eapen, G.A., Jimenez, C.A., Onn, A., Lin, E. et al. (2006). Smoking cessation after diagnosis of lung cancer is associated with a beneficial effect on performance status. *Chest, 130*(6), 1784-1790.

Beach, S.R., Schulz, R., Yee, J.L., & Jackson, S. (2000). Negative and positive health effects of caring for a disabled spouse: Longitudinal findings from the caregiver health effects study. *Psychology and Aging, 15*(2), 259-271.

Beckjord, E.B., Arora, N.K., McLaughlin, W., Oakely-Girvan, I., Hamilton, A.S., & Hesse, B.W. (2008). Health-related information needs in a large and diverse sample of adult cancer survivors: Implications for cancer care. *Journal of Cancer Survivorship, 2*(3), 179-189.

Bellizzi, K.M., & Blank, T.O. (2006). Predicting posttraumatic growth in breast cancer survivors. *Health Psychology, 25*(1), 47-56.

Bellizzi, K.M., & Blank, T.O. (2007). Cancer-related identity and positive affect in survivors of prostate cancer. *Journal of Cancer Survivorship, 1*, 44-48.

Bellizzi, K.M., Miller, M.F., Arora, N.K., & Rowland, J.H. (2007). Positive and negative life changes experienced by survivors of non-Hodgkin's lymphoma. *Annals of Behavioral Medicine, 34*(2), 188-199.

Bellizzi, K.M., Rowland, J.H., Jeffery, D.D., & McNeel, T. (2005). Health behaviors of cancer survivors: Examining opportunities for cancer control intervention. *Journal of Clinical Oncology, 23*(34), 8884-8893.

Bender, C.M., Sereika, S.M., Berga, S.L., Vogel, V.G., Brufsky, A.M., Paraska, K.K. et al. (2006). Cognitive impairment associated with adjuvant therapy in breast cancer. *Psycho-Oncology, 15*(5), 422-430.

Blanchard, C.M., Stein, K.D., Baker, F., Dent, M., Denniston, M., Courneya, K.S. et al. (2004). Association between current lifestyle behaviors and health-related quality of life in breast, colorectal, and prostate cancer survivors. *Psychology and Health, 1*(1), 1-13.

Bloom, J.R., Stewart, S.L., Chang, S., & Banks, P.J. (2004). Then and now: Quality of life of young breast cancer survivors. *Psycho-Oncology, 13*(3), 147-160.

Bower J.E. (2005). Prevalence and causes of fatigue after cancer treatment: The next generation of research. *Journal of Clinical Oncology, 23*(33), 8280-8282.

Bower, J.E. (2008). Behavioral symptoms in patients with breast cancer and survivors. *Journal of Clinical Oncology, 26*(5), 768-777.

Bower, J.E., Ganz, P.A., Aziz, N., Fahey, J.L., & Cole, S.W. (2003). T-cell homeostasis in breast cancer survivors with persistent fatigue. *Journal of the National Cancer Institute, 95*(15), 1165-1168.

Bower, J.E., Ganz, P.A., Desmond, K.A., Rowland, J.H., Meyerowitz, B.E., & Belin, T.R. (2000). Fatigue in breast cancer survivors: Occurrence, correlates, and impact on quality of life. *Journal of Clinical Oncology, 18*(4), 743-753.

Bowman, K.F., Rose, J.H., & Deimling, G.T. (2005). Families of long-term cancer survivors: Health maintenance advocacy and practice. *Psycho-Oncology, 14*(12), 1008-1017.

Braun, M., Mikulincer, M., Rydall, A., Walsh, A., & Rodin, G. (2007). Hidden morbidity in cancer: Spouse caregivers. *Journal of Clinical Oncology, 25*(30), 4829-4834.

Brown, J.R., Yeckes, H., Friedberg, J.W., Neuberg, D., Kim, H., Nadler, L.M. et al. (2005). Increasing incidence of late second malignancies after conditioning with cyclophosphamide and total-body irradiation and autologous bone marrow transplantation for non-Hodgkin's lymphoma. *Journal of Clinical Oncology, 23*(10), 2208-2214.

Burton, A.W., Fanciullo, G.J., Beasley, R.D., & Fisch, M.J. (2007). Chronic pain in the cancer survivor: A new frontier. *Pain Medicine, 8*(2), 189-198.

Burton, L.C., Newsom, J.T., Schulz, R., Hirsch, C.H., & German, P.S. (1997). Preventive health behaviors among spousal caregivers. *Preventive Medicine, 26*(2), 162-169.

Carver, J.R., Shapiro, C.L., Ng, A., Jacobs, L., Schwartz, C., Virgo, K.S. et al. (2007). American Society of Clinical Oncology clinical evidence review on the ongoing care of adult cancer survivors: Cardiac and pulmonary late effects. *Journal of Clinical Oncology.*

Cella, D., Davis, K., Breitbart, W., & Curt, G. (2001). Cancer-related fatigue: Prevalence of proposed diagnostic criteria in a United States sample of cancer survivors. *Journal of Clinical Oncology, 19*(14), 3385-3391.

Centers for Disease Control & Prevention. (2007). Cancer survivorship. Department of Health and Human Services. Retrieved July 19, 2007, from http://www.cdc.gov/cancer/survivorship/index.htm

Cook, A.M., Dzik-Jurasz, A.S., Padhani, A.R., Norman, A., & Huddart, R.A. (2001). The prevalence of avascular necrosis in patients treated with chemotherapy for testicular tumours. *British Journal of Cancer, 85*(11), 1624-1626.

Courneya, K.S., Mackey, J.R., Bell, G.J., Jones, L.W., Field, C.J., & Fairey, A.S. (2003). Randomized controlled trial of exercise training in postmenopausal breast cancer survivors: Cardiopulmonary and quality of life outcomes. *Journal of Clinical Oncology, 21*(9), 1660-1668.

Deber, R.B., Kraetschmer, N., Urowitz, S, & Sharpe, N. (2005). Patient, consumer, client, or customer: What do people want to be called? *Health Expectations, 8*(4), 345-351.

Deimling, G.T., Bowman, K.F., Sterns, S., Wagner, L.J., & Kahana, B. (2006). Cancer-related health worries and psychological distress among older adult, long-term cancer survivors. *Psycho-Oncology, 15*(4), 306-320.

Deimling, G.T., Kahana, B., Bowman, K.F., & Schaefer, M.L. (2002). Cancer survivorship and psychological distress in later life. *Psycho-Oncology , 11*(6), 479-494.

Do, K.A., Johnson, M.M., Lee, J.J., Wu, X.F., Dong, Q., Hong, W.K. et al. (2004). Longitudinal study of smoking patterns in relation to the development of smoking-related secondary primary tumors in patients with upper aerodigestive tract malignancies. *Cancer, 101*(12), 2837-2842.

Doyle, J.J., Neugut, A.I., Jacobson, J.S., Grann, V.R., & Hershman, D.L. (2005). Chemotherapy and cardiotoxicity in older breast cancer patients: A population-based study. *Journal of Clinical Oncology, 23*(34), 8597-8605.

Duncan, W., Warde, P., Catton, C.N., Munro, A.J., Lakier, R., Gadalla, T. et al. (1993). Carcinoma of the prostate: Results of radical radiotherapy (1970-1985). *International Journal of Radiation Oncology, Biology, Physics, 26*(2), 203-210.

Earle C.C. (2007). Cancer survivorship research and guidelines: Maybe the cart should be beside the horse. *Journal of Clinical Oncology, 25*(25), 3800-3801.

Edwards, B.K., Howe, H.L., Ries, L.A., Thun, M.J., Rosenberg, H.M., Yancik, R. et al. (2002). Annual report to the nation on the status of cancer, 1973-1999, featuring implications of age and aging on U.S. cancer burden. *Cancer, 94*(10), 2766-2792.

Eriksson, F., Gagliardi, G., Liedberg, A., Lax, I., Lee, C., Levitt, S. et al. (2000). Long-term cardiac mortality following radiation therapy for Hodgkin's disease: Analysis with the relative seriality model. *Radiotherapy and Oncology, 55*(2), 153-162.

Eysenbach G. (2003). The impact of the Internet on cancer outcomes. *CA: A Cancer Journal for Clinicians, 53*(6), 356-371.

Finney Rutten, L., Arora, N., Bakos, A., Aziz, N., & Rowland, J. (2004). Information needs and sources of information among cancer patients: A systematic review of research (1980-2003). *Patient Education and Counseling, 57,* 250-261.

Finney Rutten, L. J., Nelson, D. E., & Meissner, H. I. (2004). Examination of population-wide trends in barriers to cancer screening from a diffusion of innovation perspective (1987-2000). *Preventive Medicine, 38,* 258-268.

Fossa, S.D., Dahl, A.A., & Loge, J.H. (2003). Fatigue, anxiety, and depression in long-term survivors of testicular cancer. *Journal of Clinical Oncology, 21*(7), 1249-1254.

Fuchs, C.S., Giovannucci, E.L., Colditz, G.A., Hunter, D.J., Speizer, F.G., & Willett, W.C. (1994). A prospective study of family history and the risk of colorectal cancer. *New England Journal of Medicine, 331,* 1669-1674.

Ganz P.A. (2005). A teachable moment for oncologists: Cancer survivors, 10 million strong and growing! *Journal of Clinical Oncology, 23*(24), 5458-5460.

Ganz, P.A., Desmond, K.A., Leedham, B., Rowland, J.H., Meyerowitz, B.E., & Belin, T.R. (2002). Quality of life in long-term, disease-free survivors of breast cancer: A follow-up study. *Journal of the National Cancer Institute, 94*(1), 39-49.

Ganz, P.A., Hussey, M.A., Moinpour, C.M., Unger, J.M., Hutchins, L.F., Dakhil, S.R. et al. (2008). Late cardiac effects of adjuvant chemotherapy in breast cancer survivors treated on Southwest Oncology Group protocol s8897. *Journal of Clinical Oncology, 26*(8), 1223-1230.

Garces, Y.I., Schroeder, D.R., Nirelli, L.M., Croghan, G.A., Croghan, I.T., Foote, R.L. et al. (2007). Second primary tumors following tobacco dependence treatments among head and neck cancer patients. *American Journal of Clinical Oncology, 30*(5), 531-539.

Glanz, K., & Rimer B.K. (1997). *Theory at a glance: A guide for health promotion practice.* Bethesda, MD: US Dept. of Health & Human Services, Public Health Service, National Cancer Institute.

Groves, R.M., Singer, E., & Corning, A. (2000). Leverage-saliency theory of survey participation: Description and an illustration. *Public Opinion Quarterly, 64*(3), 299-308.

Harpham W.S. (1998). Long-term survivorship late effects. In A. Berger (Ed.), *Principles and practice of supportive oncology* (pp. 889-907). Philadelphia, PA: Lippincott-Raven.

Hay, J.L., Ostroff, J., Burkhalter, J., Li, Y., Quiles, Z., & Moadel, A. (2007). Changes in cancer-related risk perception and smoking across time in newly-diagnosed cancer patients. *Journal of Behavioral Medicine, 30*(2), 131-142.

Helgeson, V.S., Snyder, P., & Seltman, H. (2004). Psychological and physical adjustment to breast cancer over 4 years: Identifying distinct trajectories of change. *Health Psychology, 23*(1), 3-15.

Helgeson, V.S., & Tomich, P.L. (2005). Surviving cancer: A comparison of 5-year disease-free breast cancer survivors with healthy women. *Psycho-Oncology, 14*(4), 307-317.

Hemminki, K., Lenner, P., Sundquist, J., & Bermejo, J.L. (2008). Risk of subsequent solid tumors after non-Hodgkin's lymphoma: Effect of diagnostic age and time since diagnosis. *Journal of Clinical Oncology, 26*(11), 1850-1857.

Hesse, B.W., Arora, N.K., Beckjord, E.B., & Finney Rutten, L.J. (2008). Information support for cancer survivors. *Cancer, 112*(11 Suppl), 2529-2540.

Hewitt, M., Greenfield, S., & Stovall, E. (2006). *From cancer patient to cancer survivor: Lost in transition*. Washington, DC: The National Academies Press.

Hewitt, M., Rowland, J.H., & Yancik, R. (2003). Cancer survivors in the United States: Age, health, and disability. *Journal of Gerontology. Series A, Biological Sciences and Medical Sciences, 58*(1), 82-91.

Hodges, L.J., Humphris, G.M., & Macfarlane, G. (2005). A meta-analytic investigation of the relationship between the psychological distress of cancer patients and their carers. *Social Science and Medicine, 60*(1), 1-12.

Hoffman, R.M., Gilliland, F.D., Penson, D.F., Stone, S.N., Hunt, W.C., & Potosky, A.L. (2004). Cross-sectional and longitudinal comparisons of health-related quality of life between patients with prostate carcinoma and matched controls. *Cancer, 101*(9), 2011-2019.

Horner, M.J., Ries, L.A.G., Krapcho, M., Neyman, N., Aminou, R., Howlader et al. (Eds.). (2009). SEER Cancer Statistics Review, 1975-2006, National Cancer Institute, Bethesda, MD. http://seer.cancer.gov/csr/1975_2006/, based on November 2008 SEER data submission, posted to the SEER web site, 2009.

Huddart, R.A., Norman, A., Moynihan, C., Horwich, A., Parker, C., Nicholls, E. et al. (2005). Fertility, gonadal and sexual function in survivors of testicular cancer. *British Journal of Cancer, 93*(2), 200-207.

Humpel, N., Magee, C., & Jones, S.C. ((2007). The impact of a cancer diagnosis on the health behaviors of cancer survivors and their family and friends. *Supportive Care in Cancer.*

Hurria, A., Hurria, A., Zuckerman, E., Panageas, K.S., Fornier, M., D'Andrea, G. et al. (2006). A prospective, longitudinal study of the functional status and quality of life of older patients with breast cancer receiving adjuvant chemotherapy. *Journal of the American Geriatrics Society, 54*(7), 1119-1124.

Hurria, A., Somlo, G., & Ahles, T. (2007). Renaming "chemobrain". *Cancer Investigation, 25*(6), 373-377.

Jemal, A., Clegg, L.X., Ward, E., Ries, L.A., Wu, X., Jamison, P.M. et al. (2004). Annual report to the nation on the status of cancer, 1975-2001, with a special feature regarding survival. *Cancer, 101*(1), 3-27.

Jereczek-Fossa, B.A., Marsiglia, H.R., & Orecchia, R. (2001). Radiotherapy-related fatigue: How to assess and how to treat the symptom. A commentary. *Tumori, 87*(3), 147-151.

Kattlove, H., & Winn, R.J. (2003). Ongoing care of patients after primary treatment for their cancer. *CA: A Cancer Journal for Clinicians, 53*(3), 172-196.

Kim, Y., Baker, F., Spillers, R.L., & Wellisch D.K. (2006). Psychological adjustment of cancer caregivers with multiple roles. *Psycho-Oncology, 15*(9), 795-804.

Kim, Y., & Given, B.A. (2008). Quality of life of family caregivers of cancer survivors across the trajectory of the illness. *Cancer, 112*(11Suppl), 2556-2568.

Kim, Y., & Schulz, R. (2008). Family caregivers' strains: Comparative analysis of cancer caregiving with dementia, diabetes, and frail elderly caregiving. *Journal of Aging and Health.*

Kinsinger, D.P., Penedo, F.J., Antoni, M.H., Dahn, J.R., Lechner, S., & Schneiderman, N. (2006). Psychosocial and sociodemographic correlates of benefit-finding in men treated for localized prostate cancer. *Psycho-Oncology, 15*, 954-961.

Knobf, M.T. (2006). The influence of endocrine effects of adjuvant therapy on quality of life outcomes in younger breast cancer survivors. *Oncologist, 11*(2), 96-110.

Kushi, L.H., Byers, T., Doyle, C., Bandera, E.V., McCullough, M., Gansler, T. et al. (2006). American Cancer Society guidelines on nutrition and physical activity for cancer prevention: Reducing the risk of cancer with healthy food choices and physical activity. *CA: A Cancer Journal for Clinicians, 56*(5), 254-281.

Kwong, A., Hancock, S.L., Bloom, J.R., Pal, S., Birdwell, R.L., Mariscal, C. et al. (2008). Mammographic screening in women at increased risk of breast cancer after treatment of Hodgkin's disease. *Breast Journal, 14*(1), 39-48.

Lechner, S.C., Zakowski, S.G., Antoni, M.H., Greenhawt, M., Block, K., & Block, P. (2003). Do sociodemographic and disease-related variables influence benefit-finding in cancer patients? *Psycho-Oncology, 12*(5), 491-499.

Lykins, E.L., Graue, L.O., Brechting, E.H., Roach, A.R., Gochett, C.G., & Andrykowski, M.A. (2008). Beliefs about cancer causation and prevention as a function of personal and family history of cancer: A national, population-based study. *Psycho-Oncology, 17*, 767-974.

Lyne, M.E., Coyne, P.J., & Watson A.C. (2002). Pain management issues for cancer survivors. *Cancer Practice, 10*(Suppl 1), S27-S32.

Manfredi, C., Czaja, R., Price, J., Buis, M., & Janiszewski, R. (1993). Cancer patients' search for information. *Journal of the National Cancer Institutes Monographs, 14*, 93-104.

Mariotto, A.B., Rowland, J.H., Ries, L.A., Scoppa, S., & Feuer, E.J. (2007). Multiple cancer prevalence: A growing challenge in long-term survivorship. *Cancer Epidemiology Biomarkers Prevention, 16*(3), 566-571.

Martini, N., Bains, M.S., Burt, M.E., Zakowski, M.F., McCormack, P., Rusch, V.W. et al. (1995). Incidence of local recurrence and second primary tumors in resected stage I lung cancer. *Journal of Thoracic and Cardiovascular Surgery, 109*(1), 120-129.

Massie, M.J. (2004). Prevalence of depression in patients with cancer. *Journal of the National Cancer Institute Monograph, 32*, 57-71.

Mayer, D.K., Terrin, N.C., Menon, U., Kreps, G.L., McCance, K., Parsons, S.K. et al. (2007a), Health behaviors in cancer survivors. *Oncology Nursing Forum,* *34*(3), 643-651.

Mayer, K.M., Terrin, N.C., Menon, U., Kreps, G.L., McCance, K., Parsons, S.K. et al. (2007b). Screening practices in cancer survivors. *Journal of Cancer Survivorship, 1,* 17-26.

McDonald, S., Rubin, P., Phillips, T.L., & Marks, L.B. (1995). Injury to the lung from cancer therapy: Clinical syndromes, measurable endpoints, and potential scoring systems. *International Journal of Radiation Oncology, Biology, Physics,* *31*(5), 1187-1203.

McKinley, E.D. (2000). Under Toad days: Surviving the uncertainty of cancer recurrence. *Annals of Internal Medicine, 133*(6), 479-480.

Meyerhardt, J.A., Heseltine, D., Niedzwiecki, D., Hollis, D., Saltz, L.B., Mayer, R.J. et al. (2006). Impact of physical activity on cancer recurrence and survival in patients with stage III colon cancer: Findings from CALGB 89803. *Journal of Clinical Oncology, 24*(22), 3535-3541.

Meyerhardt, J.A., Niedzwiecki, D., Hollis, D., Saltz, L.B., Hu, F.B., Mayer, R.J. et al. (2007). Association of dietary patterns with cancer recurrence and survival in patients with stage III colon cancer. *Journal of the American Medical Association, 298*(7), 754-764.

Mellon, S., & Northouse L.L. (2001). Family survivorship and quality of life following a cancer diagnosis. *Research in Nursing and Health, 24*(6), 446-459.

Moser, R.P., McCaul, K., Peters, E., Nelson, W., & Marcus, S.E. (2007). Associations of perceived risk and worry with cancer health-protective actions: Data from the Health Information National Trends Survey (HINTS). *Journal of Health Psychology, 12*(1), 53-65.

Mullan F. (1985). Seasons of survival: Reflections of a physician with cancer. *New England Journal of Medicine, 313,* 270-273.

Mustian, K.M., Morrow, G.R., Carroll, J.K., Figueroa-Moseley, C.D., Jean-Pierre, P., & Williams, G.C. (2007). Integrative nonpharmacologic behavioral interventions for the management of cancer-related fatigue. *Oncologist, 12*(Suppl 1), 52-67.

Muzzin, L.J., Andersen, N.J., Figueredo, A.T., & Gudelis, S.O. (1994). The experience of cancer. *Social Science and Medicine, 38*(9), 1201-1208.

National Cancer Institute (NCI). (2007). Estimated US Cancer Prevalence Counts: Who Are Our Cancer Survivors in the US? Available at http://cancercontrol.cancer.gov/ocs/prevalence/index.html [accessed 7-22-2007].

National Coalition for Cancer Survivorship (NCCS). *The Organization.* National Coalition for Cancer Survivorship. Retrieved July 19, 2007, from http://www.canceradvocacy.org/about/org/

Ng, A.K., & Travis L.B. (2008). Second primary cancers: An overview. *Hematology/ Oncology Clinics of North America, 22*(2), 271-289.

Niederdeppe, J., & Levy, A.G. (2007). Fatalistic beliefs about cancer prevention and three prevention behaviors. *Cancer Epidemiology, Biomarkers & Prevention, 16*(5), 998-1003.

Nieman, C.L., Kazer, R., Brannigan, R.E., Zoloth, L.S., Chase-Lansdale P.L., Kinahan, K. et al. (2006). Cancer survivors and infertility: A review of a new problem and novel answers. *Journal of Supportive Oncology, 4*(4), 171-178.

Northouse, L.L., Mood, D., Kershaw, T., Schafenacker, A., Mellon, S., Walker, J. et al. (2002). Quality of life of women with recurrent breast cancer and their family members. *Journal of Clinical Oncology, 20*(19), 4050-4064.

Padovan, C.S., Yousry, T.A., Schleuning, M., Holler, E., Kolb, H.J., & Straube, A. (1998). Neurological and neuroradiological findings in long-term survivors of allogeneic bone marrow transplantation. *Annals of Neurology, 43*(5), 627-633.

Petrek, J.A., Senie, R.T., Peters, M., & Rosen, P.P. (2001). Lymphedema in a cohort of breast carcinoma survivors 20 years after diagnosis. *Cancer, 92*(6), 1368-1377.

Pfeilschifter, J., & Diel, I.J. (2000). Osteoporosis due to cancer treatment: Pathogenesis and management. *Journal of Clinical Oncology, 18*(7), 1570-1593.

Prosnitz, R.G., Hubbs, J.L., Evans, E.S., Zhou, S.M., Yu, X., Blazing, M.A. et al. (2007). Prospective assessment of radiotherapy-associated cardiac toxicity in breast cancer patients: Analysis of data 3 to 6 years after treatment. *Cancer, 110*(8), 1840-1850.

Pryce, J., Munir, F., & Haslam, C. (2007). Cancer survivorship and work: Symptoms, supervisor response, co-worker disclosure and work adjustment. *Journal of Occupational Rehabilitation, 17*(1), 83-92.

Reuben, S.H. (2007). *Promoting healthy lifestyles: Policy, program, and personal recommendations for reducing cancer risk.* 2006-2007 Annual Report, President's Cancer Panel.

Ries, L. A. G., Melbert, D., Krapcho, M., Stinchcomb, D. G., Howlader, N., Horner, M. J. et al. (2008). SEER Cancer Statistics Review, 1975-2005. National Cancer Institute, based on November 2007 SEER data submission [On-line]. Retrieved March 1, 2008, from http://seer.cancer.gov/csr/1975_2005/.

Robb, K.A., Williams, J.E., Duvivier, V., & Newham, D.J. (2006). A pain management program for chronic cancer-treatment-related pain: A preliminary study. *Journal of Pain, 7*(2), 82-90.

Rolland, J.S. (2005). Cancer and the family: An integrative model. *Cancer, 104*(11Suppl), 2584-2595.

Schultz, P.N., Beck, M.L., Stava, C., & Vassilopoulou-Sellin, R. (2003). Health profiles in 5836 long-term cancer survivors. *International Journal of Cancer, 104*(4), 488-495.

Shah, M., Zhu, K., Palmer, R.C., Jatoi, I., Shriver, C., & Wu, H. (2007). Breast, colorectal, and skin cancer screening practices and family history of cancer in U.S. women. *Journal of Women's Health, 16*(4), 526-534.

Sherwood, P.R., Donovan, H.S., Given, C.W., Lu, X., Given, B.A., Hricik, A. et al. (2007). Predictors of employment and lost hours from work in cancer caregivers. *Psycho-Oncology.*

Shim, M., Kelly, B., & Hornik, R. (2006). Cancer information scanning and seeking behavior is associated with knowledge, lifestyle choices, and screening. *Journal of Health Communication, 11*(Suppl 1), 157-172.

Shinn, E.H., Basen-Engquist, K., Thornton, B., Spiess, P.E., & Pisters, L. (2007). Health behaviors and depressive symptoms in testicular cancer survivors. *Urology, 69*(4), 748-753.

Short, P.F., Vasey, J.J., & Tunceli, K. (2005). Employment pathways in a large cohort of adult cancer survivors. *Cancer, 103*(6), 1292-1301.

Stasi, R., Abriani, L., Beccaglia, P., Terzoli, E., & Amadori, S. (2003). Cancer-related fatigue: Evolving concepts in evaluation and treatment. *Cancer, 98*(9), 1786-1801.

Stein, K.D., Hawkins, N.A., Smith, T.G., Zhao, L., Rodriguez, J., & Berkowitz, Z. (2008). *Health-related behavior change after cancer: Results of the American Cancer Society's Studies of Cancer Survivors (SCS)*. Podium presentation at the 10th World Congress of Psycho-Oncology, Madrid, Spain.

Stein, K.D., Syrjala, K.L., & Andrykowski, M.A. (2008). Physical and psychological long-term and late effects of cancer. *Cancer, 112*(11Suppl), 2577-2592.

Steinherz, L.J., & Yahalom, J. (2001). Cardiac toxicity. In V. T. DeVita, S. Hellman, & S. A. Rosenberg (Eds.), *Cancer: Principles and practices of oncology* (pp. 2904-2931). Philadelphia, PA: Lippincott Williams & Wilkins.

Sunga, A.Y., Eberl, M.M., Oeffinger, K.C., Hudson, M.M., & Mahoney, M.C. (2005). Care of cancer survivors. *American Family Physician, 71*(4), 699-706.

Tannock, I.F., Ahles, T.A., Ganz, P.A., & van Dam, F.S. (2004). Cognitive impairment associated with chemotherapy for cancer: Report of a workshop. *Journal of Clinical Oncology, 22*(11), 2233-2239.

Tchen, N., Juffs, H.G., Downie, F.P., Yi, Q.L., Hu, H., Chemerynsky, I. et al. (2003). Cognitive function, fatigue, and menopausal symptoms in women receiving adjuvant chemotherapy for breast cancer. *Journal of Clinical Oncology, 21*(22), 4175-4183.

Trask, P.C., Rabin, C., Rogers, M.L., Whiteley, J., Nash, J., Frierson G. et al. (2005). Cancer screening practices among cancer survivors. *American Journal of Preventive Medicine, 28*(4), 351-356.

Travis L.B. (2006). The epidemiology of second primary cancers. *Cancer Epidemiology, Biomarkers & Prevention, 15*(11), 2020-2026.

Twombly R. (2004). What's in a name? Who is a cancer survivor? [News]. *Journal of the National Cancer Institute, 19*(96), 1414-1415.

Velanovich, V., & Szymanski, W. (1999). Quality of life of breast cancer patients with lymphedema. *American Journal of Surgery, 177*(3), 184-187.

Vistad, I., Fossa, S.D., Kristensen, G.B., & Dahl, A.A. (2007). Chronic fatigue and its correlates in long-term survivors of cervical cancer treated with radiotherapy. *British Journal of Obstetrics and Gynaecology, 14*(9), 1150-1158.

Wefel, J.S., Lenzi, R., Theriault, R.L., Davis, R.N., & Meyers, C.A. (2004). The cognitive sequelae of standard-dose adjuvant chemotherapy in women with breast carcinoma. *Cancer, 100*(11), 2292-2299.

Wenzel, L., Dogan-Ates, A., Habbal, R., Berkowitz, R., Goldstein, D.P., Bernstein, M. et al. (2005). Defining and measuring reproductive concerns of female cancer survivors. *Journal of the National Cancer Institute Monograph, 34*, 94-98.

Yabroff, K.R., Lawrence, W.F., Clauser, S., Davis, W.W., & Brown, M.L. (2004). Burden of illness in cancer survivors: Findings from a population-based national sample. *Journal of the National Cancer Institute, 96*(17), 1322-1330.

13

BIOLOGICAL LITERACY

A Key to Cancer Prevention and Control in the 21st Century

Jon D. Miller
Michigan State University

Gary L. Kreps
George Mason University

To preserve democratic traditions in the 21st century, citizens of modern democratic states will need to develop and sustain literacy in a number of important domains. Citizens need to understand the history of their country, their culture, and their society; the economic policy choices for their country in a world of global competition; and a core set of scientific and technological constructs necessary to participate as citizens in the formulation of science and technology policy. Without diminishing the importance of any of the other kinds of knowledge that citizens need, this analysis focuses on the acquisition of civic scientific literacy broadly and on the development of a functional level of biological literacy to enable citizens to make informed choices about cancer prevention, early detection, treatment, and survivorship.

The case for higher levels of civic scientific literacy in modern democratic states is simple and straightforward. The great Western tradition of democratic government is built on an assumption that citizens are able to acquire the information necessary to understand important public policy issues, to understand that information at a level sufficient to make sense of competing arguments, and to reach a judgment about the policy choices that they would prefer, including those that impact healthcare and health outcomes.

Thus, the American belief has been that it is important for citizens to understand the issues and to make sense of them at some level. This belief structure has more recently penetrated traditional patriarchal practices in health care and medicine, thereby leading to greater patient autonomy and participation in health care and health decisions.

Since World War II, the world has been increasingly dominated by science and technology; these issues have occupied an increasing share of the public policy agenda. In the second half of the 20th century, new public policy disputes arose over the safety of chemical additives in foods, the sources and treatment of environmental pollution, the use of genetic modification technologies for agricultural and medical purposes, and emerging patterns of climate change on this planet. These disputes had clear and profound implications for public health and health care.

In broad terms, it can be argued that the 20th century was the century of physics and that the 21st century is the century of biology. During the 20th century, our understanding of the structure of matter expanded exponentially and produced a series of physical manifestations in the form of radios, telephones, televisions, transistors, nuclear weapons and power plants, airplanes, missiles, space craft and space stations, computers, and the Internet. Many of these new products resulted in public policy debates related to their use, safety, and regulation. Some of these issues will continue to be debated in the 21st century, but the major impact of these physics-based technologies occurred in the 20th century.

In the 21st century, human understanding of the nature and structure of life will grow exponentially and with that growth will come the opportunity for interventions of various kinds, and these opportunities will produce a growing volume of public policy disputes. The mapping of the human genome and hundreds of other genomes has provided a basic picture of the structure and interchangeability of DNA. Within the next 10 years, a comparable map of all of the proteins produced by genes in humans will provide a gene–protein matrix that will redefine health and illness. It is impossible to predict the level of human understanding of the biology of life at the end of the 21st century, but it will almost surely change how we view and participate in our own health and health care.

All of this work will produce a substantial growth in public policy discussions and disputes and opportunities for participatory medicine that will require an increasing level of biological literacy to understand, discuss, and think about these issues. In the first decade of the 21st century, U.S. presidential candidates discussed the use of embryonic and adult stem cells in biomedical research, the definition of the beginning and ending of life, and the causes and solutions for global climate change. In Europe, the political wars over genetically modified foods continue and Greenpeace and its political allies continue to expand their opposition to all forms of genetic modification.

Given the increasingly participatory nature of health care and the prospect of a public policy agenda that includes a significant number of issues that require some understanding of science generally and biology specifically, it is necessary to ask how many citizens are currently sufficiently scientifically literate or biologically literate to make sense of the kinds of issues that are presently on the American political agenda. For this purpose, we briefly examine the history of civic scientific literacy in the United States during the 1980s and 1990s and some more recent measures of biological literacy.

THE CONCEPT AND MEASUREMENT OF CIVIC SCIENTIFIC LITERACY

To understand the concept of civic scientific literacy, it is necessary to begin with an understanding of the concept of *literacy* itself. The basic idea of literacy is to define a minimum level of reading and writing skills that an individual must have to participate in written communication. Historically, an individual was thought of as literate if he or she could read and write their own name. In recent decades, there has been a redefinition of basic literacy skills to include the ability to read a bus schedule, a loan agreement, or the instructions on a bottle of medicine. Adult educators often use the term *functional literacy* to refer to this new definition of the minimal skills needed to function in a contemporary industrial society (Cook, 1977; Harman, 1970; Kaestle, 1985; Resnick & Resnick, 1977). The social science and educational literature indicates that about one fourth of Americans are not functionally literate, and there is good reason to expect that roughly this proportion applies in most mature industrial nations and a slightly higher rate in emerging industrial nations (Ahmann, 1975; Cevero, 1985; Guthrie & Kirsch, 1984; Northcutt, 1975).

In this context, civic scientific literacy is conceptualized as the level of understanding of science and technology needed to function as citizens in a modern industrial society (Miller, 1983a, 1983b, 1987, 1996, 1998, 2000, 2004; Shen, 1975). This conceptualization of scientific literacy does not imply an ideal level of understanding, but rather a minimal threshold level to follow and engage in public policy discussions involving scientific and technological issues. It is neither a measure of job-related skills nor an index of economic competitiveness in a global economy.

The initial measurements of scientific literacy in the 1980s and 1990s found evidence of two dimensions—a basic vocabulary of scientific terms and concepts and an understanding of the process or methods of science for testing our models of reality (Durant, Evans, & Thomas, 1989, 1992; Evans & Durant, 1995; Miller, 1983b, 1987, 1996, 1998, 2000, 2004). National surveys of adults in the United States show that the distinction originally found between the two factors in studies in the mid-1980s narrowed over the remaining years of the 20th century. Recent national surveys in Europe and the United States—reported later in greater detail—indicate that the vocabulary and process dimensions have become empirically inseparable.

In developing a measure of civic scientific literacy, it is important to construct a measure that will be useful over a period of years and that will be sufficiently sensitive to capture changes in the structure and composition of public understanding. If a time series indicator is revised too often or without consciously designed linkages, it may be impossible to separate the variation attributable to measurement changes from real change over time. The periodic debates over the composition of consumer price indices in the United States and other major industrial nations are a reminder of the importance of stable indicators over periods of time.

The durability problem can be seen in the early efforts to develop measures of the public understanding of science in the United States. In 1957, the National Association of Science Writers (NASW) commissioned a national survey of public understanding of and attitudes toward science and technology (Davis, 1958). Since the interviewing for the 1957 study was completed only 2 months prior to the launch of Sputnik I, it is the only measure of public understanding and attitudes prior to the beginning of the space race. Unfortunately, the four major items of substantive knowledge were radioactive fallout, fluoridation in drinking water, polio vaccine, and space satellites. Fifty years later, at least three of these terms are no longer central to the measurement of public understanding.

Recognizing this problem, Miller attempted to identify a set of basic constructs, such as atomic structure or DNA, that are the intellectual foundation for reading and understanding contemporary issues, but that will have a longer durability than specific terms, such as the fallout of strontium 90 from atmospheric testing. In a 1988 collaboration between Miller in the United States and Thomas and Durant in the United Kingdom, an expanded set of knowledge items[1] was developed that asked respondents direct questions about scientific concepts. In the 1988 studies, a combination of open- and closed-ended items were constructed that provided significantly better estimates of public understanding than had been collected in any prior national study. From this collaboration, a core set of knowledge items[1] emerged that have been used in studies in Brazil, Canada, China, Japan, Korea, India, New Zealand, and all 27 members of the European Union.

---

[1]Some writers have referred to this set of items as the "Oxford" items. This is incorrect when interpreted to mean that the items were the product of one group of scholars or one nation. To the contrary, these items were the result of a genuine international collaboration among Jon Miller, Geoffrey Thomas, John Durant, Geoffrey Evans, Donald Buzzelli, and Robert Wright.

To a large extent, these core items have provided a durable set of measures of a vocabulary of scientific constructs, but it is important to continually enrich the mix to reflect the growth of science and technology. For example, Miller's 2003, 2004, 2005, and 2007 studies of the American public have included new open-ended measures of stem cell, nanotechnology, neuron, and neuroscience and new closed-ended knowledge items concerning the genetic modification of plants and animals, nanotechnology, ecology, and infectious diseases. Through the use of Item-Response Theory (IRT), it is possible to incorporate marginal changes in the composition of a set of items and to produce comparable total scores (Zimowski et al., 1996). The IRT scoring procedure produces a standardized score with a mean of zero and a standard deviation of 1.0. For reporting purposes, the mean (computed over the full database) was set to 50 with a standard deviation of 20. In terms of individual scores on the Index of Civic Scientific Literacy (CSL), the resulting scores range from approximately zero to 100.

A score of 70 or higher is indicative of a level of understanding sufficient to understand science and technology stories in *The New York Times* Science Times section or in *Science et Vie*. Like all threshold measures, the cut point is somewhat arbitrary. It is only somewhat arbitrary because it is clear from an examination of the items that respondents are able to answer correctly that individuals with a score below the middle 60s would have a very difficult time making sense of the current debates over global climate change or embryonic stem cells. If the cut point were to be moved up or down 2 or 3 points, the basic conclusions that one would draw from this work would not change.

Using this threshold measure of CSL, the results show a steady and significant improvement in the score of American adults over the last 18 years, in sharp contrast to the performance of American secondary school students. The proportion of American adults who are able to score 70 or higher in this index grew from 10% in 1988 to approximately 25% by 2007.

THE CONCEPT AND MEASUREMENT OF BIOLOGICAL LITERACY

Inherently, biological literacy is a subset of the broader and more general measure of CSL just described. It is an important subset because of the growing number of public policy issues that involve biology, biotechnology, and the use and modification of biological processes. Apart from public policy issues, biological literacy is increasingly important to individuals in making personal and family medical decisions. For all of these reasons, it is important to construct a simple measure of biological literacy to improve our understanding of the size and composition of the real audience for biological information and messages.

Using the same set of items described above in regard to civic scientific literacy and the same analytic methods, it is possible to build a summary measure of biological literacy among American adults. A confirmatory factor analysis (using LISREL) of national studies conducted in 2003, 2005, and 2007 found a set of 21 biological science items that formed a single coherent scale of biological literacy in each of the three years (see Tables 13.1 and 13.2). Using the same procedures just described, a summary Index of Biological Literacy (BL) was constructed for 2003, 2005, and 2007.

TABLE 13.1. Percentage Correct on Selected Biology Knowledge Items, 2003, 2005, 2007.

	PERCENT CORRECT		
	2003 (%)	2005 (%)	2007 (%)
Provide a correct open-ended definition of a "stem cell."	8	13	15%
Provide a correct open-ended definition of a "molecule."	15	16	18
Provide a correct open-ended definition of "DNA."	32	32	34
Provide a correct open-ended definition of a "neuron."	—	26	—
Disagree: "Ordinary tomatoes . . . do not have genes but genetically modified tomatoes do."	52	48	49
Provide a correct open-ended definition of "what it means to study something scientifically."	29	31	29
Disagree: "Antibiotics kill viruses as well as bacteria."	48	53	55
Provide a correct open-ended definition of an "experiment."	40	50	50
Disagree: "For the first time in recorded history, some species of plants and animals are dying out and becoming extinct."	—	43	44
Agree: "More than half of human genes are identical to those of mice."	—	32	34
If some one eats a genetically modified fruit, there is a risk that the person's genes might be modified too.	58	71	—
Disagree: "The earliest humans lived at the same time as the dinosaurs."	42	51	50
Agree: "Over periods of millions of years, some species of plants and animals adjust and survive while other species die and become extinct."	—	78	—
Agree: "All plants and animals have DNA."	83	78	77
Disagree: "Humans have somewhat less than half of their DNA in common with chimpanzees."	30	38	40
Agree: "The greenhouse effect causes the Earth's temperature to rise."	63	74	—
Indicate a correct understanding of the meaning of the probability of 1 in 4.	72	71	73
Agree: "One of the effects of global warming will be that some species of plants and animals will thrive and other species will become extinct."	—	59	—
Agree: "Human beings, as we know them today, developed from earlier species of animals."	36	40	40
Today it is not possible to transfer genes from humans to animals.	50	—	—
Today it is not possible to transfer genes from animals to plants.	43	—	—
NUMBER OF CASES	1,600	1,484	1,407

Items are listed in the order of their factor loading in 2005.

TABLE 13.2. Confirmatory Factor Analysis of Biology Knowledge Items, 2003, 2005, 2007.

	FACTOR LOADINGS		
	2003	2005	2007
Provide a correct open-ended definition of a "stem cell."	.81	.84	.91
Provide a correct open-ended definition of a "molecule."	.71	.78	.76
Provide a correct open-ended definition of "DNA."	.66	.77	.74
Provide a correct open-ended definition of a "neuron."	—	.75	—
Disagree: "Ordinary tomatoes . . . do not have genes but genetically modified tomatoes do."	.82	.73	.74
Provide a correct open-ended definition of "what it means to study something scientifically."	.68	.71	.73
Disagree: "Antibiotics kill viruses as well as bacteria."	.65	.71	.62
Provide a correct open-ended definition of an "experiment."	.64	.65	.70
Disagree: "For the first time in recorded history, some species of plants and animals are dying out and becoming extinct."	—	.61	.69
Agree: "More than half of human genes are identical to those of mice."	—	.58	.58
If some one eats a genetically modified fruit, there is a risk that the person's genes might be modified too.	.64	.58	—
Disagree: "The earliest humans lived at the same time as the dinosaurs."	.53	.56	.61
Agree: "Over periods of millions of years, some species of plants and animals adjust and survive while other species die and become extinct."	—	.55	—
Agree: "All plants and animals have DNA."	.66	.54	.57
Disagree: "Humans have somewhat less than half of their DNA in common with chimpanzees."	.51	.51	.51
Agree: "The greenhouse effect causes the Earth's temperature to rise."	.48	.45	.39
Indicate a correct understanding of the meaning of the probability of 1 in 4.	.53	.44	.54
Agree: "One of the effects of global warming will be that some species of plants and animals will thrive and other species will become extinct."	—	.38	—
Agree: "Human beings, as we know them today, developed from earlier species of animals."	.45	.35	.44
Today it is not possible to transfer genes from humans to animals.	.63	—	—
Today it is not possible to transfer genes from animals to plants.	.56	—	—
NUMBER OF CASES	1,600	1,484	1,407

Items are listed in the order of their factor loading in 2005.

An examination of the pool of items shown in Table 13.1 and the distribution and loadings of these items in the three years (see Table 13.2) illustrates the utility of IRT. For years, national examinations such as the Graduate Record Examination (GRE) have been administered over a series of weeks, but for security purposes, each of the GRE examinations is composed of different sets of questions with about a 25% overlap in question usage between any two examinations. Through the use of the IRT technique, it is possible to calibrate each of the items in terms of its relationship to an underlying dimension or test domain and to calibrate and score each of the tests on a common metric even though no two sets of the examinations are identical. Using the same methods, the three national surveys in 2003, 2005, and 2007 used slightly different sets of questions and even slightly different numbers of questions, but it is relatively simple to use IRT scoring methods to produce a single summary score.

As with the previously described Index of CSL, the Index of BL ranges from approximately zero to approximately 100. Respondents with a score of 70 or higher on this Index of BL were labeled as biologically literate. In functional terms, these individuals should be able to read and understand stories and debates about biological issues in the Tuesday *New York Times*, on the Web sites of the National Institutes of Health, or in books and materials that are readily available online and in bookstores. The cut-off of 70 is not a magic number and it would make no difference in any of the arguments or conclusions in this analysis if we were to move the cut point up or down by 2 or 3 points. The essential point of the index is that those adults with higher levels of understanding of basic biological ideas and constructs will be able to make sense of new biomedical discoveries, understand public policy issues faster and more thoroughly, and make personal health decisions more effectively than individuals with lower levels of BL.

Using this approach, approximately 12% of American adults aged 18 and older qualified as biologically literate in 2003, and this number increased to 18% in 2007 (see Fig. 13.1). Given the volume of media and public debate of biomedical and biological issues in recent years, this pattern of growth is not surprising. In the next section of this analysis, we turn to an exploration of some of the factors that predict BL in the United States, but it is sufficient to note at this point that adult scientific literacy and adult BL are the result of a combination of formal instruction in regard to some basic constructs and persistent use of available adult science learning resources in the years after the end of formal schooling.

The Index of BL is a comprehensive measure and the items necessary to measure it have only been asked in sufficient number in recent years. It is possible, however, to gain some insight into the growth of public awareness of biological concepts in recent years using a simpler marker variable. Beginning in 1988, Miller and his colleagues have asked national samples of American adults to define the meaning of DNA in an open-ended format.

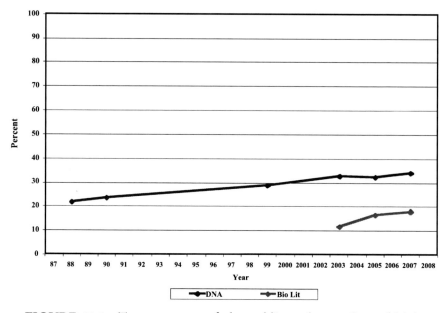

FIGURE 13.1. Two measures of the public understanding of biology, 1988–2007.

This approach is useful because it allows a respondent to provide a description in his or her own words and, in so doing, to demonstrate the scope and depth of their understanding. It does not reward guessing in a multiple-choice format and the question is administered in a manner that avoids embarrassment to respondents who have little or no familiarity with the term DNA.

This item is a good indicator of the extent to which the term DNA has become a part of our vocabulary. Individuals who first learned about DNA as students—essentially adults under the age of 40—are advantaged in that they can use this knowledge to make sense of the abundance of genetic and biological information in the news and in popular media—newspapers, magazines, online, and even in television and motion picture plots. Many adults without any formal school exposure to DNA have managed to learn about the meaning of the term and have been able to use it in making sense of more advanced biological information. In broad terms, this single item provides a measure of *general exposure to a core genetic construct* and the Index of BL provides a more *in-depth measure of the ability of an individual to understand and use biological concepts* in thinking about personal and public policy choices. As Figure 13.1 illustrates, the level of general awareness of DNA is higher than the level of cognitive ability measured by the BL index. Both general awareness and biological understanding have been growing over the last two decades.

The lines in Fig. 13.1 are plotted on a full zero to 100 metric to remind us that biological awareness and BL involve only a minority of American adults. Two of three American adults appear to be unable to define the meaning of DNA and only 18% have developed the ability to use biological constructs as a part of their thinking. We have a long way to go and all of the white space above the lines in Fig. 13.1 illustrates the magnitude of the task ahead.

SOURCES OF BIOLOGICAL LITERACY

Given the relatively low level of BL reported in the preceding section and the growing number of political and public policy issues that will require some understanding of basic biological concepts, two issues emerge:

1. What are the sources of BL for adults in the United States?
2. What can we do to enhance the BL of Americans?

This section utilizes data from the 2005 U.S. study to identify some of the primary factors associated with the acquisition and maintenance of BL among U.S. adults, and the final section of this analysis discusses some science policy and educational policy issues to address this issue.

Although nearly three decades of international education studies have found that American secondary school students do relatively poorly on standardized tests in science and mathematics (Beaton et al., 1996; Schmidt, McKnight, & Raizen, 1997), formal science instruction is still an important source of basic biology constructs that form the foundation for later and more advanced learning. Virtually all students first learn that living things are composed of cells, and current students would be expected to know that all cells contain DNA and something about its central role in the formation and operation of cells.

In recent decades, a good deal of attention has been devoted to studying and revising the elementary and secondary science and mathematics curricula in the United States. The National Science Foundation has spent more than $1 billion on precollegiate curricular issues and the performance of American secondary school students has failed to improve. The results from the Second International Mathematics and Science Study (SIMSS) and the Third International Mathematics and Science Study (TIMSS) are compelling and disappointing (Beaton et al., 1996; Schmidt et al., 1997). The poor performance of American students is not a measurement error and reflects real problems in secondary education in the United States.

At the same time, many science and education policy leaders are unaware that the United States is the only major nation to require all of its college and university students to complete 1 year of college science as a part of their baccalaureate program. C. P. Snow's (1959) famous treatise on the two cultures is about the absence of general education requirements at Oxford and Cambridge and his plea that all educated persons should know both Shakespeare and the Second Law of Thermodynamics was—in fact—a call for general education requirements in British higher education. Neither Snow nor subsequent advocates of general education have been able to change the system and British students still read in only one field for a degree, but American college students studied science at the university level throughout the 20th century and the United States ranks second in the world in the percentage of adults who are scientifically literate. We explore the role of the general education requirement at the university level on the development of biological literacy in the United States.

It is also important to examine other possible sources of BL among American adults. In the six decades since the end of World War II, the number and range of informal adult science learning opportunities in the United States has increased markedly. The number and size of science, technology, and natural history museums has increased substantially as has the number of planetariums, botanical gardens, zoos, and aquariums. In the last two decades, the availability of science and health information on television and the Internet has increased exponentially. The sale of science, health, and medical books has grown sharply in recent years. The combination of these factors provides numerous opportunities for American adults to learn about biological science after the end of formal education, and the sales and use figures indicate that many adults use these informal learning resources.

There are several factors that may encourage adults to seek biology and related science information after the end of formal schooling. One stimulus to continued science learning is individual and family health. Numerous studies show that adults who are diagnosed with cancer, for example, become active seekers of biological and biomedical information (Johnson, 1997). Another stimulus is occupational. A larger number of adults work in jobs, firms, and organizations that use a wide array of science and technology. Some individuals may need to learn more about biology and science to hold or advance in their job. The presence of minor children in a household is a third stimulus to continued adult science learning as parents seek to help with homework, science fairs, and questions from their children.

The growing number of public policy issues serves as another important stimulus to continued adult science learning. Although few adults could have studied stem cells or climate change during their years of formal education, these and related issues have been a part of current political discourse in the United States. In the United States, the continuing public policy discussions about stem cell research and global climate change permeate candidate and media discussions in the presidential primary campaigns. Events such as the recent award of the Nobel Peace Prize to Al Gore will foster greater public interest in the climate change issue and undoubtedly some adults will read news stories, buy books, or look at relevant Web sites in response to this kind of news event.

In the context of cancer, it is imperative for citizens to have basic scientific literacy and BL to make informed decisions about the best ways to prevent, detect, and respond to cancers. Cancer is complex. There are many different forms of cancer that present in distinct ways; are caused by diverse genetic, environmental, and lifestyle factors; and are detected with the use of different tests and screening procedures. Different cancer diagnoses (breast, lung, colorectal, etc.) will each necessitate specialized forms of treatment and therapy, and with the ongoing development of new and improved therapies for these cancers, it is very challenging for consumers to make good decisions about the latest and most effective ways to respond to cancer. To complicate this even further, the information available to the public about different forms of cancer is often presented in complex scientific formats, using medical and biological terminology that may be difficult for the layperson to understand. To effectively communicate relevant cancer-related information to different groups of consumers, we need to accurately assess consumers' levels of basic scientific and biological literacy, and develop communication and message strategies to match the literacy levels of key publics (Kreps, 2006). At the same time, efforts must be taken to increase citizen's levels of scientific and biological literacy to prepare them to become informed, involved, and empowered health care consumers (Parker & Kreps, 2005).

STRUCTURAL EQUATION MODELING TO PREDICT BIOLOGICAL LITERACY

To explore these possible sources of influence on the development of BL, a structural equation analysis[2] of the 2005 U.S. data set was conducted (Jöreskog & Sörbom, 1993). The analytic model included each individual's age; gender; highest level of education; number of college science courses completed; presence or absence of minor children in the household; interest in science, technology, medical, or environmental issues; personal religious beliefs; and level of use of informal science learning resources (see Fig. 13.2).

---

[2]In general terms, a structural equation model is a set of regression equations that provides the best estimate for a set of relationships among several independent variables and one or more dependent variables. For the structural analysis presented in this chapter, the program LISREL was used. LISREL allows the simultaneous examination of structural relationships and the modeling of measurement errors. For a more comprehensive discussion of structural equation models, see Hayduk (1987) and Jöreskog and Sörbom (1993). For a more detailed example of the use of this technique in the analysis of CSL, see Miller, Pardo, and Niwa (1997).

A path model is useful for examining the relative influence of variables that have a known chronological or logical order. Each individual has a gender at birth and an age based on his or her birth date. An individual's gender may influence his or her education, although this influence appears to be diminishing in the United States. For most adults, educational attainment and the number of college science courses are determined by the time that an individual reaches age 35, although more adults are returning to formal education than ever before. An individual's level of BL at any specific time may be thought of as the result of the combination of these and other factors (see Fig. 13.2). In a path model, chronological or logical causation flows from left to right.

The product of the path coefficients is an estimation of the total effect of each variable on the outcome variable—BL in this case. It is useful to look first at the total effect of each of the variables in this model, and then return to examine some of the specific path coefficients.

The number of college science courses taken is the strongest predictor of BL, with a total effect of .77 (see Table 13.3). It is important to understand this variable and its impact. The variable is a measure of the number of college science courses, including courses in both community colleges and 4-year colleges and universities. The number of courses was divided into three levels: (a) no college-level science courses, (b) one to three courses, and (c) four or more courses. Individuals with one to three courses are the students who took college science courses as a part of a general education requirement rather than as a part of a major or a supplement to a major. The use of an interval measure would have given undue weight to majors and minimized the impact of general education science courses in the analysis.

Formal educational attainment[3] is the second best predictor of adult BL (.74). This result indicates that students gain some additional value from the full range of university courses, including other general education courses in the humanities and the social sciences. The influence of formal educational attainment may also reflect a greater respect for and acceptance of academic authority as a source of knowing about the world.

The third strongest predictor of adult BL is the use of informal science learning resources[4] (.37). The measure included each individual's use of

---

[3]Educational attainment was measured with a five-category ordinal variable. The lowest level included all individuals who did not complete secondary school or obtain a General Education Development (GED) diploma. The second category included high school graduates and GED holders. The third category included respondents with an associate's degree, and the fourth category included individuals who earned a bachelor's but not graduate or professional degrees. The highest category included all individuals who completed graduate or professional degrees.
[4]The Index of Informal Science Education (ISE) includes seven separate measures of science information acquisition, described previously. A confirmatory factor analysis was performed and all seven items loaded at the .5 level or higher, indicating a common set of related activities. A factor score was computed for each respondent and converted into a zero-to-100 scale. For the purpose of this model, a five-category ordinal variable was constructed.

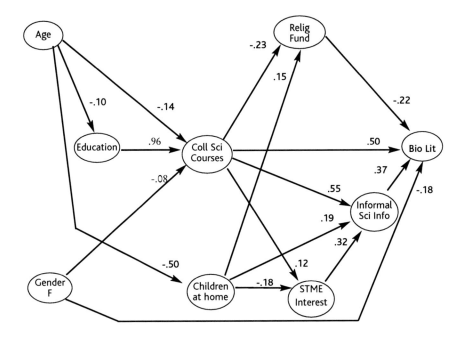

FIGURE 13.2. A path model to predict biological literacy in adults, 2005.

TABLE 13.3. Total Effect of Selected Variables on Biological Literacy, 2005

	TOTAL EFFECT
Respondent age	−.19
Gender (F)	−.25
Educational attainment	.74
College science courses	.77
Children at home	.00
Religious fundamentalism	−.22
Interest in science, technology, medical, or environmental issues	.12
Use of informal science learning resources	.37
R^2 =	.78

X^2 = 146.3; degrees of freedom = 18; Root Mean Square Error of Approximation (RMSEA) = .032; Upper confidence limit (90%) of RMSEA = .045; N =1,231.

science magazines, news magazines, science books, science television, science museums, science and health Web sites, and a public library. The magnitude of this effect indicates that informal science learning is important for adults to maintain a functional level of BL.

Gender was the fourth strongest predictor of adult BL, with a total effect of –.25 (see Table 13.3). The negative coefficient means that men were more likely to be biologically literate than women among U.S. adults. This result is counter to the stereotypic assumption that men know more about physical science and women know more about biological or life science.

Personal religious beliefs was the fifth strongest predictor of BL, with adults who hold fundamentalist religious beliefs[5] being significantly less likely to be biologically literate than other adults (–.22). In this model, religious beliefs are current religious beliefs and adults with more college science courses were significantly less likely to hold fundamentalist beliefs than other adults (–.23). Religious beliefs were not related to the use of informal science learning resources when age, gender, education, college science courses, and other variables were held constant.

Older adults were slightly less likely to be biologically literate than younger adults (–.19), holding constant differences in education, gender, college science courses, and other variables.

The level of personal interest in scientific, technical, medical, or environmental issues had a small positive effect on biological literacy (.12). The model shows that adults with more interest in these issues are more likely to be frequent users of adult science learning resources than adults with lower levels of interest in these issues (.32).

The presence of preschool or school-aged children in the home had no net effect on adult BL in the United States. Several previous U.S. studies have found very small positive effects on adult scientific literacy, but these results indicate that there is no significant residual effect on BL when all of the other independent variables in the model are held constant.

This model explains 78% of the total variance in BL among U.S. adults. This is a very good fit for the model and other indicators confirm the fit of the model. There appear to be no measurement problems with the model.

---

[5]The Index of Religious Beliefs is a count of the number of times that a respondent indicated strong agreement with the following four statements: (a) The Bible is the actual word of God and is to be taken literally, (b) There is a personal God who hears the prayers of individual men and women, (c) Human beings were created by God as whole persons and did not evolve from earlier forms of life, and (d) Humans beings as we know them developed from earlier forms of life. Individuals who scored 3 or 4 on this index were classified as fundamentalist (30%); individuals who scored 1 or 2 on the index were classified as conservative (28%); and individuals who scored zero on the scale were classified as moderate-liberal (42%). For a discussion of the impact of religious belief, see Miller, Scott, and Okamoto (2006).

DISCUSSION

These results show that about one in three U.S. adults have a general understanding that DNA is related to inherited characteristics and that DNA is associated with our health, disease, and well-being. In the context of modern learning theory, this result indicates that about one in three adults has a conceptual category—called a schema by cognitive psychologists—for genetic-based factors that may be associated with health or disease or general ability and well-being (Sternberg & Ben-Zeev, 2001). Data from the last two decades show a gradual increase in the proportion of U.S. adults who have this schema, increasing from one in five to one in three over the last two decades (see Fig. 13.1).

The development of a schema for DNA and related genetic constructs is an important first step in developing adult understanding of biological science. Many adults carry forward some understanding of a few basic biology constructs from their formal schooling. At the most basic level, most adults would know that living things are composed of cells, but it appears that only one in three adults know that each of these cells contains some DNA that controls a variety of cell functions and eventually the reproduction of the cell. For those adults with a working knowledge of the meaning of DNA, it will be possible to acquire additional information from newspapers, magazines, television shows, museum exhibits, and Internet sites and to integrate this new information into their basic DNA-genetics schema. U.S. adults are exposed to a wide array of DNA-genetic information daily through news reports and entertainment such as the *CSI* television series or the *Jurassic Park* movies, but the ability to recognize, process, and retain information from those sources depends on having a set of schemas that incorporate the individual's prior knowledge, experiences, and conclusions about any specific subject or topic.

The Index of BL is a measure of a more sophisticated understanding of some of the major constructs in modern biology—evolution through natural selection, genetic transfer through reproduction, and genetic change through random mutation or environmentally stimulated mutation. Adults who scored 70 or more on the Index of BL would be more likely to be able to recognize, process, and retain new information on these biological subjects because of their existing biological-relevant schemas. As with most adult learning, the cognitively rich get richer and the cognitively poor stay poor.

The structural analysis of the factors associated with BL in 2005 confirms this general model. Younger adults were slightly more likely to have a higher level of educational attainment and a greater exposure to college science courses. Adults with exposure to college science courses were more likely to be biologically literate, more likely to be interested in scientific and biology-related public policy issues, substantially more likely to use adult informal science learning resources, and significantly less likely to hold fundamentalist religious beliefs. This cluster of secondary benefits from college science courses contributes to the total level of adult BL.

It is useful to compare the relative influence of directly retained constructs (reflected in the direct path from college science courses to BL) and the influence of issue interest and science learning resource use on BL. The direct path from college science courses to BL had a path coefficient of .50 (see Figure 13.2). The net effect of science issue interest on BL was small[6] (.014), but the net effect of the influence of college science courses on informal science resource use was more substantial (.20). The net effect of a reduced likelihood of holding fundamentalist religious views was .05. The combination of these different sources of influence was .77, as reported in Table 13.2. By breaking down the various kinds of college science course influence, we can say that about two-thirds of the impact of college science courses was in retained constructs and that about one-third of the influence was the result of adult learning experiences of various kinds.

On balance, for those of us who have studied student and adult science learning, this model appears to be a reasonable description of today's world. We know that school learning of some basic ideas has long-lasting utility and that these conceptual building blocks are the tools with which adults seek to make sense of new complex information. And, as we enter the new electronic era, we sense that the possibilities for both school learning and adult out-of-school learning are greater than ever before. But, what, then, do these results tell us about educational and science policy choices to enhance the level of adult BL in the United States?

First, these results remind us that the roots of scientific literacy and BL are in formal schooling. The combination of decades of disappointing secondary science test results from American students and the striking power of college science courses to predict BL tell us that currently it is postsecondary education rather than secondary education that is driving the development of BL in adults. We should not be comfortable with this result. We need to recognize the disastrous condition of middle and high school science education in the United States and summon the courage to rethink that system. The idea that 7,000 independently elected school boards can develop a coherent science curriculum for this nation is absurd on its face. Even if it worked in the 19th century, it clearly does not work in the 21st century. And the continuation of our current 19th-century school funding system—based on property taxes in almost all states—is equally absurd.

Second, it is clear that our national commitment to general education requirements in colleges and universities is a critical national asset. We need

---

[6]The net effect is the product of the path coefficient from college science courses to science issue interest (.12) times the coefficient from science issue interest to information science resources use (.32) times the path coefficient from informal science resource use to BL (.37).

to recognize the wisdom of that policy and work to protect it from the numerous disciplinary and cross-disciplinary groups that seek to erode it. With the growth of community colleges, many states have mandated that transfer of community college credits to senior colleges in the same state, and in most cases, these transfers are made by eroding the general education requirement. Some community college courses would clearly qualify as a part of general education, but others would not and we need political and legislative leadership that is willing to understand this difference and act appropriately. And, we need to acknowledge that there is room for improvement in the science courses offered as a part of general education. There has been a good deal of work and improvement in these courses in recent years and we need to continue to fund that work and expand it quantitatively and qualitatively.

Third, it is clear that the importance of adult science learning resources will continue to grow in the years ahead. Most American adults will continue to work and vote for at least 50 years after their last formal degree. Although an increasing number of adults will return to school for course work periodically during their careers, it is likely that the nature of almost all of this additional work with be occupationally oriented. As noted earlier, it is likely that the number of science and biology-based issues on the political agenda will grow substantially in the decades ahead. Adults will need to use informal science resources to make sense of many of these issues. The current stem cell debate is a good illustration of this process. Few adults could have studied about stem cells in school, but millions of adults had to think about the issues raised in the media and in political campaigns. The good news is that the emerging electronic revolution is increasingly able to provide a wide array of useful and credible sources of information. The extensive use of Web-based information and communication services by patients and disease-related advocacy groups illustrates the potential of electronic resources to serve this need. It will be important to continue to monitor the quality and independence of these emerging information resources.

There can be little doubt that we stand at the beginning of an extraordinary period of growth in human knowledge of health, disease, and the nature of life itself. Before the end of the 21st century, biomedical scientists will have made major strides forward in understanding and treating many of the diseases and conditions that afflict humans today, but the speed and effectiveness of the adoption of new biomedical science will depend in part on the ability of patients and citizens to understand the basic biology that underlies this work at a level sufficient to make personal health choices and to participate in making relevant public policy decisions.

The preceding analysis is both encouraging and discouraging. There is evidence that one in three adults have developed a moderately functional understanding of DNA, and that about one in six have a reasonably sophisticated understanding of basic biological constructs. The growth in these proportions is encouraging, but the vast majority of adults remain biologically illiterate. We have a good deal of work to do, but we should not lose sight of the critical role that biological literacy will play in the quality of our personal medical decisions and in the quality of our public discourse on the biology-related issues that will populate the public policy agenda in the 21st century.

The HINTS research program provides an important source of data concerning public understandings and misunderstandings about cancer and other health-related issues. Current HINTS research findings suggest significant areas of limited BL concerning cancer. For example, in an analysis of HINTS data Viswanath et al. (2006) found confusion among lower socioeconomic status consumers about the causes of major cancers, such as lung and skin cancers. In another analysis of the HINTS data, Nguyan and Bellamy (2006) reported that Asian consumers were less aware than White consumers that not smoking or quitting smoking would reduce cancer risks. Surprisingly, Ramanadhan and Viswanath (2006) found that a significant percentage of consumers responding to HINTS who were diagnosed with cancer reported that they do not actively seek or receive health information beyond the health information given to them by health care providers. Similarly, in another analysis of HINTS data, Mayer et al. (2007) found that many cancer survivors do not actively seek health information, despite their tremendous needs for cancer information to address questions they have about side effects, calming their fears about the reoccurrence of cancer, and for improving their quality of life. These research findings illustrate the importance of developing effective evidence-based communication strategies for providing consumers, who may have limited BL, with relevant information about cancer that they can easily access and understand. HINTS research provides the evidence base needed to identify population-based limitations in BL, to learn about relevant cancer information gaps within different groups of consumers, and to design strategic targeted cancer communication interventions to promote cancer prevention and control.

REFERENCES

Ahmann, S. (1975). The exploration of survival levels of achievement by means of assessment techniques. In D.M. Nielsen (Ed.), *Reading and career education* (pp. 38-42). Newark, DE: International Reading Association.

Beaton, A.E., Martin, M.O., Mullis, I.V.S., Gonzalez, E.J., Smith, T.A., & Kelly, D.L. (1996). *Science achievement in the middle school years: IEA's Third International Mathematics and Science Study (TIMSS)*. Chestnut Hill, MA: Boston College.

Berleson, B.R., Lazarsfeld, P.F., & McPhee, W.N. (1954). *Voting: A study of opinion formation in a presidential campaign*. Chicago: University of Chicago Press.

Campbell, A., Converse, P.E., Miller, W.E., & Stokes, D.E. (1960). *The American Voter* [Unabridged edition]. New York: Wiley.

Cevero, R.M. (1985). Is a common definition of adult literacy possible? *Adult Education Quarterly, 36,* 50-54.

Cook, W.D. (1977). *Adult literacy education in the United States.* Newark, DE: International Reading Association.

Davis, R.C. (1958). *The public impact of science in the mass media.* Ann Arbor: University of Michigan Survey Research Center, Monograph No. 25.

Dillman, D. (1978). *Mail and telephone surveys: The total design method.* New York: Wiley.

Durant, J.R., Evans, G.A., & Thomas, G.P. (1989). The public understanding of science. *Nature, 340,* 11-14.

Durant, J.R., Evans, G.A., & Thomas, G.P. (1992). Public understanding of science in Britain: The role of medicine in the popular presentation of science. *Public Understanding of Science, 1,* 161-82.

Evans, G.A., & Durant, J.R. (1995). The relationship between knowledge and attitudes in the public understanding of science in Britain. *Public Understanding of Science, 4,* 57-74.

Guthrie, J.T., & Kirsch, I.S. (1984). The emergent perspective on literacy. *Phi Delta Kappan, 65,* 351-355.

Harman, D. (1970). Illiteracy: An overview. *Harvard Educational Review, 40,* 226-230.

Hayduk, L.A. (1987). *Structural equation modeling with LISREL.* Baltimore: The Johns Hopkins University Press.

Johnson, J.D. (1997). *Cancer-related information seeking.* Cresskill, NJ: Hampton Press.

Jöreskog, K., & Sörbom, D. (1993). *LISREL 8.* Chicago: Scientific Software International.

Kaestle, C.F. (1985). The history of literacy and the history of readers. In E. W. Gordon (Ed.), *Review of research in education* (Vol. 12, pp. 11-54). Washington, DC: American Educational Research Association.

Key, V.O. (1966). *The responsible electorate: Rationality in presidential voting.* Cambridge, MA: Belknap Press of Harvard University Press.

Kreps, G.L. (2006). One size does not fit all: Adapting communication to the needs and literacy levels of individuals. *Annals of Family Medicine (online commentary).* Retrieved May 19, 2009, from http://www.annfammed.org/cgi/eletters/4/3/205.

Lazarsfeld, P.F., Berleson, B., & Gaudet, H. (1948). *The people's choice: How the voter makes up his mind in a presidential campaign.* New York: Columbia University Press.

Mayer, D.K., Terrin, N.C., Kreps, G.L., Menon, U., McCance, K., Parsons, S.K. et al. (2007). Cancer survivors information seeking behaviors: A comparison of survivors who do and don't seek information. *Patient Education and Counseling, 65*(3), 342-350.

Miller, J.D. (1983a). *The American people and science policy.* New York: Pergamon Press.

Miller, J.D. (1983b). Scientific literacy: A conceptual and empirical review. *Daedalus,* *112*(2), 29-48.

Miller, J.D. (1987). Scientific literacy in the United States. In D. Evered & M. O'Connor (Eds.), *Communicating science to the public* (pp. 19-40). London: Wiley.

Miller, J.D. (1996). Scientific literacy for effective citizenship. In R.E. Yager (Ed.), *Science/technology/society as reform in science education* (pp. 185-204). New York: State University of New York Press.

Miller, J.D. (1998). The measurement of civic scientific literacy. *Public Understanding of Science, 7,* 1-21.

Miller, J.D. (2000). The development of civic scientific literacy in the United States. In D.D. Kumar & D. Chubin (Eds.), *Science, technology, and society: A sourcebook on research and practice* (pp. 21-47). New York: Plenum Press.

Miller, J.D. (2004). Public understanding of, and attitudes toward scientific research: What we know and what we need to know. *Public Understanding of Science, 13,* 273-294.

Miller, J.D., Scott, E., & Okamoto, S. (2006). Public acceptance of evolution. *Science, 313,* 765-766.

Miller, J.D., Pardo, R., & Niwa, F. (1997). *Public perceptions of science and technology: A comparative study of the European Union, the United States, Japan, and Canada.* Madrid: BBV Foundation Press.

Nguyen, G., & Bellamy, S. (2006). Cancer information seeking preferences and experiences: Disparities between Asian Americans and whites in the Health Information National Trends Survey (HINTS). *Journal of Health Communication, 11,* 173-180.

Northcutt, N.W. (1975). Functional literacy for adults. In D.M. Nielsen & H.F. Hjelm (Eds.), *Reading and career education* (pp. 43-49). Newark, DE: International Reading Association.

Pardo, R., Midden, C., & Miller, J.D. (2002). Attitudes toward biotechnology in the European Union. *Journal of Biotechnology, 98,* 9-24.

Parker, R., & Kreps, G.L. (2005). Library outreach: Overcoming health literacy challenges. *Journal of the Medical Library Association, 93*(4), 78-82.

Popkin, S.L. (1991). *The reasoning voter: Communication and persuasion in presidential campaigns.* Chicago: University of Chicago Press.

Ramanadhan, S., & Viswanath, K. (2006). Health and the information nonseeker: A profile. *Health Communication, 20*(2), 131-139.

Resnick, D.P., & Resnick, L.B. (1977). The nature of literacy: An historical exploration. *Harvard Educational Review, 47,* 370-385.

Schmidt, W.H., McKnight, C.C., & Raizen, S.A. (1997). *A splintered vision: An investigation of U.S. science and mathematics education.* Boston: Kluwer Academic.

Shen, B.J. (1975). Scientific literacy and the public understanding of science. In S. Day (Ed.), *Communication of scientific information* (pp. 44-52). Basel: Karger.

Snow, C.P. (1959). *The two cultures and the scientific revolution.* New York: Cambridge University Press.

Sternberg, R.J., & Ben-Zeev, T. (2001). *Complex cognition: The psychology of human thought.* New York: Oxford University Press.

Viswanath, K., Breen, N., Meissner, H., Moser, R., Hesse, B., Steele, W. et al. (2006). Cancer knowledge and disparities in the information age. *Journal of Health Communication, 11*, 1-17.

Zimowski, M.F.E., Muraki, E., Mislevy, R.J., & Bock, R.D. (1996). *BILOG-MG: Multiple-group IRT analysis and test maintenance for binary items*. Chicago: Scientific Software International.

III

THE FUTURE OF HEALTH COMMUNICATION AND INFORMATICS

14

THE FUTURE OF HEALTH COMMUNICATION AND INFORMATICS

Challenges and Opportunities

Lila J. Finney Rutten
National Cancer Institute

Barbara K. Rimer
University of North Carolina, Chapel Hill

Bradford W. Hesse
National Cancer Institute

A PATH NOT YET TRAVELED

In his acceptance speech to the Nobel Prize Committee on December 10, 2007, in Oslo, Norway, long-time Internet advocate Al Gore explained the importance of heeding data about the present to prepare for the future. Sometimes, without warning, the future knocks on our door, he said, and when this happens people of vision must act; but the way ahead is difficult. The outer boundary between what we know is feasible currently and what we can do seems separated by a gulf of uncertainty. Gore emphasized the point with the words of the Spanish poet, Antonio Machado: "Pathwalker, there is no path. You must make the path as you walk" (Gore, 2007).

Of course, Gore was speaking of global warming in his speech to the Nobel Prize Committee but his words echo the sentiment of many of the contributions in this last section of this book. Understanding the trends of the day will give us a hint as to where the currents in the stream of future events may be leading us; understanding what those data tell us will give us an intuition of where we are heading and how to craft the future to be the most positive and desirable one possible. As economist Charles Handy

(1989) reasoned, "the future we predict today is not inevitable. We can influence it, if we know what we want it to be. . . . We can and should be in charge of our own destinies in a time of change" (p. xi). This is the promise of looking to the future as we collect an evidence base in health communication.

Unabashedly, there is a sense of hope and optimism in the chapters included in this last section of the book. There is mutually felt recognition that if we marshal the force of the currents ahead of us we might be able to conquer some of the longstanding public health issues that have been plaguing us as a community of scientists and practitioners. Much of that optimism is refreshing, as it reflects a real sense of how the future might be channeled to improve the lives of real people, along with the lives of their loved ones. Ultimately, it is a story of people and promise—of the health care experience we all have—more than it is a story about technology (Brailer, 2005).

Despite this unyielding optimism, it should be recognized that the authors in this section of the volume are first and foremost empirical thinkers. Each one recognizes that as new technologies emerge with new solutions in hand, that same technology will introduce new problems and new challenges (Dunlop & Kling, 1991). The excitement of mass media at the height of the 20th century brought with it the seeds of an epidemic in tobacco (Davis, Gilpin, Loken, Viswanath, & Wakefield, 2008) and obesity (Johnson-Taylor, Yaroch, Krebs-Smith, & Rodgers, 2007), as described in Chapter 1. The public's enthusiasm for e-mail and computer networks brought with it an onslaught of spam and the constant threat of downloadable computer viruses (Moller & Pletson, 2008). The law of unintended consequences is an integral part of the diffusion story for any new technology or policy (Dunlop & Kling, 1991).

LOOKING FORWARD IN HEALTH COMMUNICATION

Over the past few decades, the health communication and informatics environment has changed significantly (Viswanath, 2005). Advances in technology have increased the number and variety of available communication channels and technologies, expanding population access to health information (Viswanath, 2005). Expansion of the health communication and informatics environment has been met with increasing public interest in and demand for health information (Arora et al., 2008; Rutten, Arora, Bakos, Aziz, & Rowland, 2005). These trends have shaped the very way individuals and populations engage in their health and health care (Hesse et al., 2005).

Changes witnessed over the past decades in information technology and communication will likely pale in comparison to the changes on the horizon. Opportunities for population health gain through the intersection of behavioral medicine and information technology are greater than ever. Information technology has the potential to accelerate evidence-based efforts to reduce the cancer burden by supporting communication about risk, prevention behavior, and educational advice and programs offering venues for social support and networks of care, and through the provision of personalized information and individualized care.

To realize the potential of health information technology, key challenges faced by health care consumers, providers, and researchers must be acknowledged and addressed. A key challenge in the United States to improving population health and realizing the potential of health information technology is the intense focus on treatment and illness rather than prevention and wellness. A broader perspective should seek proactively to optimize population health and health care needs across a continuum to include health management and disease prevention both within and beyond the health care setting.

Efforts to keep people healthy should begin by empowering consumers and patients alike to do all they can to protect their own health. Health information technology can play a key role in supporting and empowering people through enabling them to own and manage their health information within a larger interoperable system of data. Health information technology can support various domains of health, including social support, medication adherence, and behavioral tracking. However, health information technology should be informed by the needs of the public, patients, and health care providers.

Fundamental health care issues of cost, quality, and access should be addressed as part of health information technology initiatives. Health information technology can deliver a model to permit health care providers to deliver personalized advice, and can support health care professionals in their efforts to support patient empowerment. Health information technology can also support researchers in their efforts to discover better ways to deliver care at lower cost and with greater ease by enabling the development and implementation of research protocols.

STRUCTURE OF THE SECTION

The chapters included in this section examine the future of health communication and informatics in the context of this rapidly evolving landscape of health information technology and health communication. They cover the changing role of health care consumers, practitioners, policymakers, and researchers in response to and in anticipation of the opportunities and challenges during this time of rapid change.

Internet users in this decade have access to and use a range of information sources online, including a number of sources created and maintained by their peers rather than only credentialed experts (Hesse et al., 2005). The future of health communication depends as much on the future of the participatory web as it does on traditional communication avenues. In Chapter 15, Fox, from the PEW Internet and American Life Project and Bernhardt of the Centers for Disease Control and Prevention, describe how online health communication continues to evolve and explore how health communication, enhanced by the Internet, may progress in the future. Fox and Bernhardt trace trend lines for blogs, social networking sites, online repositories for photos and videos, wikis and other online resources, and review current Internet population statistics, including the increasing importance of understanding home broadband penetration versus dial-up access among various demographic groups. This chapter concludes with a description of some of the innovative efforts to apply the participatory web to health communication underway at the Centers for Disease Control and Prevention.

In Chapter 16, Taplin, from the National Cancer Institute, discusses important challenges to the current health care system in the United States and examines the opportunities for information technology to support improvements in health care and health care delivery. Taplin proposes challenges to the adoption of information technology in support of improved health care can be overcome by using well recognized principles from the fields of health communication and user-centered design.

The potential for population impact through health communication is greater than ever before. Large-scale efforts within the health information technology sector, coupled with greater attention to the importance of health communication in policy domains, can advance the potential to control cancer. Volckmann of Keas Inc., with colleagues from the National Cancer Institute, describe (chap. 17) the potential and impact of health information technology in shaping health communication.

CONCLUSION

Anticipating changes in health communication and the use of emerging technologies is imperative to the public health goal of disseminating important scientific findings and data to relevant audiences and supporting the important work of public health practitioners, health communicators, and scientists to improve the public's health. In this final section of the book, the contributors whose chapters have been included recognize that the purpose of collecting an evidence base in health communication is to inform the future with data from the present. What the authors in this section do is give us an intuition as to where to aim our data lens. In so doing, they help us work together in creating the best vision of the future we can collectively construct with data, purpose, and determination (Johansen, 2007).

REFERENCES

Arora, N.K., Hesse, B.W., Rimer, B.K., Viswanath, K., Clayman, M.L., & Croyle, R.T. (2008). Frustrated and confused: The American public rates its cancer-related information-seeking experiences. *Journal of General Internal Medicine, 23*(3), 223-228.

Brailer, D. (2005). Action through collaboration: A conversation with David Brailer. The national coordinator of HIT believes that facilitation, not mandates, are the way to move the agenda forward. Interview by Robert Cunningham. *Health Affairs (Millwood), 24*(5), 1150-1157.

Davis, R., Gilpin, E.A., Loken, B., Viswanath, K.V., & Wakefield, M. (Eds.). (2008). *The role of the media in promoting and reducing tobacco use* (Vol. 19). Washington, DC: U.S. Department of Health and Human Services.

Dunlop, C.E.M., & Kling, R. (1991). *Computerization and controversy: Value conflicts and social choices.* Boston: Academic Press.

Gore, A. (2007). *Nobel Lecture: Al Gore.* Retrieved June 20, 2008, from http://nobelprize.org/nobel-prizes/peace/laureates/2007/gore-lecture_en.html.

Handy, C.B. (1989). *The age of unreason.* Boston, MA: Harvard Business School Press.

Hesse, B.W., Nelson, D.E., Kreps, G.L., Croyle, R.T., Arora, N.K., Rimer, B.K. et al. (2005). Trust and sources of health information: The impact of the Internet and its implications for health care providers: Findings from the first Health Information National Trends Survey. *Archives of Internal Medicine, 165*(22), 2618-2624.

Johansen, R. (2007). *Get there early: Sensing the future to compete in the present* (1st ed.). San Francisco, CA: Barrett-Koehler.

Moller, A.N., & Pletson, C.E. (2008). *Telecommunications and media issues.* New York: Nova Science Publishers.

Rutten, L.J., Arora, N.K., Bakos, A.D., Aziz, N., & Rowland, J. (2005). Information needs and sources of information among cancer patients: A systematic review of research (1980-2003). *Patient Education and Counseling, 57*(3), 250-261.

Viswanath, K. (2005). Science and society: The communications revolution and cancer control. *Nature Reviews Cancer, 5*(10), 828-835.

15

HEALTH COMMUNICATION 2.0

The Promise of Peer Participation

Susannah Fox
Pew Internet & American Life Project

Jay M. Bernhardt
Centers for Disease Control and Prevention

The participatory web, also known as user-generated media or Web 2.0, is changing the way people gather and share information online. Today's Internet users, especially those under age 35 years, turn to a diverse range of information sources online, many of which are created and maintained by their peers, not by credentialed experts. Indeed, it is no longer useful to treat the "Internet" as a single information source when many users strongly distinguish the differences between WebMD, *The Washington Post*, a friend's blog, or a MySpace page, even though all four may be frequently used sources of health information.

This chapter reviews who uses the Internet in the United States and traces the trend lines for blogs, social networking sites, online repositories for photos and videos, wikis, and other participatory and collaborative online resources. We then explore the implications of the participatory web on health communication and contrast this "horizontal" health communication to more traditional "vertical" health communication. Finally, we illustrate strategies to apply the participatory Web to health communication by describing some of the innovative efforts underway at the Centers for Disease Control and Prevention (CDC).

TODAY'S INTERNET USERS

We begin with a review of the current demographics of the Internet population. The Pew Internet & American Life Project has sorted American adults into three broad categories related to which technology assets they own, what actions they take with these tools, and the attitudes they express toward information and communications technology.

"Elite tech users" make up 31% of all adults. They are frequent-Internet users and are likely to own cell phones, laptops, personal digital assistants, and other technological accessories. They are likely to say that technology enhances their work and personal lives.

"Middle-of-the-road tech users" comprise 20% of all adults. They may have invested in technology, but they either do not go online very often or feel burdened by this new connectivity.

Those with "few tech assets" make up 49% of all adults. Members of this group have few technology gadgets and only occasionally take advantage of the interactivity available to them. Within this group, there are 15% of adults who have neither a cell phone nor an Internet-connected computer. These are most often older adults who are likely to be satisfied with "old media" offerings such as television and print media (Horrigan, 2007).

Other Pew Internet Project studies have found that many adults who do not have Internet access say they have never been online and do not live with anyone who goes online. This group is dominated by people over age 70 years, those with less than a high school education, and those who do not have strong English skills (Fox, 2005; Fox & Livingston, 2007).

Health status is another significant factor in predicting Internet use. About one in five adults answer yes to the following question: "Does any disability, handicap, or chronic disease keep you from participating fully in work, school, housework, or other activities, or not?" Of those, 51% go online, compared to 75% of other adults. It is significant that 66% of American adults living with a disability or chronic illness are over age 50. This probably contributes to the relatively low Internet penetration rate for this group.

Once online, however, those living with disability or chronic disease are just as likely as other Internet users to search for health information online. Eight in 10 Internet users are "e-patients," people who use the Internet to gather and share health information.

One of the realities of health care is that only a minority of adults are able to connect with the information resources they require. The Health Information National Trends Survey (HINTS), sponsored by the National Cancer Institute (NCI), found a significant disparity between what people say is their preferred source of information about cancer and where they actually go to get that information. In a national survey conducted in 2003,

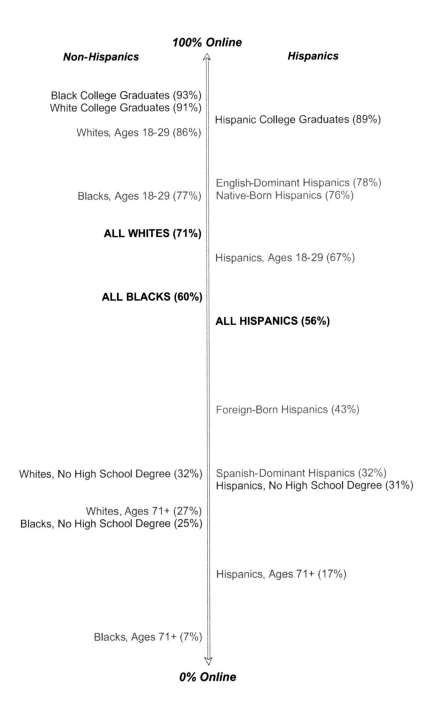

100% Online

Non-Hispanics   *Hispanics*

Black College Graduates (93%)
White College Graduates (91%)
                                    Hispanic College Graduates (89%)
Whites, Ages 18-29 (86%)

                                    English-Dominant Hispanics (78%)
                                    Native-Born Hispanics (76%)
Blacks, Ages 18-29 (77%)

ALL WHITES (71%)

                                    Hispanics, Ages 18-29 (67%)

ALL BLACKS (60%)

                                    ALL HISPANICS (56%)

                                    Foreign-Born Hispanics (43%)

Whites, No High School Degree (32%)   Spanish-Dominant Hispanics (32%)
                                    Hispanics, No High School Degree (31%)

Whites, Ages 71+ (27%)
Blacks, No High School Degree (25%)

                                    Hispanics, Ages 71+ (17%)

Blacks, Ages 71+ (7%)

0% Online

FIGURE 15.1. Internet use among Hispanics, Whites, and Blacks.

49% of adults said they would go first to a health care provider if they had a strong need to get information about cancer. In the same survey, however, 46% of people who said they had recently looked for cancer information for themselves reported that they looked online; whereas, only 11% consulted a health care professional (Rutten, Moser, Beckjord, Hesse, & Croyle, 2007).

The 2003 HINTS data also found that the highest percentage of adults (72%) reported receiving health information from television, followed closely by 68% of adults who reported that they read health information in a magazine or newspaper during the previous year. Health information on the Internet, however, was very close behind at more than 65% of adults.

The Pew Internet Project's recent research rounds out the portrait of many people's mixed-media approach to gathering health information. A 2006 survey found that 33% of e-patients took advantage of both online and offline information sources and talked with a health professional about what they found online. Those living with chronic conditions are even more likely than other e-patients to do so. Fully half of e-patients with chronic conditions talked with a health professional about what they found online during their most recent search, possibly because those living with chronic conditions are highly likely to have seen a doctor in the past year (Fox, 2006, 2007). Indeed, 8 in 10 respondents said they turn to a professional for information or assistance in dealing with health or medical issues (Fox & Jones, 2009).

So just how are these millions of e-patients connecting with health information online? A 2006 Pew Internet Project survey found that most e-patients begin their inquiries at a general search engine like Google and Yahoo, rather than at a health-related website (Fox, 2006, 2007). A 2007 study by Envision Solutions reported that these searches are probably resulting in significant exposure to user-generated health content such as blogs, discussion groups, and wikis (Johnmar, 2007). Indeed, the user-generated online encyclopedia Wikipedia appeared on the first page of results for two-thirds of the searches conducted by Envision Solutions. Forty-seven percent of Internet users have consulted Wikipedia (Pew Internet & American Life Project, 2008).

Social media is a mainstream source of health information. Of those who go online for health information, 59% have done at least one of the following activities (Fox & Jones, 2009):

- Read someone else's commentary or experience about health or medical issues on an online news group, website, or blog.
- Consulted rankings or reviews online of doctors or other providers.
- Consulted rankings or reviews online of hospitals or other medical facilities.
- Signed up to receive updates about health or medical issues.
- Listened to a podcast about health or medical issues.

Twenty percent of e-patients have taken a more active role and done at least one of the following activities:

- Tagged or categorized online content about health or medical issues.
- Posted comments, queries, or information about health or medical matters in an online discussion, listserv, or other online group forum.
- Posted comments about health on a blog.
- Posted a review online of a doctor.
- Posted a review online of a hospital.
- Shared photos, videos or audio files online about health or medical issues.

HEALTH INFORMATION USERS ON THE PARTICIPATORY WEB

The Pew Internet Project has tracked a steady increase in the percentage of Internet users who read blogs: 17% in 2004, 27% in 2005, and 32% in 2008. The current estimate is that 11% of adult Internet users keep a blog. In a special survey of bloggers conducted in 2006, most respondents said they use their blog to chronicle their personal lives, which sometimes includes health concerns (Lenhart & Fox, 2006).

For example, Dooce.com is one of the Top 50 blogs on the Web in terms of traffic.[1] In 2006, Heather Armstrong, the woman behind Dooce, first wrote about her basal cell carcinoma, which she had nicknamed "Ed." This blogger doesn't pretend to be a health educator, but she raised awareness of skin cancer among her thousands of fans as she continued to write about it.

Most bloggers have much smaller audiences, but they can be influential in their micro-local communities in the same way. Expert patients who are part of an online community are vital sources for basic home care tips, strategies for communicating with health professionals, and factors to consider when weighing treatment options (Fox, 2006; Meier, Lyons, Frydman, Forlenza, & Rimer, 2007). Health care bloggers serve another role, writing about personal experiences, health news, business developments, or policy (Johnmar & Kruglyak, 2006). These e-patients can serve as "someone like me" who can give "just-in-time" advice that many people are looking for online.

Social networking sites are another potential source for personal stories about health. Sites like MySpace, Facebook, Orkut, Twitter, and LinkedIn allow users to create profiles and connect to other people in a personal net-

---

[1]Dooce.com is ranked no. 49 as of August 4, 2009, on Technorati's list of Top 100 Blogs: http://technorati.com/pop/blogs/.

work that can number in the hundreds or even thousands. Social network profiles are often messy, silly, heartfelt collages of photos, music, videos, and links to other sites. Internet users catalogue and categorize their interests and experiences, forming affinity groups by linking to the Ovarian Cancer National Alliance profile, for example. Of online teens, 55% have created a social network profile on a site like MySpace or Facebook (Lenhart & Madden, 2007), as have 35% of Internet users age 18 and older (Lenhart, 2009).

The photo site Flickr is another example of how people categorize their own photos and put them online for public display. A search for the word "chemo" yields more than 10,000 photos, including one of a young girl awaiting her weekly treatment, which will be administered via the port that appears as a lump on her bare chest. Where else could you see such an intimate moment? Where else could someone get a clear picture of what weekly chemo actually looks like? Fully 37% of Internet users have uploaded photos to a public site, 28% of Internet users have tagged or categorized content online such as photos, news stories, or blog posts.

Video sites like YouTube are another example of a Web 2.0 site with unintended consequences for health communication. Sixty-two percent of Internet users have visited a video-sharing site such as YouTube (Madden, 2009). News and comedy are the most popular types of video, but one in five Internet users have watched an educational clip online (Madden, 2007). For example, searching YouTube for the phrase "how to use an inhaler" yields dozens of instructional videos in both English and Spanish.

HEALTH COMMUNICATION 2.0

The participatory online encyclopedia, Wikipedia (2008), defines Web 2.0 as "a trend in web design and development (and) a perceived second generation of web-based communities and hosted services . . . which aim to facilitate creativity, collaboration, and sharing among users." The next generation of health communication—what we call Health Communication 2.0—builds on peer-to-peer engagement popularized on the participatory web. Health Communication 2.0 involves the electronic exchange of health information between individuals and organizations in a manner that is interactive, collaborative, and participatory.

Traditional health communication (i.e., Health Communication 1.0) often involves the one-way delivery of health information from expert sources to nonexpert receivers through mass communication channels (e.g., televised public service announcements) or through interpersonal channels (e.g., physicians to patients). This form of health communication can be considered "vertical" communication from the highly regarded expert at the top to the layperson below.

From the earliest examples of health communication through the present, there are countless examples of traditional health communication intervention campaigns that fit this model of vertical, top–down interventions. Although many of these campaigns can be considered successful, several literature reviews of evaluated health communication campaigns have found these to have limited or moderate effects on behavior (Snyder & Hamilton, 2002; Snyder, Hamilton, Mitchell, Kiwanuka-Tondo, Fleming-Milici, & Proctor, 2004).

Although there are numerous explanations and hypotheses for the limited effects of vertical health communication, there are two moderating factors related to how the information is presented and received that are important to this discussion. First, the effectiveness of health communication messages is influenced by how much receivers are personally involved in the messages and find them to be personally relevant (Petty, Priester, & Brinol, 2002). Perceived personal relevance of messages leads to higher-

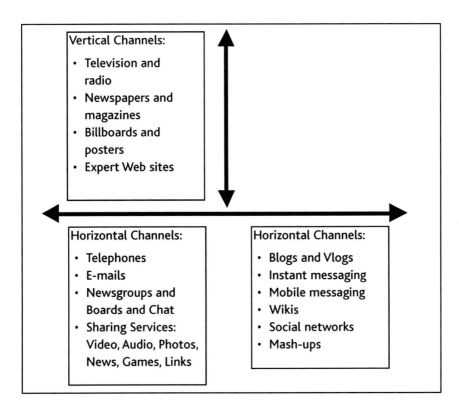

FIGURE 15.2. Vertical and horizontal communication channels.

order cognitions, or elaboration, according to the Elaboration Likelihood Model, when compared with messages perceived to be less relevant, which are often processed more peripherally (Petty & Cacioppo, 1986). Numerous experimental studies have found that the persuasive effects of centrally processed messages are stronger and more enduring than messages that are peripherally processed (O'Keefe, 1990). Vertical health communication messages, particularly those delivered through mass media, often consist of static messages that are "pushed" to passive receivers. Vertical health communication campaigns, in essence, become a game of hit-or-miss, where health messages will vary in degrees of perceived relevance among members of diverse intended audiences.

The effectiveness of a health communication message also can be influenced by receiver perceptions about the message source. Numerous source factors can moderate message effects among receivers, including perceived source credibility, trust, and likability (O'Keefe, 1990). Many vertical health communication campaigns involve messages delivered from a self-identified expert source, such as a doctor, a scientist, the government, or an advocacy organization. Other vertical campaigns may use celebrity sources or peer sources, but these campaigns face the same hit-or-miss challenge as they have perceived personal relevance to the receiver. Diverse message receivers may or may not find static sources credible, trustworthy, or likable, and the campaign messages may therefore be less persuasive and, therefore, effective for behavior change.

By leveraging the power of the participatory web, Health Communication 2.0 will revolutionize public health by accelerating the proliferation of "horizontal" health communication. Horizontal health communication means exchanging health information between "real people" who seek out or "pull" health information when, where, how, and from whom they want it. This is not a new phenomenon. Humans have always exchanged health information through their interpersonal networks, especially among their families and close friends. The first mass-media horizontal channel for exchanging health information was the telephone. A more recent and more popular channel for exchanging health information is e-mail. Today, people are leveraging all the participatory, new media channels for exchanging health information—including Web-based chat, blogs, bulletin boards, text messaging, social networks, media-sharing networks, wiki, e-games, and virtual worlds. In the future, many more sophisticated participatory channels for exchanging health information will develop that allow for deeper exchanges and engagements, and that "mash-up" data from multiple sources in real time. Although many people believe that electronic personal health records (PHR) will revolutionize health, the "killer app" related to PHRs that will accelerate their spread is likely to be one that combines highly relevant personal health information with interpersonal social networks of like-minded, and possibly like-healthy people.

The two factors that moderate the impact of vertical health communication—perceived personal message relevance and perceived relevant sources—are likely to be greater in horizontal health communication because individual receivers play a much more central role in selecting how they are exposed to health communication messages. Although the communicator may have the best intentions, whether a message is considered relevant to a receiver is a function of the receiver's sense of the importance of the problem as opposed to the expert communicator's sense of an issue's importance or immediacy (Rothschild, 1987). Because individuals who are highly interested in a topic often use electronic media to seek out topic-specific information (Dutta-Bergman, 2004), many will continue searching until they find information they consider to be highly relevant. People who are similar or who have had similar experiences are already online sharing their stories, opinions, and health information; searchers are likely to find these stories highly relevant.

The supply of available online health information has already surpassed demand and this growth shows no signs of slowing. Today's health information consumers already are struggling with content overload. In this environment, factors such as source familiarity and perceived personal relevance will become critical predictors of whether information is attended to or simply goes unheard amid the noise (Della, DeJoy, & Lance, 2008).

Online health consumers also intentionally avoid and ignore messages they perceive to be inconsistent with their values and perspectives (Della, Eroglu, Bernhardt, Edgerton, & Nall, 2008), thereby reinforcing their personal viewpoints while preventing exposure to new or opposing information (Atkin, 1985; Sanbonmatsu, Posavac, Kardes, & Mantel, 1998). In this context, the participatory web offers great potential for reaching and influencing our intended audiences. Health information received from sources that are perceived to be similar may be seen as more real and relevant to receivers than advice that comes from an expert who has not personally had the same experiences.

Numerous studies suggest that source perceptions can affect message impact (O'Keefe, 1990), and perceived source similarity can moderate the effects of observational and vicarious learning (Bandura, 1986). Annual consumer research conducted by Edelman also demonstrates that "people like me" are the most trusted source among Americans and many other developed countries, especially when compared with governments or private companies (Edelman, 2008). Many will see health information exchanged horizontally between real people on the participatory web as more trusted and will have a greater impact than vertical health communication from experts. Health Communication 2.0 will take place among naturally forming social networks on the Web among like-minded people (or "friends") whose network self-selection results in health information exchanges that are highly relevant and that come from sources that are credible and trustworthy. In this context, horizontal health communication messages and may be more effective than vertical health communication campaigns.

APPLYING HEALTH COMMUNICATION 2.0

As with traditional health communication, audience analysis and intervention goals are the two most important drivers for Health Communication 2.0 planning and implementation. There are many audiences and issues for which new media and the participatory web will not be appropriate or ideal, as the Pew Internet Project's typology illustrates, and this will remain an ongoing challenge in reaching many vulnerable populations (Horrigan, 2007). It is worth noting, however, that even in these "low-tech" situations, the Health Communication 2.0 strategies and tactics of audience participation, collaboration, and involvement can improve the effectiveness of any intervention or campaign.

For those issues and audiences where Health Communication 2.0 may be appropriate, professionals should remember to apply appropriate theories, models, and best practices to intervention development, and to start slowly by pilot testing different participatory web strategies and applications. This is the approach employed at the CDC under the leadership of the E-Health Marketing Division in the National Center for Health Marketing. The examples given here illustrate the CDC's efforts in the context of Health Communication 2.0.

For decades, the CDC has used traditional health communication interventions and campaigns to protect and promote people's health in the United States and around the world. Because of the CDC's very high name recognition and credibility among the US public (Porter/Novelli, 2007), vertical "top–down" communication from experts is still an important and worthwhile strategy to employ, especially when trying to increase knowledge or awareness, or when responding to a public health emergency. However, when the goal is to impact or change more complex behaviors, the CDC is now pursuing a communication strategy that combines and integrates vertical and horizontal health communication to maximize the impact of health communication. This nexus between horizontal and vertical communication is what Edelman called the "sweet spot" and this is where the CDC will aim its health communication and social marketing efforts now and in the future (Edelman, 2007).

The CDC's health communication activities in promoting National Influenza Vaccination Week in 2006 and 2007 represent this hybrid strategy. In addition to its traditional health communication intervention consisting of television, radio, and print messages encouraging vaccine use, the CDC implemented several new media and participatory strategies. For example, in 2006 the CDC conducted its first online seminar (or webinar) for influential bloggers who write about influenza, parenting, or child health to encourage seasonal flu vaccine for children. The main focus of this event was the communication strategies that have proven to be most effective in encouraging vaccination uptake. These bloggers subsequently blogged about the CDC's science on vaccinations using the communication strategies they learned and the messages spread across the Web horizontally. The CDC created several podcasts about influenza protection. Podcasts are short video and audio messages designed to be accessible and interesting to consumers. These podcasts were promoted widely through numerous electronic channels. Perhaps most creatively, the CDC partnered with an online virtual world, called "Whyville," which has more than 2 million teen and pre-teen players. In this Web-based simulation, the CDC promoted virtual vaccinations to players and then introduced the "Why-Flu" in the virtual world which affected players who had not been vaccinated. As a result, the CDC engaged hundreds of thousands of at-risk users and taught them about influenza and the importance of seasonal flu vaccination.

The CDC has launched numerous other participatory web products that leverage Health Communication 2.0 principles. Examples include podcasts, electronic greeting cards, interactive games, tag clouds, and widgets and gadgets, all of which undergo audience-centered usability testing before launch. Even within the CDC's most "vertical" channel, the CDC.gov Web site, extensive efforts over several years have increased interactivity and user participation. For example, the CDC has added RSS feeds and e-mail alerts to many critical pages so users can subscribe for automated updates with content changes or important new information that becomes available. This approach seeks to balance "pull" messages that people actively seek, with "push" messages that are sent to people to whom they are most relevant and when they may have a greater impact. The CDC has also embraced social networks and currently has a MySpace page and ongoing partnerships with several other networks including DailyStrength and Sermo. The CDC has many other Health Communication 2.0 strategies on the horizon, including mobile messaging and increased public engagement through Web dialogues. By evolving its communication and marketing strategies to meet the changing capabilities of technology and the rising demands from e-patients, the CDC is committed to using horizontal models and Health Communication 2.0 principles to deliver relevant health information through new channels.

CONCLUSION

Internet users, especially young people, are no longer just surfing the Web. They are shaping it. They download, upload, mash it up, and make it their own. And their peers rely on that new content to make choices about what movie to see, what products to buy, and what health decisions they will make on a daily basis.

Health Communication 2.0 offers great potential to reach elite tech users, and other online health users, because it combines the strongest aspects of mass communication and interpersonal communication with messages that will be seen as trustworthy and highly relevant. In today's world of health information clutter and overload, it is imperative to consider the relative strengths and challenges of vertical and horizontal health communication and to strike a balance so as to have the most positive impact on each intended audience.

Because Health Communication 2.0 is still in its infancy, additional research is urgently needed to explore and understand how people seek and process health information on the participatory web and how best to package and place that information for maximum impact. Surveys such as HINTS and the ongoing work by Pew Internet & American Life should begin tracking health information on the participatory web. We also recommend that researchers continue to track the small but significant group of adults—often older and in poorer health—who are offline in an online world. We need to consider how the principles of participation, collaboration, and interactivity can make health communication activities targeted to these audiences more effective as well.

REFERENCES

Atkin, C. (1985). Informational utility and selective exposure. In D. Zillman & J. Bryant (Eds.), *Selective exposure to communication.* Hillsdale, NJ: Erlbaum.

Bandura, A. (1986). *Social foundations of thought and action: A social cognitive theory.* Englewood Cliffs, NJ: Prentice Hall.

Della, L.J., DeJoy, D.M., & Lance, C.E. (2008). Promoting fruit and vegetable consumption in different lifestyle groups: Recommendations for program development based on behavioral research and consumer media data. *Health Mark Quarterly, 25*(1-2), 66-96.

Della, L.J., Eroglu, D., Bernhardt, J.M., Edgerton, E., & Nall, J. (2008). Looking to the future of new media in health marketing: Deriving propositions based on traditional theories. *Health Mark Quarterly, 25*(1-2), 147-174.

Dutta-Bergman, M.J. (2004). Primary sources of health information: Comparisons in the domain of health attitudes, health cognitions, and health behaviors. *Health Communication, 16,* 273-288.

Edelman, R. (2007). Edelman Trust Barometer. Accessed May 2009, from http://www.edelman.com/trust/2007/trust_final_1_31.pdf.

Edelman, R. (2008). Trust Barometer. Accessed May 2009, from http://www.edelman. co.uk/trustbarometer/

Fox, S. (2005). *Digital Divisions.* Washington, DC: Pew Internet & American Life Project.

Fox, S. (2006). *Online health search 2006*. Washington, DC: Pew Internet & American Life Project.

Fox, S. (2007). *E-Patients with chronic conditions*. Washington, DC: Pew Internet & American Life Project.

Fox, S., & Jones, S. (2009). *The social life of health information*. Washington, DC: Pew Internet & American Life Project.

Fox, S., & Livingston, G. (2007). *Latinos online*. Washington, DC: Pew Internet/Pew Hispanic Projects.

Horrigan, J. (2007). *A typology of information and communication technology users*. Washington, DC: Pew Internet & American Life Project.

Johnmar, F. (2007). *Diving deeper into online health search*. New York: Envision Solutions, LLC.

Johnmar, F., & Kruglyak, D. (2006). *Taking the Pulse of the Healthcare Blogosphere*. New York: Envision Solutions and the Medical Blog Network.

Lenhart, A. (2009). *Adults and social network websites*. Washington, DC: Pew Internet & American Life Project.

Lenhart, A., & Fox, S. (2006). *Bloggers*. Washington, DC: Pew Internet & American Life Project.

Lenhart, A., & Madden, M. (2007). *Teens, privacy & online social networks*. Washington, DC: Pew Internet & American Life Project.

Madden, M. (2007). *Online video*. Washington, DC: Pew Internet & American Life Project.

Madden, M. (2009). *The audience for online video-sharing sites shoots up*. Washington, DC: Pew Internet & American Life Project.

Meier, A., Lyons, E.J., Frydman, G., Forlenza, M., & Rimer, B. (2007). How cancer survivors provide support on cancer-related internet mailing lists. *Journal of Medical Internet Research, 9*(2).

O'Keefe, D.J. (1990). *Persuasion: Theory and research*. Thousand Oaks, CA: Sage.

Petty, R.E., & Cacioppo, J.T. (1986), The elaboration likelihood model of persuasion. In L. Berkowitz (Ed.), *Advances in experimental social psychology* (Vol. 19, pp. 123-205). New York: Academic Press.

Petty, R.E., Priester, J.R., & Brinol, P. (2002). Mass media attitude change: Implications of the elaboration likelihood model of persuasion. In J. Bryant & D. Zillman (Eds.), *Media effects: Advances in theory and research*. Mahwah, NJ: Erlbaum.

Pew Internet & American Life Project. Survey, December 2008

Rothschild, M.L. (1987). *Advertising: From fundamentals to strategies*. Lexington, MA: D.C. Heath.

Rutten, L.F., Moser, R.P., Beckjord, E.B., Hesse, B.W., & Croyle, R.T. (2007). *Cancer communication: Health Information National Trends Survey 2003 and 2005.* Washington, DC: National Cancer Institute. NIH Pub. No. 07-6214.

Sanbonmatsu, D.M., Posavac, S.S., Kardes, F.R., & Mantel, S. (1998). Selective hypothesis testing. *Psychonomic Bulletin and Review, 5*, 197-220.

Snyder, L.B., & Hamilton, M.A., (2002). A meta-analysis of US health campaign effects on behavior: Emphasize enforcement, exposure, and new information and beware the secular trend. In R.C. Hornik, (Ed.), *Public health communication: Evidence for behavior change*. Mahwah, NJ: Erlbaum.

Snyder, L.B., Hamilton, M.A., Mitchell, E.W., Kiwanuka-Tondo, J., Fleming-Milici, F., & Proctor, D. (2004). A meta-analysis of the effect of mediated health communication campaigns on behavior change in the United States. *Journal of Health Communication, 9*(Suppl. 1), 71-96.

Wikipedia. (2008). Web 2.0. http://en.wikipedia.org/wiki/Web_2.0

16

TAKING HINTS

Understanding Users Needs in Order to Achieve the Potential of Information Technology in Cancer Care Delivery

Stephen Hunt Taplin

Holly Massett

Sarah Lillie

Christy Mylks

National Cancer Institute

Health care in the United States is not achieving its potential (Committee on Quality Health Care, 2001; IOM, 1999). Although the United States spends more than $94 billion for biomedical research (Moses, Dorsey, Matheson, & Thier, 2005), and has the highest per capita expenditure on health care in the developed world, it has the lowest life expectancy at birth (Ginsburg, 2008), a relatively slow rate of decline in mortality from treatable conditions (Nolte & McKee, 2008), and patients get recommended therapies about half the time (Asch et al., 2006). This failure of our health care in general extends to cancer care specifically. A 1999 Institute of Medicine (IOM) report concluded that "for many Americans with cancer, there is a wide gulf between what could be construed as the ideal and the reality of their experience with cancer care" (p. 2). A key reason for this chasm in cancer care is our health care system; isolated providers operating within a fragmented network of offices, organizations, hospitals, and mechanisms of reimbursement (Bodenheimer, 2006; IOM, 1999). Successfully addressing this fragmentation and ensuring high-quality cancer care for those facing cancer concerns will require increasing communication throughout the health care system.

THREE PERSPECTIVES ON CANCER CARE NEEDS

Communication across the health care system is a particular challenge for cancer care: Multiple providers are involved in care across a continuum of needs from prevention and detection through diagnosis, treatment, survivorship, and end-of-life care (Zapka, Taplin, Solberg, & Manos, 2003). Figure 16.1 describes this continuum of care and highlights the problem that one patient needs to communicate with multiple providers at different stages of care across the continuum. Those providers, in turn, need to communicate with each other. The figure also demonstrates that it is the sum of these interactions and care that leads to reducing morbidity and mortality from cancer, so solving the communication issues of our fragmented system of health care is critical to delivering high-quality care (Zapka et al., 2003).

This continuum of cancer care occurs within a network of providers and reimbursement and implies at least three perspectives on what is needed to deliver cancer care: (a) that of individuals seeking cancer care; (b) that of providers offering cancer care; and (c) that of the "system" responsible for coordinating and reimbursing cancer care (Hesse & Shneiderman, 2007).

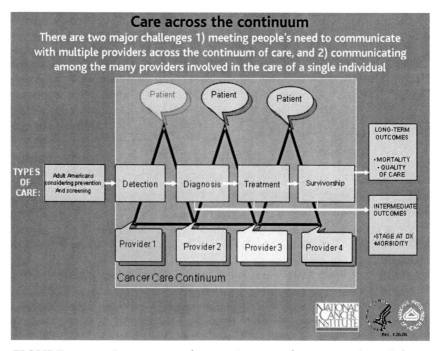

FIGURE 16.1. Care across the continuum of cancer (adapted from Zapka et al., 2003).

These three perspectives on cancer care reflect three different but overlapping worlds: the world of the general population who seeks a physician's care an average of four times per year but spends the vast majority of their time outside the health care system (Schappert & Burt, 2006), the medical world of providers concerned with improving an individual's health while dealing with multiple patients and an overwhelming amount of information; and the world of insurers, regulators, and administrators who manage the health care system. Each world sees the challenge of communication and improving cancer care from slightly different perspectives because each has different needs that must be met during the delivery of care. Patients need information about health, health risk, disease, an accurate accessible current health record, and help with scheduling appointments and completing follow-up plans. Providers need help managing their practice, and the ever-increasing amount of information relevant to their patients' health and disease. The system as a whole needs data to provide better service, monitor productivity, evaluate performance, and manage reimbursement (IOM et al., 1999, p. 8; Hazelwood, 2008). Table 16.1 presents a more detailed summary of potential functional needs across the cancer care continuum from each of these three perspectives.

There is no single information system that links these three worlds and meets all their respective needs. Traditionally, patients seek information through mass media, books, friends, and consultations with the physician. They use the telephone to schedule appointments and at times to access their providers for advice. Physicians typically record notes on paper; one study found physicians use paper more than 75% of the time (Wears & Berg, 2005). Physicians usually consult by telephone and correspond by letter. The only information technology that links patients, providers, and the system is for managing insurance status, claims submission, and reimbursement, not medical care.

TABLE 16.1. Potential Needs of Groups Across the Cancer Continuum

	PLACE IN THE CANCER CARE CONTINUUM				
	PREVENTION	DETECTION	DIAGNOSIS	TREATMENT	SURVIVORSHIP
INDIVIDUALS IN THE GENERAL POPULATION NEED . . .	**ACROSS THE CONTINUUM** • Easily scheduled health care appointments • Access health information appropriate to their stage in the continuum • Access a care plan appropriate to their stage in the continuum				
	• Track and easily access personal and family health history, including past screening results • Access understandable age-, gender-, and risk-appropriate prevention guidelines • Learn about healthy behaviors such as exercise, diet • Conduct personal risk assessment	• Store and access test results • Fully understand test results • Access information and resources to aid in decision making (medical, financial, coverage implications)	• Access comparative films • Access a repository for test results and their explanations • Access resources for explaining test result implications (medical, financial, coverage implications) • Transfer records, test results, and some tests • Find assistance with determining financial options	• Access recommendations on how to increase compliance/ treatment adherence • Find information on treatment choices: who, what, where, when • Find information on treatment and symptom management • Consult the treatment care plan for next steps • Access to information that supports their decision making	• Access to a plan regarding 'what to do now' and how to act on it successfully • Find information on how to move forward and focus on life quality • Understand survival expectations • Connect to survivor networks as needed

PROVIDERS OF CARE NEED TO …				
• Facilitate scheduling appointments (within primary care, at referral sites)	• Facilitate scheduling appointments (within primary care, at referral sites)	• Facilitate scheduling appointments (within primary care, at referral sites)	• Facilitate scheduling appointments (within primary care, at referral sites)	• Access a follow-up plan for coordinating care among several potential providers
• Use inreach reminders for age, gender, and risk-appropriate recommendations	• Report an accurate result	• receive results of all tests	• Link to other providers	• Facilitate acceptance of the patient's care and life options
• Access patient risk summaries	• Obtain patient history	• Report results and explanations to their patients	• Create a care plan	• Clarify the provider who is responsible for care and/or the health care problem at any point in time
• Quick access to family and patient history	• Document results	• Plan next steps for multiple individuals and document each	• Decide who is responsible for care	
• Use decision support regarding risk, referral	• Recommend next steps (who, what)	• Access treatment options	• Manage patient's expectations	
	• Use decision support	• Prepare patients for their tests and results	• Access information that supports their decision support	
	• Access a plan	• Educate the staff, patients, and themselves about evolving care		
	• Track completion of steps in the plan	• Access information that supports their decision process		

TABLE 16.1. Potential Needs of Groups Across the Cancer Continuum *(continued)*

| | PLACE IN THE CANCER CARE CONTINUUM | | | | |
	PREVENTION	DETECTION	DIAGNOSIS	TREATMENT	SURVIVORSHIP
SYSTEMS OF CARE NEED	ACROSS THE CONTINUUM - • Guidelines for care and metrics of quality • Tracking of individual care and rules for who is falling outside the guidelines • Accurate mailing and phone information for patients and providers • Financial tracking and management • Clarity regarding coverage and policies for patients and providers				
	• Management of outreach reminders and correspondence with patients • Monitoring of adherence to care recommendations • Measure care quality • Accurate patient summaries available to providers	• Assurance that communication has been initiated when appropriate • All test results and relevant information from referral sites • Facilitated information exchange and care hand off	• Plans for next steps in the care of individuals • Work with insurance • An easy to understand summary of diagnosis • Provide information on diagnosis	• Access to clinical trial information • Coordination of care among providers and patients • Compliance/treatment adherence	• Coordination of resources for long-term survivors • Coordinated care

- Facilitate referrals
- Ensure evidence-based guidelines used

- Tracking of referrals and adherence
- Facilitated next steps

- Veted educational information for patients that is easily accessible and understandable
- Provide notifications

- Give feedback to providers, patients, and patients' family
- Access to data

HEALTH INFORMATION TECHNOLOGY IS SEEN AS A POTENTIAL SOLUTION

Solutions that successfully address the competing communication and informational needs previously described are required in order to improve the cancer care in our country. Much hope rests on health information technology (health IT; Anderson, 2007; The White House, 2004). Health IT refers to the full range of information technology available in the health arena, including the Internet, e-mail, home telemedicine, personal health records (PHRs), and comprehensive electronic health record (EHR) systems (Blumenthal & Glaser, 2007; Tang, 2006). PHRs are accessed by individuals to enter and store their relevant medical history in an electronic format that can be transferred to their physician online or through a small card or flashdrive. EHRs are primarily accessed and controlled by the medical providers and staff. EHRs store information regarding the health of a subject of care to be processed by a computer, facilitating at least the following four functions:

1. recording health information and data,
2. managing test results,
3. managing the direct entry of pharmacy orders,
4. providing information to assist physicians with medical decisions (Blumenthal et al., 2006).

EHR systems are a foundational technology because their characteristics determine what functions can be met within an office and how the people in that office will be able to communicate with patients, other providers, and reimbursement agencies.

In 2004, President George Bush put forth a plan to improve the delivery of health care to all Americans by encouraging the adoption of EHR systems that would reduce medical errors and inefficiencies, facilitate coordination among health care providers, and ultimately improve patient outcomes (Transforming Health Care, 2004). The President's vision emphasized EHRs and called for ubiquitous health IT that allowed for communication among primary and specialty providers, pharmacists, and physicians; we emphasize EHRs, but recognize that additional health IT is important to improving people's health. It also is clear from a 2008 strategic plan to achieve the President's vision that it will take the substantial commitment of multiple groups to make progress (Office of the National Coordinator for Health Information Technology, 2008).

Two sources of information provide national estimates regarding progress toward the vision of ubiquitous health IT: The Health Information National Trends Survey (HINTS; Nelson et al., 2004), and the National Ambulatory Medical Care Survey (NAMCS; Hing, Burt, & Woodwell,

2007). HINTS focuses on how the general population obtains cancer information, and NAMCS includes the use of EHRs by physicians and hospitals. Both are rigorously designed to sample their respective target populations. Although they provide the best sources of national information regarding use of health IT and EHRs, they do not provide information on what users want. This is not necessarily a limitation of the studies, but a reality that users may not be able to anticipate what they want from a new technology until they have used it. Achieving the vision of ubiquitous interoperable health IT must therefore anticipate that progress will require iterations of success and failure as users gain experience with what exists in health IT and can better express what they need.

HINTS data do show that the general public is seeking health information through the Internet. This technology that existed for many years as an academic resource evolved tremendously during the 1990s into a tool available to commercial interests and the public (Hesse & Shneiderman, 2007). HINTS demonstrates that the Internet is growing more important to people who are seeking health information (Nelson et al., 2004; Rutten, Moser, Beckjord, Hesse, & Croyle, 2007). HINTS shows that 73% of Americans have access to the Internet and 52% used it to obtain health information in 2005 compared with 29% in 2003 (Rutten et al., 2007). Providers of care also have been quick to adopt the Internet for assistance with cancer care (Huang & Penson, 2008); physicians are able to find information on medical associations' Web sites, read journal articles, and easily follow the research of other physicians in their field. In a survey of physicians attending continuing education courses, 71% reported using the Internet regularly for medical and professional updating (Podichetty, Booher, Whitfield, & Biscup, 2006).

Although seeking information on the Internet is a function that the general population and providers may use independently, technologies that link the general population to their health care providers are important in health care delivery. HINTS does not provide information about these less widely-used systems. E-mail is a good example of a linking IT, but it is more eagerly accepted by the general population than by physicians. The general population thinks e-mail, in addition to the Internet, will potentially provide them with greater access to health care providers and oncology care (Katzen, Solan, & Dicker, 2005; Virji et al., 2006). One study looked at the feasibility of e-mail access to pediatricians during routine care over a 2-year period; 93% of families who were offered the service accepted it, and 37% used it (Rosen & Kwoh, 2007). The authors found that as a result of using the e-mail system, parents reported a better understanding of their child's medical tests, and physicians provided responses 57% faster than they did using the telephone. According to a 2001 Harris poll, 74% of people want to use e-mail to communicate directly with their physician, and 77% want e-mail reminders when they are due for a medical visit or some type of medical care

(Pizzi, 2007). E-mail appeals to the general population who want increased communication with medical providers.

In contrast, providers are much less eager to use e-mail because their time is not reimbursed even though they are providing care (Brooks & Menachemi, 2006; Eggert & Protti, 2006). In one random sample of 120 e-mails from 112 patients to 69 physicians through a PHR system, 22% had enough medical information to justify a medical encounter (Tang, Black, & Young, 2006). But even if the reimbursement issues were addressed, concerns are high enough about confidentiality and inappropriate advice that some have called for the FDA to establish regulations before e-mail is widely used (Brooks & Menachemi, 2006; Rannefeld, 2004). Communication among providers might also occur by e-mail, but security concerns exist there as well (Brooks & Menachemi, 2006; Rannefeld, 2004). It does not appear that e-mail will be quickly adopted by providers without addressing these concerns.

Another linking technology is the PHR system. Its lack of adoption demonstrates a general problem, that is, all linking technologies are influenced by medical providers' adoption of IT. PHR systems have been widely discussed, but not widely adopted (Tang, 2006). Although approximately 125 PHR products currently exist and 6 of 10 Americans support the creation of secure online PHRs (Markle Foundation, 2005), very few people (approximately 1%) use them (Steinbrook, 2008). Unlike Internet use that can operate independent of a provider, PHRs, scheduling appointments, and communicating medical advice require a connection to the activities of a medical provider's office and their EHR. The characteristics of the communication and record-keeping of that office will therefore influence the adoption of linking technologies by the general public. The problem is that providers are slowly adopting EHR systems (Brooks & Menachemi, 2006).

SLOW ADOPTION OF ELECTRONIC HEALTH RECORDS

Despite high optimism that EHR systems can improve the health care system in the United States, there seems to be a consistent story of unmet potential. EHR systems have been available for more than 40 years, since Lawrence Reed established the COSTAR system to replace paper records at a Boston health maintenance organization (Himmelstein & Woolhandler, 2005), and commercial versions of EHR systems have existed for more than 20 years (HIStalk, 2006). But by 2007 and 2008, a national survey of physicians found that only 4% were using fully functional EHR systems with the four characteristics described above (DesRoches, Campbell, & Sowmya, 2008). Between 13% and 25% of practices have adopted a rudimentary EHR system (Burt & Sisk, 2005; DesRoches, Campbell, & Sowmya, 2008; Hing et al., 2007; Shields et al., 2007; Simon, Rundall, & Shortell, 2005). Of physician practices with 10 or fewer providers, only 11.3% reported having rudimentary EHR systems, and these practices account for 88% of outpatient visits in the United States (Lee, Cain, Young, Chockley, & Burstin, 2005). A survey of practices in Massachusetts showed that only half of the practices had an interest in adopting EHR systems (Simon et al., 2008). In a comprehensive review of the literature of the impact of health information technology on quality, efficiency, and costs of medical care, only four organizations around the United States accounted for 25% of the reports (Chaudhry et al., 2006). Their reports showed the expected improvement in quality and efficiency, but the low levels of adoption suggest that few Americans reap the benefits (Chaudhry et al., 2006). For EHR systems to become a tool for quality improvement, the health field needs to better understand the conditions that would promote their use.

BARRIERS TO ADOPTION WITHIN THE DIFFUSION OF INNOVATION FRAMEWORK

The conditions to promote the diffusion of a new technology are described in Everett Rogers' (2003) classic Diffusion of Innovation framework. According to Rogers, an innovation is more likely to diffuse successfully and be adopted widely if it meets five major criteria: (a) relative advantage (it should be better than what it is expected to replace); (b) compatibility (it should be consistent with existing values, past experiences, and the needs of the potential user); (c) complexity (it should be easy to understand, implement, and use); (d) observability (other people should be able to easily see its results and value); and (e) trialability (there should be the capacity to test it on a limited basis). Although not all criteria are necessary for an innovation to diffuse, meeting them greatly influences the likelihood of successful adoption. Additionally, not all criteria are of equal weight; the first two (relative advantage, compatibility) are particularly important.

We already have discussed how the Internet is being adopted widely by the general population and physicians to gather information. In fact, it easily meets the requirements of a successful innovation according to the Diffusion of Innovations. For lay individuals and health care providers, the Internet has an easy advantage over books, articles, discussions with friends, and telephone or personal contact with colleagues and experts. The search engine, Google, provides a mechanism to quickly examine a complex array of topics and identify potentially relevant sources of information. There are lay and professional Web sites that can be accessed for in-depth information, support, and discussion. Information-seeking by people facing health challenges has been shown to be an effective way of coping with health challenges, and the Internet provides quick answers (Rutten et al., 2007). The ease of access to information is compatible with the values and needs of users. Although there is some complexity accessing the Internet, it is now available in libraries, and search engines simplify the task of finding relevant information. Internet access can be demonstrated and talked about with others, and once on the Internet, people can easily experiment with a variety of information sources and searches so it is observable and trialable. It is therefore not surprising that the Internet is being adopted widely by the general public and health care providers.

RELATIVE ADVANTAGE OF EHR ADOPTION

The story of adoption of EHR systems is different than it is for the Internet, and it is not occurring rapidly. At the root of the problem of EHR adoption is the different perspectives of the general population, providers, and the health care system as whole. The general population may recognize a relative advantage in EHR systems to the extent that they create new ways of accessing information and health care providers. A recent randomized trial of an automated laboratory test management system with imbedded patient notification of results showed increased patient satisfaction among those receiving electronic notification (Matheny et al., 2007). In another randomized trial, patients with hyperlipidemia were given one visit-independent e-mail in addition to their office visit and achieved better lipid control (Lester, Grant, Barnett, & Chueh, 2006). In a survey, oncology patients expressed a clear desire to access their physicians through e-mail for routine, but not emergent, care (Katzen et al., 2005). A summary conclusion by parents involved in a pediatric study was that e-mail "brings the doctor into our home" (Rosen et al., 2007).

The desire to bring the doctor into the home is consistent with the 2005 HINTS showing more people want to go to their physician first for cancer information compared with 2003 (23.5% vs. 11%) and a larger proportion of people saying their physician was their "preferred source of cancer information" (67.2% vs. 62.4%; Rutten et al., 2007). Although we have shown earlier that more people are using the Internet for health information, it appears to be reinforcing rather than detracting from the role of the physician. So, the question is whether the physicians and the health care system can accommodate the demand and use the opportunities that IT creates. Information technologies like e-mail and electronic scheduling replace the telephone in a novel way and open new means of communication. But in each case they are best used if there is an EHR that facilitates the scheduling, gathers specific data, and documents any communication with providers.

There is a clear relative advantage for IT from the perspective of patients, but whether EHR systems offer a relative advantage in communication and documentation over paper records is less clear for health care providers (Baron, Fabens, Schiffman, & Wolf, 2005; Blumenthal & Glaser, 2007; Wears & Berg, 2005). The paper record is simple, flexible, and completely reliable in the moment. With a paper record, providers can write notes, document their plans, and move on to the next patient. The paper record has worked for generations to take care of individual patients in the isolation of a physician's office, and it will continue to work for that narrow purpose. Despite the historic use of paper, there are many providers who recognize this record has problems, including often-missing critical information that affects the care of patients (Smith et al., 2005). Providers also recognize the potential for failure to follow-up after abnormal test results, and many are not satisfied with the current paper processes (Murff, 2003). So it is not surprising that there is evidence from a 2007 Internet survey, and a 2008 national survey, that health care providers identify two consistent motivators for adopting EHR systems: the need to improve clinical processes and workflow efficiency, and the potential to improve quality of care (DesRoches, Campbell, & Sowmya, 2008; Medical Records Institute, 2007).

Part of the motivation for EHR systems is that they may offer a way to do things paper records cannot do, such as assist with decisions and check medication interactions and dosages. Although there is evidence that computerized clinical decision-support systems improved physician decision making, the ones that worked best automatically prompted providers and were developed by the physicians themselves (Garg et al., 2005). Whether physicians in general should expect decision-support systems to help them is much less clear. In fact, 75% of information system projects in health care failed (Wears & Berg, 2005). Another study looking at computerized prescriber order entry suggested that these systems often facilitated medication errors (Koppel et al., 2005). Moving to EHR systems may not meet the expectations of improving decisions and medication administration without more work to improve their functioning.

There also are expectations that EHR systems will improve efficiencies within and between practices (Chaudhry et al., 2006). Efficiencies are defined as using fewer resources (laboratories, x-ray, hospital beds, etc.) for care and using less physician time. By either metric, EHR systems are associated with savings (Chaudhry et al., 2006). However, achieving these ends within a practice requires a change in the organization of the office and the activities of daily practice as much as the adoption of EHR systems (Blumenthal & Glaser, 2007). One effort to improve cancer screening showed how providers needed to consider and redesign the flow of patients through their office, the delegation of tasks, and the communication among the participants in care (Taplin, Galvin, Payne, Coole, & Wagner, 1998).

Simply implementing an information system will not be adequate to achieve efficiencies within a practice.

Just as achieving efficiencies within a practice requires redesigning fundamental interactions, so does achieving efficiencies across organizations. But even before those issues are addressed, there are imposing technical problems. Current EHR systems rarely communicate across offices or institutions, and the standards to achieve this level of communication have not been realized (Anderson, 2007; Hamm, Knoop, Schwarz, Block, & Davis, 2007; Hayrinen, Saranto, & Nykanen, 2008; Jian et al., 2007; Vishwanath & Scamurra, 2007). One effort to create 145 communities with a standard information infrastructure that allows for communication across institutions has been floundering because of the complexity of achieving standards and maintaining funding from participating institutions (Adler-Milstein, McAfee, Bates, & Jha, 2008). It is not obvious that adoption of an EHR system is going to improve efficiency between practices either.

Finally, even if efficiencies and improved decision support could be achieved, there is a large start-up cost that must borne by the providers being asked to implement EHR systems and this barrier must be overcome (Anderson, 2007; Baron, 2007; Vishwanath & Scamurra, 2007; Wears & Berg, 2005). Implementing an EHR system costs about $32,000 per full time equivalent (FTE) physician, and about $1,500 per physician per month for maintenance (Gans, Kralewski, Hammons, & Dowd, 2005). One researcher noted that one of the least appreciated but most important barriers among physicians for adopting an EHR system is the cost–benefit tradeoff for making the transition from paper to automation (Vishwanath & Scamurra, 2007). The potential for negative as well as positive consequences, and the huge costs leave clinicians uncertain whether they want to pay the price to achieve the touted advantages of EHR systems (Blumenthal et al., 2006).

Organized systems of care, insurance companies, and society as a whole are more likely to see the relative advantage and adopt EHR systems, because such systems could meet their needs for aggregate information on costs and for large-scale tracking and improvement to quality of care (Blumenthal & Glaser, 2007; IOM, 1999). The federal government is encouraging the adoption of health information technology through a program testing performance-based reimbursement and information technology incentives (Hazelwood, 2008). But the adoption of EHR systems and information technology that go beyond reimbursement tracking is now becoming a more important priority (Office of the National Coordinator for Health Information Technology, 2008). It is clear from the societal perspective that we need to control costs and achieve the potential of our health care knowledge (The White House, 2004). The federal strategic plan for health IT includes language emphasizing the establishment of standards and mechanisms to exchange population health information and to export it to organizations and agencies (Office of the National Coordinator for

Health Information Technology, 2008, p. 32). From the systems' perspective, an IT structure that allows the monitoring of reimbursement and quality has a relative advantage over the current system that primarily manages reimbursement.

COMPATIBILITY OF EHR ADOPTION

Perspective also matters in compatibility (an innovation's consistency with existing values and preferences), and again the providers have a view less amenable to EHR adoption. The general population wants personalized information and independence; access to health information and their health care providers through the Internet provides both. In a randomized trial of general versus personalized information, cancer patients preferred information about their own laboratory results over general information about cancer (Jones et al., 1999). Internet Web sites that link patients to providers also are valued, and may be especially important to people who have difficulty reaching or communicating with their physicians (Zickmund et al., 2008).

Physicians are concerned about the practical aspects of EHR implementation, including maintenance and the need to continue caring for their patients. The values of physicians were demonstrated in a concept-mapping exercise with 58 physicians invited to attend a seminar on health information sponsored by the Buffalo Academy of Medicine (Vishwanath & Scamurra, 2007). Their concerns included five major areas:

1. customization (inability to make the EHR do what the physician wanted),
2. costs (costs of software but also cost of conversion, maintenance, and interface with legacy systems),
3. logistics (lack of national standards for EHRs) and regulatory concerns,
4. return on investment (lost practice time during conversion and when the EHR breaks down), and
5. integration (lack of support staff for the EHR system, loss of productive time) (Vishwanath & Scamurra, 2007).

All these values put EHRs in a negative light from the perspective of providers.

Leaders within systems value the ability to monitor care and reimbursement. Managed care organizations have been leaders with respect to the implementation of EHR and PHR systems because they perceive the potential to improve care and reduce costs of care (Wallace, 2007). A Medicare project has a similar incentive (Hazelwood, 2008). President Bush's EHR initiative reflects the perception that the system as a whole will benefit. The challenge of EHR adoption that systems face is that most patients are seen by physicians in small practices, who demonstrate the concerns expressed in Buffalo (Wears et al., 2005). Furthermore, these concerns are only part of the challenge because nurses have critical needs that also affect adoption. Leaders must listen to the needs of all providers who they are asking to adopt EHRs (Geibert, 2006).

COMPLEXITY, OBSERVABILITY, TRIALABILITY OF EHR ADOPTION

Although EHR systems have advantages for the health care system as a whole and for the general public frustrated with its access to providers, there are severe barriers from the standpoint of providers regarding relative advantage and compatibility. These barriers alone could explain the slow adoption of EHRs, but when Rogers' remaining three criteria are examined further, barriers to the adoption of EHRs emerge. The general public and systems may continue to have different perspectives on these three issues, but this review suggests that the major barriers to adoption grow out of the perspective of the providers. These provider barriers also are seen when considering complexity, observability, and trialability.

The complexity of using an EHR system with data-entry standards and layers of information present one of those barriers (Anderson, 2007; Baron et al., 2005; Smith & Haque, 2006). Clean white space on paper that is almost always available is simple, and its replacement with EHR systems that break down, aren't interoperable with other systems, and will have a long learning curve, present a complex alternative (Baron et al., 2005; Chaudhry et al., 2006). Another barrier is that it is difficult to observe the success of others who have adopted EHR systems. One major systematic review of health information technology found that the benchmark institutions for health information technology all used internally developed systems that are therefore not available to others (Chaudhry et al., 2006). The report also makes the explicit point that there is little evidence about how to make the transition from paper to EHR systems even if one is available (Chaudhry et al., 2006). Care providers don't have the opportunity to see success of EHR adoption and, in fact, consistently hear about the challenges (Hartzband, 2008; Wears & Berg, 2005). Finally, the ability to test an innovation in a limited way is typically not possible with information systems. The cost of adoption is huge, and it is not surprising that providers are skeptical of purchasing an EHR system that might become obsolete, that cannot "do it all," and that cannot be returned (Anderson, 2007; Vishwanath & Scamurra, 2007).

TRANSLATING NEEDS INTO EFFECTIVE HEALTH INFORMATION TECHNOLOGY SYSTEMS

From the standpoint of the Diffusion of Innovations, it is clear that information technology has potential to improve care while facing some major barriers to adoption. Using EHR systems as an example, there is no doubt that providers recognize the limitation of the paper record and that EHRs could help individuals, providers, and health care organizations in the cancer care continuum (Chaudhry et al., 2006; Murff, 2003; Smith & Haque, 2006). Regardless of the limitations, EHR systems use is increasing, and even those who note the pitfalls report they would not go back to paper (Baron, 2007). The question now is how to ensure that when diffusion is complete, it achieves the ends of improving the health care of the nation (Hesse & Shneiderman, 2007).

We suggest that until EHR systems are specifically built around the needs, culture, and workflow of the general public and health care providers, they will struggle to meet Rogers' requirements for adoption and diffusion, and will struggle to be a tool for improving health care. There is no easy way forward. Financial incentives, concerns about regulation, and establishing standards for interoperability must all be addressed to see that EHR adoption is compatible with the values of providers. But beyond these primary barriers, the relative advantage and workflow compatibility of EHR systems must become more apparent, and their complexity reduced, for all intended users (the general population and providers, not just the larger system).

One way to make progress in addressing these factors critical to diffusion of EHR systems is to encourage health information technology developers to include user-centered design (UCD) methods in their EHR development processes. As described below, these methods are targeted at uncovering, understanding, and accommodating technology users' needs and the realities of their usage situations.

USER CENTERED DESIGN PRINCIPLES

UCD (also called human-centered design) is a formal methodology for gathering information from a technology's intended users about actual usage and users' needs and preferences throughout the design and development process (Norman & Draper, 1986; Mao, Vredenburg, Smith, & Carey, 2005). UCD includes both conducting research to gain insight into users' needs, workflow, communication patterns, and sociocultural environment, and accounting for them in the design. Better understanding of users' needs, workflow, and work cultures is a win for both health IT users and the developers if all the users' (the general population, providers, and the system) perspectives are considered and affect the design. That way the product is better and implementation goes faster. UCD also includes letting users test and evaluate the resulting designs to be sure they address those needs before developing the final product. In this manner, UCD can help improve the adoptability of health information technology systems in three main ways:

1. Providing reality-based insights into the settings and people the technology will serve.
2. Incorporating these insights into existing design and development processes and evaluating the resulting designs with users in time to make changes.
3. Providing a way for designers and stakeholders (such as clinicians consulting on a technology project) to understand and learn both what is needed and what is possible.

The recent strategic planning document to achieve the 2004 health informatics initiative emphasizes establishing "mechanisms for multi-stakeholder priority-setting and decision-making" (Office of the National Coordinator for Health Information Technology, 2008). This is an important acknowledgment of the perspectives outlined here, but we are suggesting that to actually provide the data for the decisions that will be made, attention needs to be paid to methods of identifying how information technology will be used by care providers now and in the future.

It has been noted that surveys provide an important starting point for understanding the use of information technology, and we have used the two national surveys specifically designed to track its use (Hing et al., 2007; Nelson et al., 2004). But surveys alone will not achieve better EHR systems, because self-reported needs and behavior are notoriously unreliable (Wears & Berg, 2005). The advantage of UCD is that it focuses on what people actually do, rather than what they say they do; this knowledge is a key to understanding how to design for complex situations such as health care. Because health care involves many people and roles and includes communications and cultural mores, it takes trained observers and interviewers to understand them. It has been said that at a high level, health information technology systems fail because they reflect a naïve model of how health care actually takes place (Nemeth, Feifer, Stuart, & Ornstein, 2008). By focusing on observing end-users doing work in real settings and having them test-drive design prototypes, UCD also provides insights into the many unconscious subtasks being performed throughout the day. Rounding out information technology developers' lists of requirements with UCD methods provides rich information, including information users cannot describe about themselves and their work culture because it is automatic or intuitive to them.

UCD follows an iterative process; in this way UCD could address relative advantage, complexity, trialability, observability, and some aspects of compatibility. UCD allows developers and users to refine a design concept and get input from users until it reduces complexity for those using the system and demonstrates an observable relative advantage. Once designers incorporate the needs identified by UCD methods into their processes and use it to create designs, design prototypes can be evaluated by the method of onsite usability testing with real users, addressing the trialability of a system. Finally, the crucial interaction between health information technology users and information technology developers allows them to understand each other's jargon, information requests, and technical capabilities. Applying UCD evaluation methods with design prototypes will help developers get information based on users trying out the system to complete realistic tasks; the realistic usage can likewise prompt users to consider new possibilities now that they can visualize what an EHR is and what it can do. There is, therefore, a need to recognize that EHR systems will go through several cycles as users see what is being offered and express what they want.

THE CHALLENGE IS PUTTING UCD INTO PRACTICE

UCD may offer a way forward through the development of EHR systems that address issues relevant to the Diffusion of Innovations, but this design process is dependent on data and observation. This is challenging in a world where practices are spread throughout the United States, and vendors are selling specific products with a standard design to people implementing them in different locations and times. The dispersed implementation means that no single purchaser can necessarily influence the basic underlying design, and the vendors are not compelled or inspired to accommodate changes that may well reflect fundamental needs in practice. The vendors have no way of distinguishing among idiosyncratic requests and ones that reflect a need for current or future practice so there may be a tendency to be inflexible. It is no accident that the most successful EHR systems have been developed by the organizations using them (Chaudhry et al., 2006). But we are moving into a period of commercial EHRs. The challenge is to develop EHR systems that provide some local flexibility while basing fundamental designs on systematic research and pooled observations of what users need. This is likely to take a considerable amount of time and expense unless those promoting adoption can identify ways of creating small pilots and tests that provide quick responses on small aspects of a system.

Designers need to watch people using EHR systems, and users need to talk with designers about their needs. We can learn from HINTS, but we need more information from users to address the design issues that will give

EHR systems a relative advantage. That also requires better information about what care providers need, and how their needs can be met during the transition from paper to EHR systems. As more EHR systems are implemented across the country, there may be more opportunity for observation and more information about how the transitions are made most efficiently. Unfortunately, more evidence about what is needed and how providers use EHR systems does not mean design will be improved. We also need a national forum for interaction between users and designers so that the systematic observations influence design. The eHealth Initiative that convenes affected parties offers one such private forum. The new strategic plan for EHR adoption could offer another if its governance body of all the stakeholders in health care delivery can offer a means to encourage the incorporation of evolving health care needs into EHR designs (Office of the National Coordinator for Health Information Technology, 2008).

CONCLUSION

There are tremendous expectations that health information technology is the critical tool for closing the gap between what is known and what is practiced. Despite those expectations, adoption of certain health information technology, such as EHR systems, has been slow. In this review we argue that the successful adoption of information technology will require physicians' support and an understanding of the common needs of all users including patients, providers, administrators, and leaders in the system. Many physicians see the limitations in the current paper record and want to improve quality; there is a need to facilitate rather than force their transition to information technology because these physicians are still caring for the nation. The push to adopt EHR systems is asking providers to do what one anonymous physician said was comparable to redesigning an airplane while it is in flight. Care needs to be taken so that we do it right.

We are suggesting that a user-centered approach that includes both people seeking health care and providers delivering health care is going to be critical to the development of EHR systems that will be adopted and used to successfully improve cancer care. This UCD process begins with surveys like HINTS that enable understanding of current use. But then systematic observation, discussion, and an iterative process of small improvements and prototypes are needed well before systems are fully developed. In this way, UCD could address relative advantage, complexity, trialability, observability, and some aspects of compatibility, and may get us closer to an EHR system that is adopted and therefore can contribute to improvements in the quality of health care.

ACKNOWLEDGMENT

This work represents the opinion of the authors and cannot be construed to reflect the views of the National Cancer Institute or the federal government.

REFERENCES

Adler-Milstein, J., McAfee, A. P., Bates, D. W., & Jha, A. K. (2008). The state of regional health information organizations: Current activities and financing. *Health Affairs, 27,* w60-w69.

Anderson, J. G. (2007). Social, ethical and legal barriers to e-health. *International Journal of Medical Informatics, 76,* 480-483.

Asch, S. M., Kerr, E. A., Keesey, J., Adams, J. L., Setodji, C. M., Malik, S. et al. (2006). Who is at greatest risk for receiving poor-quality health care? *New England Journal of Medicine, 354,* 1147-1156.

Baron, R. J. (2007). Quality improvement with an electronic health record: Achievable, but not automatic. *Annals of Internal Medicine, 147,* 549-552.

Baron, R. J., Fabens, E. L., Schiffman, M., & Wolf, E. (2005). Electronic health records: Just around the corner? Or over the cliff? *Annals of Internal Medicine, 143,* 222-226.

Blumenthal, D., DesRoches, C., Donelan, K., Ferris, T., Jha, A., Kaushal, R. et al. (2006). *Health information in the United States: The information base for progress.* Robert Wood Johnson Foundation.

Blumenthal, D., & Glaser, J. P. (2007). Information technology comes to medicine. *New England Journal of Medicine, 356,* 2527-2534.

Bodenheimer, T. (2006). Primary care—will it survive? *New England Journal of Medicine, 355,* 861-864.

Brooks, R. G., & Menachemi, N. (2006). Physicians' use of email with patients: Factors influencing electronic communication and adherence to best practices. *Journal of Medical Internet Research, 8,* e2.

Burt, C. W., & Sisk, J. E. (2005). Which physicians and practices are using electronic medical records? Survey data show limited use of these information tools. *Health Affairs, 24,* 1334-1343.

Chaudhry, B., Wang, J., Wu, S., Maglione, M., Mojica, W., Roth, E. et al. (2006). Systematic review: Impact of health information technology on quality, efficiency, and costs of medical care. *Annals of Internal Medicine, 144,* 742-752.

Committee on Quality Health Care In America, & Institute of Medicine (2001). *Crossing the quality chasm: A new health system for the 21st century.* Washington, DC: National Academy Press.

DesRoches, C.M., Campbell, E.G., Sowmya, R.R., Donelan, K., Levy D.E., Rosenbaum S. et al (2008). Electronic health records in ambulatory care—A national survey of physicians. *NEJM, 359,* 50-60.

Eggert, C., & Protti, D. (2006). Clinical electronic communications: A new paradigm that is here to stay? *Healthcare Quarterly, 9,* 88-96.

Gans, D., Kralewski, J., Hammons, T., & Dowd, B. (2005). Medical groups' adoption of electronic health records and information systems. *Health Affairs, 24*, 1323-1333.

Garg, A. X., Adhikari, N. K., McDonald, H., Rosas-Arellano, M. P., Devereaux, P. J., Beyene, J. et al. (2005). Effects of computerized clinical decision support systems on practitioner performance and patient outcomes: A systematic review. *Journal of the American Medical Association, 293*, 1223-1238.

Geibert, R. C. (2006). Using diffusion of innovation concepts to enhance implementation of an electronic health record to support evidence-based practice. *Nursing Administration Quarterly, 30*, 203-210.

Ginsburg, J. A. (2008). Achieving a high-performance health care system with universal access: What the United States can learn from other countries. *Annals of Internal Medicine, 148*, 55-75.

Hamm, R. A., Knoop, S. E., Schwarz, P., Block, A. D., & Davis, W. L. (2007). Harmonizing clinical terminologies: Driving interoperability in healthcare. *Medinfo, 12*, 660-663.

Hartzband, P. (2008). Off the record—avoiding the pitfalls of going electronic. *New England Journal of Medicine, 358*, 1656-1658.

Hayrinen, K., Saranto, K., & Nykanen, P. (2008). Definition, structure, content, use and impacts of electronic health records: A review of the research literature. *International Journal of Medical Informatics, 77*, 291-304.

Hazelwood, A. (2008). Improving quality of health care through pay-for-performance programs. *The Health Care Manager, 27*, 104-112.

Hesse, B. W., & Shneiderman, B. (2007). eHealth research from the user's perspective. *American Journal of Preventive Medicine, 32*, S97-103.

Himmelstein, D. U., & Woolhandler, S. (2005). Hope and hype: Predicting the impact of electronic medical records. *Health Affairs, 24*, 1121-1123.

Hing, E. S., Burt, C. W., & Woodwell, D. A. (2007). Electronic medical record use by office-based physicians and their practices: United States, 2006. *Advance Data*, 1-7.

HIStalk. (2006). *An exclusive interview with Andy Ury, President and CEO of Practice Partner*. Retrieved June 2, 2008, from http://histalk.blog-city.com/an_exclusive_interview_with_andy_ury_president_and_ceo_of_pr.htm

Huang, G. J., & Penson, D. F. (2008). Internet health resources and the cancer patient. *Cancer Investigation, 26*, 202-207.

Institute of Medicine, & Commission on Life Sciences National Research Council. (1999). *Ensuring quality cancer care*. Washington, DC: National Academy Press.

Jian, W. S., Hsu, C. Y., Hao, T. H., Wen, H. C., Hsu, M. H., Lee, Y. L. et al. (2007). Building a portable data and information interoperability infrastructure-framework for a standard Taiwan electronic medical record template. *Computer Methods and Programs in Biomedicine, 88*, 102-111.

Jones, R., Pearson, J., McGregor, S., Cawsey, A. J., Barrett, A., Craig, N. et al. (1999). Randomised trial of personalised computer based information for cancer patients. *British Medical Journal, 319*, 1241-1247.

Katzen, C., Solan, M. J., & Dicker, A. P. (2005). E-mail and oncology: A survey of radiation oncology patients and their attitudes to a new generation of health communication. *Prostate Cancer and Prostatic Diseases, 8*, 189-193.

Koppel, R., Metlay, J. P., Cohen, A., Abaluck, B., Localio, A. R., Kimmel, S. E. et al. (2005). Role of computerized physician order entry systems in facilitating medication errors. *Journal of the American Medical Association, 293,* 1197-1203.

Lee, J., Cain, C., Young, S., Chockley, N., & Burstin, H. (2005). The adoption gap: Health information technology in small physician practices. Understanding office workflow can help realize the promise of technology. *Health Affairs, 24,* 1364-1366.

Lester, W. T., Grant, R. W., Barnett, G. O., & Chueh, H. C. (2006). Randomized controlled trial of an informatics-based intervention to increase statin prescription for secondary prevention of coronary disease. *Journal of General Internal Medicine, 21,* 22-29.

Mao, J. Y., Vredenburg, K., Smith, P. W., & Carey, T. (2005). The state of user-centered design practice. *Communications of the ACM, 48,* 105-109.

Markle Foundation. (2005). *Attitudes of Americans regarding personal health records and nationwide electronic health information exchange.* Retrieved May 20, 2008, from http://www.markle.org/downloadable_assets/research_release_101105.pdf

Matheny, M. E., Gandhi, T. K., Orav, E. J., Ladak-Merchant, Z., Bates, D. W., Kuperman, G. J. et al. (2007). Impact of an automated test results management system on patients' satisfaction about test result communication. *Archives of Internal Medicine, 167,* 2233-2239.

Moses, H., III, Dorsey, E. R., Matheson, D. H., & Thier, S. O. (2005). Financial anatomy of biomedical research. *Journal of the American Medical Association, 294,* 1333-1342.

MRInstitute. (2007). *Medical Record Institute's Ninth Annual Survey of Electronic Medical Records Trends and Usage 2007.* Retrieved June 2, 2008, from http://www.medrecinst.com/MRI/emrsurvey.html

Murff, H. J. (2003). Primary care physician attitudes concerning follow-up of abnormal test results and ambulatory decision support systems. *International Journal of Medical Informatics, 71,* 137-149.

Nelson, D. E., Kreps, G. L., Hesse, B. W., Croyle, R. T., Willis, G., Arora, N. K. et al. (2004). The Health Information National Trends Survey (HINTS): Development, design, and dissemination. *Journal of Health Communication, 9,* 443-460.

Nemeth, L. S., Feifer, C., Stuart, G. W., & Ornstein, S. M. (2008). Implementing change in primary care practices using electronic medical records: A conceptual framework. *Implementation Science, 3,* 3.

Nolte, E., & McKee, C. M. (2008). Measuring the health of nations: Updating an earlier analysis. *Health Affairs, 27,* 58-71.

Norman, D. A., & Draper, S. W. (1986). *User-centered design: New perspectives on human-computer interaction.* Hillsdale, NJ: Lawrence Erlbaum Associates.

Office of the National Coordinator for Health Information Technology. (2008). *The ONC-coordinated Federal Health IT Strategic Plan: 2008-2012.* Washington, DC: U.S. Department of Health and Human Services.

Pizzi, R. (2007). *Telehealth market to expand, report claims.* Retrieved May 15, 2008, from http://www.healthcareitnews.com/story.cms?id=7705

Podichetty, V. K., Booher, J., Whitfield, M., & Biscup, R. S. (2006). Assessment of internet use and effects among healthcare professionals: A cross sectional survey. *Postgraduate Medical Journal, 82,* 274-279.

Rannefeld, L. (2004). The doctor will e-mail you now: Physicians' use of telemedicine to treat patients over the Internet. *Journal of Law and Health, 19,* 75-105.

Rogers, E. M. (2003). *Diffusion of innovations* (5th ed.). New York: Free Press.

Rosen, P., & Kwoh, C. K. (2007). Patient-physician e-mail: An opportunity to transform pediatric health care delivery. *Pediatrics, 120,* 701-706.

Rutten, L. F., Moser, R. P., Beckjord, E. B., Hesse, B. W., & Croyle, R. T. (2007). *Cancer Communication: Health Information National Trends Survey* (Rep. No. NIH Pub No. 07-6214). Washington, DC: National Cancer Institute.

Schappert, S. M., & Burt, C. W. (2006). Ambulatory care visits to physician offices, hospital outpatient departments, and emergency departments: United States, 2001-02. *Vital and Health Statistics Series, 13,* 1-66.

Shields, A. E., Shin, P., Leu, M. G., Levy, D. E., Betancourt, R. M., Hawkins, D. et al. (2007). Adoption of health information technology in community health centers: Results of a national survey. *Health Affairs, 26,* 1373-1383.

Simon, J. S., Rundall, T. G., & Shortell, S. M. (2005). Drivers of electronic medical record adoption among medical groups. *Joint Commission Journal on Quality and Patient Safety, 31,* 631-639.

Simon, S. R., McCarthy, M. L., Kaushal, R., Jenter, C. A., Volk, L. A., Poon, E. G. et al. (2008). Electronic health records: Which practices have them, and how are clinicians using them? *Journal of Evaluation in Clinical Practice, 14,* 43-47.

Smith, C. A., & Haque, S. N. (2006). Paper versus electronic documentation in complex chronic illness: A comparison. *AMIA. Annual Symposium Proceedings,* 734-738.

Smith, P. C., Araya-Guerra, R., Bublitz, C., Parnes, B., Dickinson, L. M., Van Vorst, R. et al. (2005). Missing clinical information during primary care visits. *Journal of the American Medical Association, 293,* 565-571.

Steinbrook, R. (2008). Personally controlled online health data—the next big thing in medical care? *New England Journal of Medicine, 358,* 1653-1656.

Tang, P. C. (2006). Personal health records: Definitions, benefits, and strategies for overcoming barriers to adoption. *Journal of the American Medical Informatics Association, 13,* 121-126.

Tang, P. C., Black, W., & Young, C. Y. (2006). Proposed criteria for reimbursing eVisits: Content analysis of secure patient messages in a personal health record system. *AMIA. Annual Symposium Proceedings,* 764-768.

Taplin, S. H., Galvin, M. S., Payne, T., Coole, D., & Wagner, E. (1998). Putting population-based care into practice: Real option or rhetoric? *The Journal of the American Board of Family Practice, 11,* 116-126.

The White House (2004). *Promoting innovation and competitiveness—transforming health care: The President's health information technology plan.* Washington, DC: The White House.

Virji, A., Yarnall, K. S., Krause, K. M., Pollak, K. I., Scannell, M. A., Gradison, M. et al. (2006). Use of email in a family practice setting: Opportunities and challenges in patient- and physician-initiated communication. *BMC Medicine, 4,* 18.

Vishwanath, A., & Scamurra, S. D. (2007). Barriers to the adoption of electronic health records: Using concept mapping to develop a comprehensive empirical model. *Health Informatics Journal, 13,* 119-134.

Wallace, P. J. (2007). Reshaping cancer learning through the use of health information technology. *Health Affairs, 26,* w169-w177.

Wears, R. L., & Berg, M. (2005). Computer technology and clinical work: Still waiting for Godot. *Journal of the American Medical Association, 293,* 1261-1263.

Zapka, J. G., Taplin, S. H., Solberg, L. I., & Manos, M. M. (2003). A framework for improving the quality of cancer care: The case of breast and cervical cancer screening. *Cancer Epidemiology, Biomarkers & Prevention, 12,* 4-13.

Zickmund, S. L., Hess, R., Bryce, C. L., McTigue, K., Olshansky, E., Fitzgerald, K. et al. (2008). Interest in the use of computerized patient portals: Role of the provider-patient relationship. *Journal of General Internal Medicine, 23*(Suppl 1), 20-26.

17

FROM SICK CARE TO HEALTH CARE

The Transformative Effect of the Health Information Revolution

Linsey Volckmann
Keas, Inc.

Lila J. Finney Rutten
National Institute of Health

Bradford W. Hesse
National Institute of Health

BACKGROUND

One of the purposes of implementing a biennial survey as an evidence base in health communication is to monitor changes in populations as they are influenced by structural alterations in the information environment over time. The Behavioral Risk Factors Surveillance System (BRFSS), conducted by the Centers for Disease Control and Prevention (CDC), offers a prime example of how subtle changes in behavior can lead to epidemic health problems when plotted over years of administration. The BRFSS is an ongoing surveillance program funded by the CDC to combine state-level population estimates of self-reported health behavior into a portrayal of national patterns of risk (CDC, 2006). In the 1980s, the BRFSS began including questions related to height and weight from which analysts could construct a body mass index (BMI). Figure 17.1 portrays patterns for the self-reported BMI for states included in the BRFSS assessment from 1985 to 2004 (CDC, 2007b).

What the BRFSS maps make explicit is how a shift in American culture, undoubtedly influenced by communication media and advertising (Johnson-Taylor, Yaroch, Krebs-Smith, & Rodgers, 2007), can lead to shifts

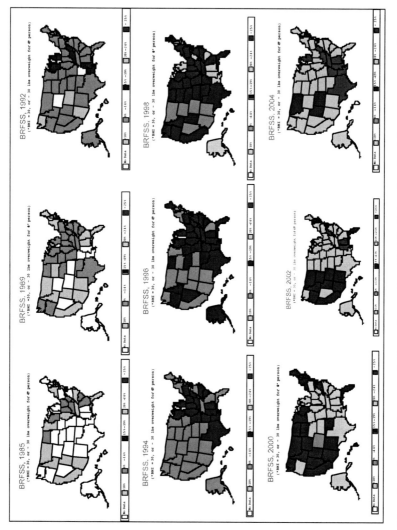

FIGURE 17.1. Mapping the obesity trend: Data from the CDC's Behavioral Risk Factor Surveillance System (BRFSS) illustrating how self-reported body mass index (BMI) increased nationally from 1985 to 2004.

in behavior and ultimately to physical health. The so-called obesity epidemic alone will begin claiming untold lives and will consume an increasingly large part of individuals' health care dollars in the future if left unchecked (President's Cancer Panel, 2007). The recurring population survey was an important tool in the public health professional's armamentarium because it collected the necessary data to chart the course of a chronic disease epidemic over time. It made explicit what nutritional and media experts had suspected for years. In short, it served as a type of "macroscope" (Litt, Tran, & Burke, 2002) for population scientists, allowing them to explore the influences of structural transformations on the beliefs, behaviors, and capacities of individual Americans working in the "real world" and their ability to thrive and survive.

In this chapter, we look at how other changes in the health information environment could be utilized to improve individual and population health. The implications of these changes, we believe, can help guide the focus of the Health Information National Trends Survey (HINTS) macroscope in the coming years.

FROM SICK CARE TO HEALTH CARE

As many health-systems researchers lament, a reactionary health care system focused myopically on treatment alone can fail to keep the population truly healthy. The prevalence of obesity is but one, of many, striking examples: In the United States obesity has reached epidemic proportions with dramatic increases in the prevalence of overweight and obese adults and children. Among adults aged 20 to 74 years the prevalence of obesity increased from 15% (in the 1976–1980 National Health and Nutrition Examination Survey [NHNES]) to 32.9% (in the 2003–2004 NHNES). Similar increases have been observed among children and teens. These trends are of public health concern because being overweight or obese increases the risk of several diseases including hypertension, dyslipidemia, type 2 diabetes, cardiovascular disease, gallbladder disease, osteoarthritis, and certain cancers. Despite national health objectives for the year 2010 aimed at reducing the prevalence of obesity to less than 15%, available data suggests that the situation is worsening.

The current health care system in the United States is heavily focused on treating disease rather than promoting health (Gebbie, Rosenstock, & Hernandez, 2003). This architecture is based on episodic crisis care, rather than on lifetime health management. As a result, care tends to be fragmented, generic, confusing, and ineffective. The focus on treatment over prevention overwhelms care capacity causing frustration levels to rise among both patients and their providers, leading to the deterioration of individual health and escalating costs. Health care costs for treating preventable diseases currently account for 70% of total health care spending, and total health care spending now constitutes nearly 16% of the U.S. gross domestic product (GDP). Furthermore, U.S. health care spending is expected to increase at similar or higher rates over the next decade, reaching roughly $4 trillion by 2015, representing 20% of the nation's GDP (Borger et al., 2006).

These data illustrate the tremendous toll, both in human lives and financial capital, of poor health behaviors and chronic disease, and of a poor health system that is failing to deliver the necessary tools and services required to keep people healthy and manage illness. Initiatives focused on behavior modification, and the development of effective, evidence-based tools and services that can reduce or prevent harmful behaviors, are crucial for improving the nation's health, and lowering health care costs.

ENGINEERING SUPPORT FOR HEALTHY BEHAVIOR

Much of population health is determined by people's behavior (Institute of Medicine [U.S.], 2001). Using the case of cancer alone, estimates suggest that as much as 50% to 70% of current cancer deaths could be eliminated through changes in lifestyle (i.e., through smoking cessation, improved diet and exercise, and staying current with screening recommendations; President's Cancer Panel, 2007). Yet, despite an increased understanding of the prominent role of behavior and lifestyle choices in health outcomes and advances in behavioral research, more than 500,000 Americans will lose their battle with cancer this year, and roughly 1.5 million will be diagnosed (American Cancer Society, 2008). The enormity of this type of disease burden necessitates the identification of new ways to reach consumers with targeted, scientifically driven messages and evidence-based behavioral interventions. Innovative channels must be identified to speed the delivery and increase the scalability of scientific research and evidence-based interventions.

Advances in information technology offer the promise of health tools and services that can speed the delivery, increase the scale and scope, and improve the effectiveness and efficiency of evidence-based health information and behavioral research (Atienza et al., 2007; Hesse, 2005). Across the continuum from health to illness and death, health information technology is becoming a central component of high-quality health care, working behind the scenes to improve the experience that health care consumers have (Brailer, 2005). It can play a role in raising awareness of health risks and solutions, engage consumers by providing the motivation and skills needed to reduce health risks, help individuals find support from other people in similar situations, affect or reinforce attitudes and risk perceptions, and enable the consumer to self-manage his or her own care (Eysenbach, 2001; Ferguson, 2000; Gustafson, Brennan, & Hawkins, 2007).

This chapter highlights noted trends in the application of information technology to health and health care, and explores the transformative effect that "health information technology" tools and services can have on health communication, health delivery, and more generally, on the health care approach—both now and in the future. The central argument of this chapter is that the use of advances in information technology is crucial for transforming the health care industry from sickness to health through the provision of an infrastructure to support a health system that guides and facilitates effective, efficient, lifetime health management.

THE TRANSFORMATIVE INFLUENCE OF HEALTH IT: TODAY

One of the big questions confronting designers of HINTS in its earliest days was whether or not use of the Internet for online health information would persist as a phenomenon. Early reports suggested that when Americans went online they actively searched for health information, and suggestions were that as the technology became customary it would drive more active use of the channel to support personal health decision making. Figure 17.2 is an extract from the 2007 HINTS data report (Rutten, Moser, Beckjord, Hesse, & Croyle, 2007) illustrating the spread of health information-seeking in the previous 12 months for those who reported being online. The figure does show a dramatic increase in health information-seeking for those online from 2003 to 2005, with a marked spread of online information-seeking throughout much of the southeast portion of the United States. Increases were also noted for other types of online health behaviors such as e-mailing physicians and purchasing pharmaceuticals (Beckjord et al., 2007). People who have been touched by disease are especially likely to search online for health information, as the "activating" influence of dealing with a health condition becomes an emotional motivator for proactive use of information resources (Beckjord, Finney Rutten, Arora, Moser, & Hesse, 2008; Hesse, Arora, Beckjord, & Finney Rutten, 2008; Mayer et al., 2007).

This rise in proactive use of eHealth information is just one of the patterns in health behavior beginning to emerge today. Other trends that are just beginning to emerge within health care include a rise in social connections between people with similar health concerns and a change in business process as seen in other industries. We discuss each of these current trends below.

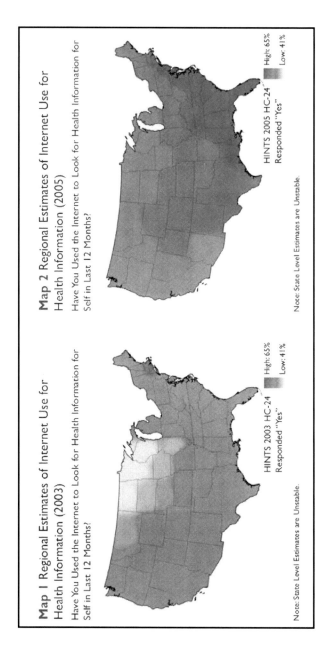

Map 1 Regional Estimates of Internet Use for Health Information (2003)

Have You Used the Internet to Look for Health Information for Self in Last 12 Months?

HINTS 2003 HC-24
Responded "Yes"

High: 65%
Low: 41%

Note: State Level Estimates are Unstable.

Map 2 Regional Estimates of Internet Use for Health Information (2005)

Have You Used the Internet to Look for Health Information for Self in Last 12 Months?

HINTS 2005 HC-24
Responded "Yes"

High: 65%
Low: 41%

Note: State Level Estimates are Unstable.

FIGURE 17.2. Spread of health information-seeking within the past 12 months for those who reported being online in HINTS 2003 and 2005.

Creating Architectures for Participation

In recent years, the proliferation of online health information technology services has enabled consumers to engage proactively in their health and health care. This type of "architecture for participation" (Conn, 2007) has facilitated a rapid increase in the number of people looking for health information online, and has allowed consumers to engage, at their convenience, in a variety of other online health-related activities. According to a recent report from the Pew Internet & American Life Project, 79% of Internet users, approximately 95 million American adults, report having searched online for health information. Furthermore, among those who found the Internet to be an important resource during a loved one's health crisis, 58% reported that the single most important information identified was something they found online. Finally, 86% of Internet users with chronic conditions (20% of the adult population) report using the Internet to research health-related issues (Fox, 2007).

Research suggests that the population is engaging in a range of online health behaviors. People are proactively engaging in "e-prescribing;" cost and quality information-seeking; e-mailing with doctors; online diet, nutrition, and exercise services; alternative therapy research; and the like (Beckjord et al., 2007). And it is not just the younger generation, or "wealthy" subset, taking part. There is an indication that usage of online resources is climbing in every age group and economic strata, although the gap across levels of education in technology use and health literacy appears to be widening (Rutten, Moser et al., 2007). These data give some credence to the claim that many people are using the Internet, and the services provided therein, to define, develop, and determine their own health strategies. The result of these trends is the advent of a "socio-technical" (Coiera, 2004) health care system, driven uniformly by people, practice, and technology; a system created by the patient for the patient through effective use of Web-based information technology.

Creating Communities of Health

As discussed by Fox and Bernhardt (Chap. 15, this volume), the social networking revolution that has engaged tens of millions of Internet users and effectively altered human interaction has come to health care, and is taking the search for health information, support, and advice to a whole new level. Internet technologies and software programs are making it easier than ever for consumers to find timely, personalized health information online, and patients are leveraging these technologies to build more sophisticated virtual communities that enable them to share information, build a personal network of friends, seek support and advice from "people like them," and manage their personal health issues (Frost & Massagli, 2008; Landro, 2006). At the same time, traditional Web sites that once offered cumbersome pages of static data are developing blogs, podcasts, and customized search engines to deliver the most relevant and timely health information, direct to the consumer (patient), in a format that is convenient, easy to use, and dynamic (Boulos, Maramba, & Wheeler, 2006; Savel, Goldstein, Perencevich, & Angood, 2007).

These same technologies are making it possible for advocacy groups, government agencies, and healthcare providers to update their health communication services. Traditionally reliant on static tools and delivery channels such as pamphlets, magazines and journals, these organizations are diversifying their communication approach by embedding messages on new technology platforms and tools that have the ability to reach a broad range of consumers with relevant health news, and personalized health-promotive messages, reminders, and alerts (Viswanath, 2005). Some organizations are even experimenting with three-dimensional online computer worlds that use surrogates known as avatars to allow consumers to virtually interact with their research and health-promotive findings (Boulos, Hetherington, & Wheeler, 2007).

Efforts to advance public health require meeting people where they are; with millions of people spending significant amounts of time online and in online health communities, the effective utilization of social networks and virtual worlds are providing new, advanced opportunities to influence consumer health and related decision making. From the perspective of health promotion and population health management, the move to an information technology-based communication "system" holds largely untested promises of improving efficiencies in reaching underserved groups, enabling real-time intervention and message delivery, advancing the monitoring and tracking of associated outcomes and morbidities, and ultimately translating health knowledge into health outcomes (CDC, 2007a). The long-term success of these networks remains unknown, as their services and structure depend entirely on consumer engagement and active, ongoing use.

Changes in Business Process

Finding new pathways to improve population health by engineering a safer and more supportive health information environment is a national priority for the United States (Brailer, 2005; Institute of Medicine, 2001; U.S. Department of Health and Human Services, 2008). The transformation of the health care industry from a focus on disease and treatment, to a focus on prevention and good health will take time, and will require a clear under-standing of system-wide obstacles in order to produce change. To ensure effectiveness and efficiency, the public, private, and not-for-profit sectors are teaming up to actively leverage the expertise, insights and best practices of leading innovators from various fields to explore how best to integrate information technology into existing infrastructures to engage patients in their health and health care. "Bridging the gap" between private corpora-tions and foundations, government agencies, and nongovernment organiza-tions to support and sustain cross-disciplinary research in public health will leverage the strengths and potential of each of these sectors in such a man-ner as to support an infrastructure that will encourage consumers to fully engage in their health and health care management.

Prior research has demonstrated significant gains in health and reduc-tions in disease when individuals actively engage in their health (Wagner, 2004). The actively engaged patient is more efficient in their use of health resources, more confident in their health system, demands higher quality care, and shows greater improvements in life expectancy and health status (Wanless, 2002). A challenge for the current health care system in the United States is to fully engage the patient in his or her own health; however, advances in information technologies applied to best-practice examples of consumer engagement in other industries, show promise for enabling fully engaged patients who co-create and manage their own health and health services.

The UK's National Health Service (NHS) provides an example of looking to other industries for support in their efforts to activate and engage the consumer for the benefit of public health. A 2002 financial analysis of the cost of U.K. health services showed the massive growth of health costs facing the U.K. system if it did not invest in reducing demand as well as improving supply. In response to these realities, Harry Cayton, director of the NHS, conceived what he termed "the flat-pack" patient. Cayton's conceptualization of a fully engaged, flat-pack patient comes from the home products retail industry, specifically, derived from the Swedish company IKEA, whose approach to self-assembly furniture has forever changed the way consumers engage in development and delivery of home products. The IKEA model can be described as follows: People buy a box containing all the necessary parts for anything from a bookcase to a bed frame. They carry it home and assemble it themselves following the simple instructions (in seven languages) provided. The customer becomes a partner in the manufacturing process, saving the company time, money, and space, and in return, the company can reduce its prices. What is more, many customers find satisfaction in investing some personal time and ener-gy in constructing their own furniture, and as such, remain loyal IKEA customers. In essence, the IKEA model streamlines consumer demand, improves efficiency, and increases customer engagement and satisfaction by giving consumers control, and in making the services and tools provided more responsive to individual needs and preferences (Cayton, 2006).

Application of the flat-pack model to health care engages consumers in their health, thereby allowing them to assemble their own care and receive targeted, real-time assistance. The U.K.'s NHS is on track to enable patients to self-manage their own health and health care by providing the tools, services, information, and support necessary to make the right choices, at the right time with the assistance of responsive health professionals (Cayton, 2006; Wanless, 2002).

Another applicable model relevant to the effective engagement of consumers in personal management and preventive practices comes from the financial industry: the automated teller machine (ATM). The ATM and associated "wealth management" services and tools are globally ubiquitous, with access points available for users in most countries around the world. The worldwide diffusion of the ATM allows people to use the ATM to pull, aggregate, and manage personal, financial data. The data is computable and convenient, and wealth care organizations and professionals offer tools and services necessary to facilitate active, ongoing management of an individual's past, current, and future financial state.

The parallels with Health 2.0 are obvious, and many energetic entrepreneurs are exploring the seemingly limitless opportunities and challenges in applying applicable industry models to the world of health. While many of the services developed to date provide useful tools, the data and services remain highly fragmented (i.e., personal health records, electronic health records, tailored search engines, patient and doctor communities, diet and exercise tools, etc.). As such, it is imperative that new health information technology innovations aggregate data across communities, disciplines, and sectors and integrate services into complete, consumer-centered solutions (just as the ATM and e-commerce have done for personal finance). The result will be an interoperable system of care that is much more valuable to consumers and essential to impact health care in meaningful ways.

Leveraging the expertise, insights, and experiences of other industries and disciplines, and facilitating public–private collaboratives to support and sustain cross-disciplinary research in public health, has and will continue to engender mutually beneficial ways to create lasting opportunities in health prevention, management, and care. However, to end the fragmentation and episodic nature of today's system and to shift the paradigm from sickness to health, it is necessary that all stakeholders look to one another for help and advice concerning how to effectively and efficiently engage consumers in the process of care. All stakeholders must begin to actively explore how to best interact with advances in technologies for improved delivery and seamless integration of health tools and services.

THE TRANSFORMATIVE EFFECT OF HEALTH IT: TOMORROW

The Patient-Centered Approach

Health care seems to be the industry with the most compelling reasons to embrace a strong consumer (patient) service focus, but unfortunately as the system has grown more complex and fragmented—and as providers feel the pressure to see more patients in less time—care has become centered on the needs of the system at the expense of the patient (Kohn, Corrigan, & Donaldson, 2000).

The result of this system-centric approach has been staggering: The United States is dead last in providing timely and effective health care to its citizens; and although most countries saw preventable deaths decline by an average of 16% in 2008, the United States saw only a 4% dip. Considering the exorbitant level of U.S. health care spending, it is clear that U.S. spending is misdirected. Priorities are misaligned, and people are dying because of it. As a result, leading innovators and policymakers are actively calling to put the patient at the center, and using advances in information technology to sculpt policies, tools and services that support patients as "health managers" and active participants in the health care process (Hibbard, 2004).

Care that is truly patient-centered considers patients' cultural traditions, their personal preferences and values, their family situations, and their lifestyles. It makes the patient and their loved ones an integral part of the care team who collaborate with health care professionals in making clinical decisions (Epstein & Street, 2007; Institute of Medicine, 2001). Patient-centered care puts responsibility for important aspects of self-care and monitoring in the patients' hands—along with the tools and support they need to carry out that responsibility.

This patient-centered approach is not yet fully instantiated, but is gaining momentum and will likely motivate significant change in varied aspects of health care in the foreseeable future (Cunningham, 2003). Effective utilization of information technology tools and services is essential (Gustafson, 2007; Hesse & Shneiderman, 2007). Not every patient is the same, and patients do not necessarily want, use, or resonate with the same systems and services. Health professionals need the resources and tools to deliver the right help and advice to patients, at the right time, in the right way, and in the right (most convenient) place. Information technology can provide user (patient) data, the technical tools needed to make intelligent use of that data, and connective channels through which health patients can engage.

Using Information Technology to Integrate Research, Medical Science, and the Consumer

We live in a time of unparalleled scientific and technologic opportunity. The pace at which we accumulate new knowledge and engineer advanced systems has never before been so great (Hesse, 2005). Thus, unprecedented opportunities to accelerate progress in health care and health care delivery are at hand. As we work to take full advantage of these evolving opportunities, it is increasingly important to integrate behavioral research, medical science, and technology as effectively as possible to have the broadest, most profound population impact. In the face of such opportunity, the key question becomes one of how to translate the use of information technology tools in conjunction with state of science health information into improved health outcomes for the population (Kerner et al., 2005; Nieva et al., 2006).

Medical science and behavioral research have contributed significantly to the growing evidence base in health prevention, promotion, communication, diagnosis, and treatment. Continued research in these areas offers promise for new health advancements with even greater utility and efficiency in the years to come. Currently, we are faced with a challenge in the dissemination and translation of health research. To be timely and effective, medical science and behavioral research need to move from the laboratory into practice quickly, easily, and efficiently to meet patient and population health needs. Currently, it can take an average of 17 years to turn 14% of original research findings to the benefit of patient care (Clancy, Fraser, & Palmer, 2006).

Looking to the future, it is important to explore how connective technologies can enable the translation and application of both current and emerging science, and advance the delivery of timely, tailored, scalable, evidence-based health solutions to a broad range of consumers. Two examples of ways in which information technology can integrate medical science and behavioral research, and translate information into better health outcomes, are highlighted here:

1. Information technology tools can help fill current gaps in medical practice such as the management of conflicting medical advice and expert opinions, the gathering and intelligent analysis of patient data, and the translation of that data into services that help and advise patients in the management of their own and their families care.
2. Currently, it is expensive, time-consuming, and inefficient to test new drugs, protocols, behavioral measures, behavioral theories, and other health-related interventions. In addition to having full understanding of health content, researchers are required to

understand new health concepts, develop new protocols and measures, analyze data test hypotheses, innovate ways to track and evaluate outcome variables, and build their own management and delivery systems. Information technology can give practitioners the tools they need to quickly and easily deploy into the test phase, aggregate and analyze large pools of data, conduct real-time evaluation and data tracking, and eventually disseminate research findings quickly, easily and inexpensively to key audiences.

In effect, integration of information technology into medical and research communities has the potential to affect the greatest level of discovery, in the shortest time, in a way that can directly translate into population health benefits. If we can harness the power of the health community through information technology—even 1 of every 100 of the physicians and researchers currently practicing today—that would be tens of thousands of people contributing on an ongoing basis to helping people improve their lives, leveraged by the power of the Internet and other innovate technologies. The effect would be a profound transformation in the health care system, and in enormous improvements in the health of our population.

CONCLUSION

This chapter argued that effective utilization of advances in information technology, applied to health, can have a transformative affect on health care—both now and in the future—and can facilitate the necessary paradigm shift our nation so badly needs—a shift from treatment of sickness to management of health over a lifetime. To maximize finite health care resources, it is essential to identify and utilize tools with the broadest reach, scale, and scope. We cannot afford to miss the opportunities at hand; scientists and practitioners must stay in step with innovations that may increase the relevance, application, and speed of delivery of science to all in need. Creating an evidence base to analyze the effects of these changes, and to inform their progress, should be a focus in public health.

REFERENCES

American Cancer Society. (2008). *Cancer Facts & Figures: 2008*. Atlanta, GA: Author.

Atienza, A.A., Hesse, B.W., Baker, T.B., Abrams, D.B., Rimer, B.K., Croyle, R.T. et al. (2007). Critical issues in eHealth research. *American Journal of Preventive Medicine, 32*(5 suppl), S71-74.

Beckjord, E.B., Finney Rutten, L.J., Arora, N.K., Moser, R.P., & Hesse, B.W. (2008). Information processing and negative affect: Evidence from the 2003 Health Information National Trends Survey. *Health Psychology, 27*(2), 249-257.

Beckjord, E.B., Finney Rutten, L.J., Squiers, L., Arora, N.K., Volckmann, L., Moser, R.P. et al. (2007). Use of the internet to communicate with health care providers in the United States: Estimates from the 2003 and 2005 Health Information National Trends Surveys (HINTS). *Journal of Medical Internet Research, 9*(3), e20.

Borger, C., Smith, S., Truffer, C., Keehan, S., Sisko, A., Poisal, J. et al. (2006). Health spending projections through 2015: Changes on the horizon. *Health Affairs, 25*(2), w61-73.

Boulos, M., Hetherington, L., & Wheeler, S. (2007). Second Life: An overview of the potential of 3-D virtual worlds in medical and health education. *Health Information and Libraries Journal, 24*(4), 233-245.

Boulos, M., Maramba, I., & Wheeler, S. (2006). Wikis, blogs and podcasts: A new generation of Web-based tools for virtual collaborative clinical practice and education. *BMC Medical Education, 6*(1), 41.

Brailer, D. (2005). Action through collaboration: A conversation with David Brailer. The national coordinator of HIT believes that facilitation, not mandates, are the way to move the agenda forward. Interview by Robert Cunningham. *Health Affairs (Millwood), 24*(5), 1150-1157.

Cayton, H. (2006). The flat-pack patient? Creating health together. *Patient Education and Counseling, 62*(3), 288-290.

Centers for Disease Control and Prevention (CDC). (2006). *Behavioral risk factor surveillance system: About the BRFSS—overview.* Atlanta, GA: Centers for Disease Control and Prevention.

Centers for Disease Control and Prevention (CDC). (2007a). Second Life let's CDC be everywhere—all at once [Electronic Version]. Retrieved January 11, 2007, from http://www.cdc.gov/about/ stateofcdc/everywhere/secondLife.htm

Centers for Disease Control and Prevention (CDC). (2007b). *U.S. obesity trends 1985-2006.*

Clancy, C., Fraser, I., & Palmer, C. (2006, June 1). *Turning research to ACTION through delivery systems.* Paper presented at the 1st annual meeting of AHRQ, Washington, DC.

Coiera, E. (2004). Four rules for the reinvention of health care. *Bmj, 328*(7449), 1197-1199.

Conn, J. (2007). Health 2.0: The next generation of web enterprises [Electronic Version]. *Modern Health Care Online.* Retrieved December 20, 2007, from www.modernhealthcare.com

Cunningham, R. (2003). The Mental Health Commission tackles fragmented services: An interview with Michael Hogan. *Health Affairs*, hlthaff.w3.440.

Epstein, R., & Street, R. (2007). *Patient-centered communication in cancer care: Promoting healing and reducing suffering* (NIH Publication No. 07-6225). Bethesda, MD: National Cancer Institute.

Eysenbach, G. (2001). What is e-health? *Journal of Medical Internet Research, 3*(2), E20.

Ferguson, T. (2000). Online patient-helpers and physicians working together: A new partnership for high quality health care. *Bmj, 321*(7269), 1129-1132.

Fox, S. (2007). *E-patients with a disability or chronic disease.* Washington, DC: Pew Internet & American Life Project.

Frost, J.H., & Massagli, M.P. (2008). Social uses of personal health information within PatientsLikeMe, an online patient community: What can happen when patients have access to one another's data. *Journal of Medical Internet Research, 10*(3), e15.

Gebbie, K.M., Rosenstock, L., & Hernandez, L.M. (2003). *Who will keep the public healthy? Educating public health professionals for the 21st century.* Washington, DC: National Academy Press.

Gustafson, D.H., Brennan, P.F., & Hawkins, R. (2007). *Investing in e-health: What it takes to sustain consumer health informatics.* New York: Springer.

Hesse, B.W. (2005). Harnessing the power of an intelligent health environment in cancer control. *Studies in Health Technology Information, 118*, 159-176.

Hesse, B.W., Arora, N.K., Beckjord, E.B., & Finney Rutten, L.J. (2008). Information support for cancer survivors. *Cancer, 112*(11S), 2529-2540.

Hesse, B.W., & Shneiderman, B. (2007). eHealth research from the user's perspective. *American Journal of Preventive Medicine, 32*(5 suppl), S97-103.

Hibbard, J.H. (2004). Perspective: Moving toward a more patient-centered health care delivery system. *Health Affairs,* hlthaff.var.133.

Institute of Medicine. (2001). *Crossing the quality chasm: A new health system for the 21st century.* Washington, DC: National Academy Press.

Institute of Medicine (U.S.). (2001). *Health and behavior: The interplay of biological, behavioral, and societal influences.* Washington, DC: National Academy Press.

Johnson-Taylor, W.L., Yaroch, A.L., Krebs-Smith, S.M., & Rodgers, A.B. (2007). What can communication science tell us about promoting optimal dietary behavior? *Journal of Nutrition Education and Behavior, 39*(2 suppl), S1-4.

Kerner, J.F., Guirguis-Blake, J., Hennessy, K.D., Brounstein, P.J., Vinson, C., Schwartz, R.H. et al. (2005). Translating research into improved outcomes in comprehensive cancer control. *Cancer Causes Control, 16*(suppl 1), 27-40.

Kohn, L.T., Corrigan, J., & Donaldson, M.S. (2000). *To err is human: Building a safer health system.* Washington, DC: National Academy Press.

Landro, L. (2006, December 29). Social networking comes to healthcare. *Wall Street Journal.*

Litt, J.S., Tran, N.L., & Burke, T.A. (2002). Examining urban brownfields through the public health "macroscope." *Environmental Health Perspectives, 110*, 183-193.

Mayer, D.K., Terrin, N.C., Kreps, G.L., Menon, U., McCance, K., Parsons, S.K. et al. (2007). Cancer survivors information seeking behaviors: A comparison of survivors who do and do not seek information about cancer. *Patient Education and Counseling, 65*(3), 342-350.

Nieva, V., Murphy, R., Ridley, N., Donaldson, N., Combes, J., Mitchell, P. et al. (2006). From science to service: A framework for the transfer of patient safety research into practice. In *Advances in patient safety: From research to implemen-tation*. Washington, DC: National Academies of Science, Institute of Medicine.

President's Cancer Panel. (2007). *Promoting healthy lifestyles: Policy, program, and personal recommendations for reducing cancer risk*. Washington, DC: U.S. Department of Health and Human Services.

Rutten, L.F., Moser, R.P., Beckjord, E.B., Hesse, B.W., & Croyle, R.T. (2007). *Cancer Communication: Health Information National Trends Survey* (No. NIH Pub. No. 07-6214). Washington, DC: National Cancer Institute.

Savel, R.H., Goldstein, E.B., Perencevich, E.N., & Angood, P.B. (2007). The iCritical care podcast: A novel medium for critical care communication and education. *Journal of American Medical Informatics Association, 14*(1), 94-99.

Tenenbaum, M. (2007). Health 2.0: Marty Tenenbaum's vision for an accelerator of Health 2.0 [Electronic Version]. *The Health Care Blog*. http://www.thehealth-careblog.com (accessed February 2, 2008).

U.S. Department of Health and Human Services. (2008). *The ONC-coordinated fed-eral health IT strategic plan: 2008-2012*. Washington, DC: Author.

Viswanath, K. (2005). Science and society: The communications revolution and can-cer control. *Nature Reviews. Cancer, 5*(10), 828-835.

Wagner, E.H. (2004). Chronic disease care. *Bmj, 328*(7433), 177-178.

Wanless, D. (2002). *Securing our future health: Taking a long-term view*. London: HM Treasury.

CONCLUSION

18

BUILDING THE EVIDENCE BASE IN COMMUNICATION

Next Steps

Gary L. Kreps
George Mason University

Lila J. Finney Rutten
National Cancer Institute

THE EVIDENCE BASE FOR CANCER COMMUNICATION

Cancer communication is the study and application of strategically designed messages delivered through a broad array of channels and media. The goal of cancer communication is to convey relevant health information to targeted audiences who confront cancer (cancer patients/survivors and their supporters, health care providers and administrators, health researchers, at-risk populations, policymakers, and many others), promote recommended cancer prevention and control behaviors, encourage the adoption of cancer screening and early detection activities, facilitate the delivery of the best available cancer care, and enhance quality of life (Kreps & Chapelsky Massimilla, 2002; Kreps & Viswanath, 2001). Cancer communication is an important translational area of applied research and intervention that should ideally provide clear direction to enlightened cancer control practices and policies (Kreps, 2003). However, translational cancer communication research demands strong, valid, and revealing evidence to guide cancer control efforts (Kreps, Viswanath, & Harris, 2002).

There is tremendous demand for timely, accurate, relevant, and persuasive information about cancer prevention, treatment, and control to inform cancer prevention and control activities (Kreps & Sivaram, 2008). Strategic communication is the primary social process for promoting informed decision making that can help reduce cancer morbidity and mortality. Yet the process of cancer communication is exceedingly complex. Influencing strongly held health beliefs and changing entrenched health behaviors is no simple matter. Although most health promotion practices, policies, and interventions are based on good intentions, they too often are developed with limited data about the target audiences, the social barriers that influence health behaviors, the communication processes and channels that are likely to be most influential with targeted audiences, and the necessary systemic community for sustaining cancer control activities (Kreps et al., 2002).

CANCER COMMUNICATION
ACROSS THE CONTINUUM OF CARE

The continuum of cancer care described by Zapka, Taplin, Solberg, and Manos (2003) includes the following phases: risk assessment, primary prevention, early detection/cancer screening, diagnosis, treatment, long-term surveillance during survivorship, and end-of-life care. This continuum provides a useful framework for examining communication within the context of cancer. There are complex cancer communication demands for communicating cancer-risk information, promoting cancer prevention, and encouraging early detection. Communication around cancer risk, efficacy and possible implications of screening exams, and conveying information about the benefits and potential burdens of screening exams is essential for informing the public (Brown, 1991; Wolf & Becker, 1996). What are effective strategies for conveying information about risk? How do we know what the best available cancer prevention and early detection strategies are for different at-risk populations? How can we determine the best ways to communicate with different groups of consumers who are at risk for cancer that will allow us to effectively reach and influence their adoption of cancer prevention and early detection behaviors? How much do consumers already know about cancer prevention and detection? What are their current beliefs and attitudes about cancer? Are they predisposed to follow cancer prevention and early detection recommendations? What messages will be most motivating to different groups of consumers? What information sources will be most credible to different groups of consumers? Answers to these questions are needed to guide effective cancer prevention and early detection efforts.

Individuals who are diagnosed with cancer desperately need specific information about the nature of their cancers, where they can get the best cancer care, and what promising courses of treatment are available to them. Communicating effectively with those who have just been diagnosed with cancer is tremendously challenging. The stigma and fear associated with a cancer diagnosis, the complexity of medical information around cancer treatment options, and uncertainty regarding the course of the disease and treatment exacerbates communication challenges (Siminoff, Radvin, Colabianchi, & Saunders-Sturm, 2000). These newly diagnosed patients often experience shock. They are likely to be scared. They may not believe their cancer diagnosis. These feelings of vulnerability, uncertainty, and loss of self that are often experienced by newly diagnosed cancer patients (McWilliam, Brown, & Stewart, 2000), coupled with evidence suggesting that patients who have their informational and support needs met are likely to experience less disruption in quality of life and more favorable health outcomes (Rose, 1990; Schain, 1990), underlie the importance of effective, evidence-based communication. Furthermore, where indications for treatment are not always straightforward, communication about available treatments, clinical trials, and the treatment risks and benefits is essential in cancer care. How much do patients already know about cancer, and how much of the information they have is accurate? How well do they understand health care concepts, terminology, and procedures? Are they ready to really make sense of and respond to diagnostic, prognostic, and treatment information? Reliable and accurate information is needed to answer these and many more questions to guide the best cancer care.

Cancer care physicians depend on strategic communication to acquire full and accurate patient diagnosis and history information to enable them to recommend the best forms of cancer treatment. These physicians also need to use their communication skills to coordinate cancer treatment activities with many other health care providers (specialists, pharmacists, nurses, therapists, and various support personnel), as well as with representatives of health care delivery systems where cancer care is provided. They also need to communicate effectively and sensitively with patients' family members and home caregivers who typically perform important roles in cancer care and survivorship. However, communicating effectively with these different audiences is challenging and relevant information is needed to coordinate efforts in the treatment of cancer.

It is common for cancer survivors to experience late and or long-term complications of cancer treatment of a physiologic and/or psychosocial nature (Campbell, Marbella, & Layde, 2000; Fernsler & Fanuele, 1998; Gotay & Muraoka, 1998; Hancock & Hoppe, 1996). Therefore, cancer survivors and their supporters have tremendous health information needs related to making decisions about managing health after cancer treatment, coping with the many side effects from cancer treatments (such as pain, fatigue, depression, and nausea), reintegrating into personal and professional lives after cancer, and selecting strategies for reducing the chances for reoccurrence of cancer (Mayer et al., 2007). Cancer survivors need social support for coping with the many uncertainties they face to help promote their quality of life. Yet, there are many complexities in providing relevant information and support to cancer survivors. Evidence is needed to guide strategic communication efforts with different groups of cancer survivors and their caregivers. Furthermore, there is a great need for improved communication during the end of life; such improvements have beey recommended consistently (Hanson, Danis, & Garrett, 1997; Steinhauser et al., 2000). Policymakers also depend on relevant information about the communication demands confronting health care consumers and providers to develop appropriate infrastructure, legislation, and support to promote cancer prevention, detection, treatment, control, and survivorship. What are the most serious current barriers to cancer prevention, early detection, the delivery of cancer care, and effective cancer survivorship that face different groups of consumers? What are the unique cancer-related information needs of different groups of consumers? What are these consumers' preferences for accessing cancer-related information and care? Accurate information about these issues can help guide the development of strategic cancer communication policies and practices to promote cancer prevention, treatment, control, and survivorship.

INNOVATING THE HINTS RESEARCH PROGRAM

This volume describes how the Health Information National Trends Survey (HINTS) research program has been developed to begin building an important comprehensive evidence base for guiding cancer communication efforts. The HINTS research program has already provided a wealth of data about the cancer-related beliefs, attitudes, and behaviors of the American public. The biennial repeated administration design of HINTS is beginning to provide interesting trend data about changes in public responses to cancer that track variations in public access to cancer-related information, health information gaps, as well as cancer information needs by different publics. Ideally, the HINTS research program will provide data to inform the development of far-reaching communication interventions to promote cancer prevention and control. Yet, there are also many challenges that must be met for the HINTS research program to gather the accurate and comprehensive information needed to inform cancer communication policy and practices. The HINTS research program must be strategically refined and innovated to maximize its potential for building the information base for effective cancer communication.

The chapters in this volume identify a number of evolving methodological challenges confronting the HINTS research program, such as declining response rates to surveys, the complexities of analyzing trends in space and time, and the need to make HINTS data interoperable with other data sets in an online, collaborative science environment. The national scope of the HINTS data set makes it difficult to make accurate predictions and applications to specific groups and regions across the United States based on the biennial survey data, suggesting the need for supplemental HINTS-based studies with targeted populations to augment the national HINTS data. Targeted samples, particularly with vulnerable at-risk populations who may be underrepresented in the national HINTS data, could provide very useful supplementary information to guide interventions with these groups. Moreover, translational strategies need to be developed to encourage applications of HINTS research program data to guiding cancer communication policy and practices.

The National Cancer Institute (NCI) already has helped to expand the evidence base from the HINTS research program by making the national HINTS data set easily available online to researchers who are encouraged to conduct secondary analyses with these data. Secondary analysis studies have been tracked and conferences have been held to promote forums for cancer communication researchers to network and discuss the implications of supplementary studies. Developing networks of HINTS researchers (invisible colleges) for supplemental HINTS research will geometrically expand the influences and outcomes of HINTS-related research. Researchers are being encouraged to expand collection of HINTS data with different populations using the national survey HINTS questions and also probing beyond the initial questions to expand depth of analysis. New research questions can supplement the HINTS dataset by adding additional information and identifying new implications from these data.

There are many strategies for enhancing the collection of HINTS data for guiding cancer communication interventions. For example, cognitive interviewing is a promising strategy that can be used to assist HINTS researchers in collecting deep and meaningful health information. The use of geographic information systems can help to increase the abilities of HINTS researchers to compare and contrast health information needs and practices across geographic regions. The implications of using new technologic devices in HINTS research, such as cell phones, for survey practice, applying novel sampling approaches to reach diverse respondents, and the capacity to use small area estimation procedures to increase the precision of survey estimates at the local level can enhance and expand HINTS research. It is important to develop strategies for increasing the methodological sophistication of HINTS research through the use of both quantitative and qualitative methods, innovative survey design and scale development, formative evaluation strategies, diverse multimodal survey delivery platforms, and multimethodological designs.

New strategies need to be developed to disseminate HINTS data broadly to different audiences that need evidence to guide cancer communication
efforts, such as to members of the health research community, the public
health promotion community, to health care providers, to cancer patients/
survivors/advocates, and to health policymakers. The HINTS Web site is a
primary channel for disseminating data about HINTS (see http://hints.can-
cer.gov/). HINTS research reports, fact sheets and brochures, the HINTS
survey instrument, data set, and research tools, as well as HINTS research
program publications, presentations and announcements are easily available
on this Web site. Additional communication channels (including other
online channels, as well as print and electronic media) can be strategically
utilized to promote dissemination and use of HINTS research data to guide
evidence-based cancer control interventions. An independent evaluation of
the HINTS program was conducted in 2007 to assess reach and utility of the
HINTS program; results of this evaluation informed the development of a
HINTS dissemination plan that was initiated in 2008.

Future HINTS-related research should be designed to increase the depth
of information available on a number of important cancer-related issues. For
example, more in-depth data should be gathered concerning the critical cancer information-searching/seeking problems and opportunities that confront
different audiences, the interrelationships among different communication
channels in providing relevant cancer information, the specific information
needs of cancer survivors, and the influences of critical audience variables
(such as income, education, race, ethnicity, health status, age, residence, gender, culture, language, disability, literacy, social power) on health communication practices. It is important to learn more about the motivations and
goals different audiences have for seeking information about cancer. Future
HINTS research can provide more information about message exposure to
different audiences and implications for cancer information dissemination.

A key area that is particularly ripe for expansion in the HINTS research
program is the impact of health information dissemination on health disparities and health knowledge gaps. It is important to expand the collection of
data examining communication inequalities, unequal access to information,
differences in processing information, and differences in using information
(decision making, adopting health behaviors, screening, access to care, and
quality of survivorship). HINTS data that provides in-depth analyses of key
cultural issues have the potential to stimulate innovative intervention strategies targeted toward disadvantaged populations. However, to achieve these
goals, new strategies must be developed to increase ethnic and minority
response in HINTS research. Studies may need to be conducted using specific native languages for diverse Asian, Hispanic, and African populations.
Supplemental questions that examine the specific health information needs
and concerns of these populations are needed to enable HINTS research to
help reduce and eventually eliminate cancer-related health disparities. For

example, efforts are underway by the NCI to implement dedicated Spanish-language HINTS data-collection activities in Puerto Rico in collaboration with the Puerto Rico Cancer Center of the University of Puerto Rico. These efforts promise to provide revealing data about the cancer information needs of vulnerable populations who currently suffer from serious disparities in cancer-related health outcomes.

Continued efforts need to be taken to ground future HINTS research in revealing scientific theories and models, as well as to connect HINTS research to additional relevant databases and research programs to expand both scientific and applied impact. More needs to be done to track and examine important trends data about the changing nature of health information dissemination and use. Key implications of HINTS data need to be identified for future generations of health care consumers, noting changing information trends. HINTS researchers also need to identify the best strategies for effectively disseminating cancer risk information to diverse audiences to reduce problems of information overload and feelings of fatalism about cancer risks among the public. With these innovations, the expanding HINTS research program has the potential to serve as a powerful evidence base for directing far-reaching cancer communication interventions, practices, and policies.

REFERENCES

Brown, H. G. (1991). The messages primary care physicians should convey to their patients about mammography. *Women's Health Issues, 1*, 74-77.

Campbell, B. H., Marbella, A., & Layde, P. M. (2000). Quality of life and recurrence concern in survivors of head and neck cancer. *Laryngoscope, 110*, 895-906.

Fernsler, J., & Fanuele, J. S. (1998). Lymphomas: Long-term sequelae and survivorship issues. *Seminars in Oncology Nursing, 14*, 321-328.

Gotay, C. C., & Muraoka, M. Y. (1998). Quality of life in long-term survivors of adult-onset cancers. *Journal of the National Cancer Institute, 90*, 656-667.

Hancock, S. L., & Hoppe, R. T. (1996). Long-term complications of treatment and causes of mortality after Hodgkin's disease. *Seminars in Radiation Oncology, 6*, 225-242.

Hanson, L. C., Danis, M., & Garrett, J. (1997). What is wrong with end-of-life care? Opinions of bereaved family members. *Journal of the American Geriatric Society, 45*(11), 1339-1344.

Kreps, G. L. (2003). Opportunities for health communication scholarship to shape public health policy and practice: Examples from the National Cancer Institute. In T. Thompson, R. Parrott, K. Miller, & A. Dorsey (Eds.), *The handbook of health communication* (pp. 609-624). Hillsdale, NJ: Erlbaum.

Kreps, G. L., & Chapelsky Massimilla, D. (2002). Cancer communications research and health outcomes: Review and challenge. *Communication Studies, 53*(4), 318-336.

Kreps, G. L., & Sivaram, R. (2008). The central role of strategic health communication in enhancing breast cancer outcomes across the continuum of care in limited-resource countries. *Cancer, 113*(58), 2331-2337.

Kreps, G. L., & Viswanath, K. (2001). Communication interventions and cancer control: A review of the National Cancer Institute's health communication intervention research initiative. *Family and Community Health, 24*(3), ix-xiii.

Kreps, G. L., Viswanath, K., & Harris, L. M. (2002). Advancing communication as a science: Opportunities from the federal sector. *Journal of Applied Communication Research, 30*(4), 369-381.

Mayer, D. K., Terrin, N. C., Kreps, G. L., Menon, U., McCance, K., Parsons, S. K. et al. (2007). Cancer survivors information seeking behaviors: A comparison of survivors who do and don't seek information. *Patient Education and Counseling, 65*(3), 342-350.

McWilliam, C. L., Brown, J. B., & Stewart, M. (2000). Breast cancer patients' experiences of patient-doctor communication: A working relationship. *Patient Education and Counseling, 39*, 191-204.

Rose, J. H. (1990). Social support and cancer: Adult patients' desire for support from family, friends, and health professionals. *American Journal of Community Psychology, 18*, 439-464.

Schain, W. S. (1990). Physician–patient communication about breast cancer: A challenge for the 1990s. *Surgical Clinics of North America, 70*, 917-935.

Siminoff, L. A., Ravdin, P., Colabianchi, N., & Saunders-Sturm, C. M. (2000). Doctor-patient communication patterns in breast cancer adjuvant therapy discussions. *Health Expectations, 3*, 26-36.

Steinhauser, K. E., Clipp, E. C., McNeilly, M., Christakis, N. A., McIntyre, L. M., & Tulsky, J. A. (2000). In search of a good death: Observations of patients, families, and providers. *Annals of Internal Medicine, 132*(10), 825-832.

Wolf, A. M. D., & Becker, D. (1996). Cancer screening and informed patient discussions: Truth and consequences. *Archives of Internal Medicine, 156*, 1069-1072.

Zapka, J. G., Taplin, S. H., Solberg, L. I., & Manos, M. M. (2003). A framework for improving the quality of cancer care: the case of breast and cervical cancer screening. *Cancer Epidemiology, Biomarkers and Prevention, 12*(1), 4-13.

ABOUT THE AUTHORS

Erik M. Augustson received his PhD in Clinical Psychology from the University of New Mexico. He performed his clinical internship at the University of Alabama at Birmingham School of Medicine and also completed a 2-year post doctoral fellowship in Behavioral Medicine with a focus on Chronic Pain. He then served as an Assistant Professor within the medical school and was Director of Psychological Services in the Chronic Pain Center. Dr Augustson left UAB in 2000 to pursue additional training at the National Cancer Institute and was selected for the Cancer Prevention Fellowship Program. He completed an MPH with a focus in Epidemiology from Johns Hopkins School of Public Health and two additional years of research at NCI. Since 2001, he has worked in the National Cancer Institute's Tobacco Control Research Branch where he was involved in a wide variety of research and dissemination activities, including working closely with the NCI Smoking Cessation Quitline. He currently serves as a Behavioral Scientist and Health Science Administrator within TCRB.

Jay M. Bernhardt (PhD, University of North Carolina at Chapel Hill, 1999; MPH, University of Medicine and Dentistry of New Jersey, 1994) is the Director of the National Center for Health Marketing (NCHM) at the US Centers for Disease Control and Prevention in Atlanta, Georgia. NCHM's signature programs include the Morbidity and Mortality Weekly Report (MMWR), Guide to Community Preventive Services, "CDC-INFO" toll free hotline, CDC's website (CDC.gov) and new media, the Joint Information Center of the CDC Emergency Operations Center, CDC's consolidated graphic design and writer/editor staffs, and coordination of CDC's external partnerships and strategic alliances. Before joining the CDC in August 2005, Dr. Bernhardt was an Assistant Professor of Behavioral Sciences and Health Education at the Rollins School of Public Health at

Emory University and the Founding Director of the Emory Center for Public Health Communication. Prior to that, he was an Assistant Professor of Health Promotion and Behavior at the University of Georgia. Dr. Bernhardt's research and instruction have focused on health communication, social marketing, and new media, with an emphasis on information technology, e-health, and strategic communication. He has published more than 40 articles and chapters in respected volumes and scholarly journals including the American Journal of Public Health, Journal of Health Communication, and the British Medical Journal.

Kelly D. Blake (ScD, Harvard School of Public Health, 2009) is a research assistant at the Dana-Farber Cancer Institute. She is also a freelance science writer and editor. Her research interests include public opinion and public health policy, risk communication, and media studies, specifically examining how information access gaps contribute to health disparities in underserved populations. Before pursuing her doctoral degree, she was a science writer and editor in the Division of Cancer Control and Population Sciences at the National Cancer Institute (NCI), National Institutes of Health. At NCI, she served as the division's lead for press and communication projects, and managed the publication process for several print and electronic publications and Web sites. Before joining NCI, Kelly was a public health educator, conducting screening and disease prevention programs in rural communities in West Virginia. Before that, she was a health communication research fellow at the Centers for Disease Control and Prevention. She earned a doctoral degree from the Harvard School of Public Health, master's degree in community health education from West Virginia University and a bachelor's degree in journalism from Marshall University.

David Cantor (PhD, University of Illinois, 1985) is an Associate Director for Survey Methodology at Westat and a research professor at the Joint Program for Survey Methods at the University of Maryland, College Park. He has over 20 years of experience conducting survey research and policy evaluation studies. He has published on a wide variety of topics in survey methodology, including non-response, respondent recall, respondent conditioning, the effects of incentives on surveys and the effects of different modes of interviewing. At the JPSM he teaches courses on data collection methods, questionnaire design and organizational surveys.

Patricia A. Cavazos-Rehg (PhD, State University of New York at Buffalo, 2004) is a Research Instructor at Washington University School of Medicine (WUSM) in St. Louis, Missouri. She is currently a scholar in the K12 Multidisciplinary Clinical Research Development Program (MCRCDP) at WUSM. She teaches courses in research methods, health communication, and health disparities. Her research agenda involves the investigation of the interrelationships between various dimensions of risk behaviors, health problems (e.g. substance abuse and cancer), and mental health status among underserved populations.

Elliot J. Coups received his PhD in social/health psychology from Rutgers University, completed a postdoctoral fellowship in cancer prevention and control at Memorial Sloan-Kettering Cancer Center, and is currently an Associate Member in the Division of Population Science, Fox Chase Cancer Center. Dr. Coups' primary area of research focuses on understanding and promoting health-related behaviors among cancer survivors. His research in this area has included documenting the prevalence of health behaviors among survivors of varying cancers, identifying the prevalence and correlates of physical activity among lung cancer survivors, and testing the feasibility of an Internet-based weight loss intervention for colorectal cancer survivors. Dr. Coups also conducts research to identify the prevalence, patterns, and correlates of behavioral risk factors for cancer among the general adult population. His research has been supported by grants from the National Cancer Institute and the Lance Armstrong Foundation.

Corinne Crammer, PhD, MDiv, MM received her undergraduate degree from Northwestern University, with a major in history. She subsequently received a master's degree in management with majors in accounting and marketing from Northwestern University's Kellogg Graduate School of Management. She then passed the examination in Illinois to be a Certified Public Accountant. After working in real estate development in Chicago for a number of years, Dr. Crammer returned to school and earned a Master in Divinity degree at Yale University. She moved to Atlanta to attend Emory University, and in 2006 she received a doctorate from the Graduate School of Arts and Sciences.

Dr. Cramer is involved in a wide range of activities and projects, primarily related to the outreach and dissemination of the work of the Behavioral Research Center. Her responsibilities involve providing information to the staff of the Society's National Home Office and Divisions about psychosocial oncology and the work of the Behavioral Research Center. She has served as Chair of the Planning Committee for the 2008 Cancer Survivorship Research Conference.

William W. Davis (PhD, University of Wisconsin—Madison, 1974) is a statistician with more than 30 years of experience in statistical consultation and analysis in academia, government, and industry. His areas of interest include survey design and analysis, small area estimation, and Bayesian methods. In his current position at the National Cancer Institute, he assists researchers in the design and analysis of surveys such as the Health Information National Trends Survey, the California Health Interview Survey, and the

Tobacco Use Supplement to the Current Population Survey. Also, he collaborates with government and university researchers in publishing the findings from these and other surveys.

Jennifer S. Ford, PhD is an Assistant Attending Psychologist in the Department of Psychiatry and Behavioral Sciences and the Department of Pediatrics at Memorial Sloan-Kettering Cancer Center in New York City. Her research focuses on psychosocial adjustment and health behaviors of pediatric, adolescent and young adult cancer survivors. She has been funded by the National Cancer Institute, Langeloth Foundation, T. J. Martell Foundation, Society of MSKCC, and Lance Armstrong Foundation for her research. She currently has a Mentored Research Scholar Grant in Applied and Clinical Research from the American Cancer Society focused on identity development and adaptation of adolescent cancer survivors. Using developmental and social ecological perspectives, this work is directed towards understanding how adolescent cancer survivors adapt and respond to the demands of cancer survivorship, over time. Her clinical practice at MSKCC is focused on providing psychotherapy to pediatric, adolescent and young adult cancer survivors.

Susannah Fox is an associate director of the Pew Internet & American Life Project, an initiative of the Pew Research Center, a nonpartisan, nonprofit "fact tank" that provides information on the issues, attitudes, and trends shaping America and the world. Fox leads the Project's research on the impact of the internet on health and health care and is a contributor to e-patients.net. Prior to joining the Project, she was the editor of the website for U.S. News & World Report and a researcher during the start-up phase of RealNetworks.

Jennifer Hay, Assistant Attending Psychologist at Memorial Sloan-Kettering Cancer Center in the Department of Psychiatry and Behavioral Sciences, is a clinical psychologist and behavioral science researcher in cancer prevention and control. She has a primary interest in understanding the health behavior change process, particularly uptake and maintenance of cancer screening and sun protection behaviors. She has ongoing research programs examining the role of cancer risk perception — including perception of genomic information — in motivating cancer prevention and control behavior in individuals and families from the general population as well as moderate-risk families.

Bradford W. Hesse (PhD, University of Utah, 1988) is Chief of the Health Communication and Informatics Research Branch at the National Cancer Institute (NCI). Dr. Hesse serves as the Program Director the Centers of Excellence in Cancer Communication Research (CECCRs) and as the Program Officer for the Health Information National Trends Survey

(HINTS). He also serves in an advisory capacity for the NCI's User Centered Informatics Research laboratory, and is a standing member of the American Psychological Association's Electronic Resources Advisory Committee. Trained as a psychologist, Dr. Hesse has spent most of his career working to improve the ways in which mediated communication environments can be utilized to support behaviors in positive ways. His work has taken him into the areas of human-computer interaction, medical informatics, health psychology, media psychology, interpersonal communication, health communication, and artificial intelligence. In 1989 he took his interest in "Tech Psych" to Silicon Valley, where he co-founded the Center for Research on Technology at the American Institutes for Research. While at the American Institutes for Research, he conducted studies on various aspects of computer-supported collaborative work for government (Departments of Education, Labor, Defense, & Social Security) and for corporate sponsors (Apple Computer, Microsoft, Adobe, Netscape, Xerox, IBM, and Hewlett Packard). He also taught classes in human factors, social psychology, research methods, statistics, and systems design through a joint appointment with the University of San Francisco. In 1999, he joined the survey research firm Westat to expand his studies into evaluations of knowledge and behavior at the population level. He was recruited to join the NCI formally in 2003. His research has since focused on using advances in communication science and technology to improve health outcomes, sustain high quality of life, and reduce the nation's burden from cancer.

Jeffrey Kerwin (PhD, University of Georgia, 1991) is a senior study director at Westat, a social science research firm in Rockville, MD. Since joining Westat in 1993, he has directed studies, both qualitative and quantitative, on a wide variety of topics. Dr. Kerwin specializes in the social and cognitive aspects of survey methods, and has worked to improve the methodology of data collection in numerous federal surveys, such as the American Community Survey, the National Health and Nutrition Survey, and the Health Information National Trends Survey. He has conducted a large number of cognitive interviewing tasks for purposes of detecting and correcting problems in survey questionnaires. He designed and regularly conducts for Westat staff a general training on cognitive interviewing methods. Dr. Kerwin worked in the Office of Research and Methodology at the National Center for Health Statistics for two years before joining Westat.

Sarah Kobrin, PhD, MPH has been working in the field of cancer control for more than 15 years; she is currently a Program Director in the National Cancer Institute's Applied Cancer Screening Research Branch. Dr. Kobrin manages the Behavioral Research Program's Theories Project, including the Web site "Health Behavior Constructs: Theory, Measurement, and Research" and a workshop "Stimulating Advances in Behavioral Theory:

Applications to Cancer Screening." Her areas of interest include health behavior theory; risk perception; decision making under uncertainty; and measurement, particularly in regard to breast and prostate cancer screening. Her research includes development of a scale, based on attitudes rather than beliefs, to assess perceptions of breast cancer risk. With a team at NCI, she led development of a measure of the process of decision making about screening with the PSA test for prostate cancer. Prior to moving to the NCI in December 2003, Dr. Kobrin was a Walther Post-Doctoral Fellow at the Duke University Cancer Prevention and Control Program. She trained at the University of North Carolina at Chapel Hill School of Public Health.

Gary L. Kreps (PhD, University of Southern California, 1979) is the Eileen and Steve Mandell Professor of Health Communication at George Mason University, where he is Chair of the Department of Communication and Director of the Center for Health and Risk Communication. Gary's research focuses on health communication, health promotion, risk prevention, health care service delivery, and social change. He has published more than 40 scholarly books and edited volumes, and more than 220 scholarly articles and chapters concerning the applications of communication knowledge in society. He has received many awards for his scholarship including the Pfizer Professorship of Clear Health Communication, the Robert Lewis Donohew Outstanding Health Communication Scholar Award, the Future of Health Technology Award, the Distinguished Achievement Award for Outstanding Contributions in Consumer Health Informatics and Online Health, and the Gerald M. Phillips Distinguished Applied Communication Scholarship Award. Before joining the George Mason University faculty, he served for five years as the founding Chief of the Health Communication and Informatics Research Branch at the National Cancer Institute (NIH). Before that he served as the founding Dean of the School of Communication at Hofstra University, Executive Director of the Greenspun School of Communication at UNLV, and as a professor at Northern Illinois, Rutgers, Indiana, and Purdue Universities.

Sarah Lillie is a doctoral student in the Department of Health Behavior and Health Education at the University of Michigan at Ann Arbor School of Public Health. She was a Cancer Research Training Award Fellow at the National Cancer Institute in the Applied Research Program and in the Behavioral Research Program. She received her master's of public health in health behavior and health education from the University of North Carolina at Chapel Hill and graduated with a bachelor's degree in sociology from Vassar College.

Michael W. Link, PhD is Chief Methodologist/VP for Methodological Research at The Nielsen Company. He has a broad-base of experience in survey research, having worked in academia (Survey Research Laboratory at the University of South Carolina, 1989-1999), not-for-profit research (RTI International, 1999-2004), government (Centers for Disease Control and Prevention, 2004-2007), and the private sector (Nielsen, 2007-present). He received his PhD in Political Science from the University of South Carolina. Dr. Link's research efforts are centered around developing methodologies for confronting many of the most pressing issues facing survey research, including techniques for improving survey participation and data quality (use of advance letters and answering machine messages, impact of call screening technologies, effect of Do Not Call registries), methodological issues involving use of multiple modes in data collection (web, mail, CATI, and field), and obtaining participation from hard-to-survey populations (linguistically isolated, racial and ethnic groups). His current research efforts are focused on the use of address based sampling (ABS) as an alternative to random digit-dialed techniques for general population surveys and on the uses of electronic measurement strategies as replacements for some types of self-reported data.

Dr. Holly A. Massett is the associate director of the Office of Market Research and Evaluation at the National Cancer Institute where she oversees both the user-centered informatics research and market research activities within the Institute. Holly has more than 15 years of professional experience in consumer research, dissemination and social marketing, and evaluation. Her expertise is in conducting qualitative and quantitative research to better inform the development and design of products and programs to maximize their efficacy and acceptability by their intended audiences and end-users. These products include: user-centered design methodologies to develop e-health patient-centered technologies and web-based tools, interviews and observations to conduct needs assessments and workflow analyses, focus groups and triads to create health communication messages and materials for both traditional and new media, and large-scale national surveys to establish baseline measures and assess long-term impact of programs. Prior to NCI, she worked at RTI International as a senior research scientist, and at Porter Novelli as the director of Research for the Health and Social Marketing Division. She received her PhD from the University of Maryland in health communication research. Dr. Massett has reported findings of her research in peer-reviewed journals and at professional conferences.

Jon D. Miller is the John A. Hannah Professor of Integrative Studies at Michigan State University. This endowed chair was named in honor of John Hannah, a long-serving President of Michigan State University who had a strong commitment to interdisciplinary teaching and research. Jon is the Director of the Longitudinal Study of American Youth (LSAY), now located at Michigan State University. The LSAY began in 1987 with national samples of 7 th and 10 th grade public school students and has followed these students since 1987. The LSAY data base is the longest longitudinal study of students and young adults ever conducted in the United States. Jon is a Fellow of the American Association for the Advancement of Science and recently completed his second six-year term on the AAAS Committee on the Public Understanding of Science and Technology. He was a Sigma Xi National Lecturer for two years between 1989 and 1991. Jon's expertise in the measurement and analysis of the public understanding of science and technology is recognized internationally. He served as President of the International Council for the Comparative Study of the Public Understanding of Science and Technology for six years. He has served as a consultant to the European Commission, the National Institute of Science and Technology Policy in Japan, and the China Association for Science and Technology.

Richard P. Moser, PhD is a Research Psychologist within the Office of the Associate Director, Behavioral Research Program, at the National Cancer Institute (NCI). He is the data coordinator for the Health Information National Trends Survey (HINTS), provides analytic support for in-house research projects, helps lead evaluation activities for the division, serves as the liaison between the cancer prevention fellowship and the Division of Cancer Control and Population Sciences (DCCPS) at the NCI, and performs his own research. His research interests include statistical methodology, health cognitions, and end-of-life issues. Before joining the NCI, he worked at the Palo Alto VA hospital performing alcoholism research, taught statistics at several Bay Area psychology graduate schools and consulted for the statistical software company SPSS. He obtained his doctorate in Clinical Psychology from the Pacific Graduate School of Psychology in 1996.

Christy Mylks is an independent consultant who conducts user research and manages the User-Centered Informatics Research Lab at the National Cancer Institute of the U. S. National Institutes of Health. Working with fellow communications experts, scientists, and program managers, she applies her 10+ years experience in user-centered design (UCD) methods, human-computer interaction, and eHealth technologies to improving medical, health, and bioinformatics applications for the Institute. She attained her BA from The College of William and Mary and pursued graduate work in Human Factors, Cognitive Psychology, and Human Computer Interaction at both George Mason University and the University of Maryland. For several years she led the board of the DC Usability Professionals Association. More recently she has been overseeing NCI's user-centered field research at cancer hospitals to collect and disseminate best practices for clinical trials recruiting.

William Rakowski (PhD, Penn State, 1977) is a professor in the Department of Community Health and Program in Public Health at Brown University. He teaches courses about intervention planning and about behavioral/social science theories of health behavior. His research since the late 1980's has emphasized factors associated with the utilization of cancer screening tests. Dr. Rakowski led the adaptation of constructs from the "stages of change" Transtheoretical Model to screening mammography. His work has included adapting theory-based definitions of stage-based constructs, instrument development to assess construct reliability and validity, and interventions to evaluate theory-based interventions. Dr. Rakowski's research also analyses population-level datasets to examine the correlates of cancer screening. This research has used the National Health Interview Survey, the Behavioral Risk Factor Surveillance System, and the Health Information and National Trends Survey.

Barbara K. Rimer is Dean of the School of Public Health and Alumni Distinguished Professor of Health Behavior and Health Education School of Public Health at the University of North Carolina at Chapel Hill. Dr. Rimer received an MPH (1973) from the University of Michigan, with joint majors in Health Education and Medical Care Organization, and a DrPH (1981) in Health Education from the Johns Hopkins School of Hygiene and Public Health. Previously, she served as Deputy Director for Population Sciences at UNC Lineberger Comprehensive Cancer Center at UNC-Chapel Hill (2003-2005), Director of Cancer Control and Population Sciences, National Cancer Institute (1997-2002); Professor of Community and Family Medicine at Duke University (1991-97); and Director of Behavioral Research and a full member at the Fox Chase Cancer Center in Philadelphia (1981-91). Dr. Rimer has conducted research in a number of areas, including informed decision-making, long-term maintenance of behavior changes, interventions to increase adherence to cancer prevention and early detection, dissemination of evidence-based interventions and use of new technologies for information, support and behavior change. She was one of the first researchers to test the impact of stepped interventions for cancer control. She currently leads an NIH-funded study to increase regular use of mammography and recently led a project funded by the Robert Wood Johnson Foundation to assess the impact of cancer-related mailing lists on cancer patients/survivors and caregivers.

Louis Rizzo (PhD, Statistics, University of Chicago 1989) is a senior statistician at Westat. He has published papers in the Journal of the American Statistical Association, Survey Methodology, and Public Opinion Quarterly on survey methodology and analysis. He has extensive experience on national studies in health, education, transportation, and social research, contributing to state-of-the-art methodologies in the survey research realm.

Alexander Rothman received his BA in psychology and political theory from Wesleyan University and his PhD in psychology from Yale University and is currently a professor in the department of psychology at the University of Minnesota. Dr. Rothman's primary program of research concerns the application of social psychological theory to illness prevention and health promotion and is comprised of a synthesis of basic research on how people process and respond to health information with the development and evaluation of theory-based interventions to promote healthy behavior. He has published a series of articles that examine how people evaluate and process risk-relevant information and has helped to identify the conditions under which people are receptive to information about personal vulnerability. He has also conducted and published several theory-based interventions that test the influence of different forms of persuasive health messages on the performance of a range of health behaviors such as screening mammography and sun screen utilization. In recognition of his work, Dr. Rothman received the 2002 Distinguished Scientific Award for Early Career Contribution to Psychology in the area of Health Psychology from the American Psychological Association.

Lila J. Finney Rutten, MPH, PhD received her MPH from Harvard University, and her PhD in Psychology from Miami University. Dr. Rutten joined NCI as a Cancer Prevention Fellow in 2001. She later moved into the role of Behavioral Scientist for the Health Communication and Informatics Research Branch, contracted by Scientific Applications International Corporation (SAIC). Dr. Rutten oversees the Health Information National Trends Survey (HINTS), supports other Branch initiatives including the Centers for Excellence in Cancer Communication (CECCR), and pursues her own program of research in population surveillance of behavioral and communication constructs.

Tenbroeck Smith received a bachelor's degree in psychology at Rutgers University, with coursework in advanced mathematics and computer science. He has developed applications using Active Server Pages, Visual Basic, and SQL Server. He received his MA in psychology from Georgia State University in 1996, where he taught undergraduate statistics. Before coming to the Society, he managed population-based studies at the Georgia SEER cancer registry.

Tenbroeck provides operational and strategic support to the vice president of the Behavioral Research Center (BRC) at the American Cancer Society as well as pursuing independent research. He works on major initiatives such as the 2008 Cancer Survivorship Research Conference and preparing for advisory committee meetings. He also supervises masters-level statistical staff. As co-investigator of the Society's Studies of Cancer Survivors—a study of the quality of life and adjustment of cancer survivors—Tenbroeck leads data cleaning and consolidation and produces peer-reviewed manuscripts. In support of the Society's 2015 challenge goals, he developed nationwide measures of hospice utilization among those dying of cancer using Medicare data. Tenbroeck is a member of the Society of Behavioral Medicine and a reviewer for the journals Cancer and Psycho-Oncology. His research interests include cancer survivorship, quality of life, programs for cancer patients and survivors, end-of-life issues, the application of information technology, patient reported outcomes, and survey methodology.

Michael Stefanek received his MS and PhD in Psychology (1984) from Virginia Polytechnic and State University and his MA in Behavior Therapy and Analysis from Southern Illinois University in 1976. He completed his Pre-doctoral internship at Johns Hopkins in the Division of Medical Psychology. His research has focused on psychosocial and behavioral oncology, and he has published extensively on issues related to women at high risk of developing breast cancer and other psychosocial areas. Michael Stefanek, PhD, has been Vice President of Behavioral Research and Director of the Behavioral Research Center of the American Cancer Society (ACS) since April, 2006. Prior to that, Dr. Stefanek was Chief of the Basic Biobehavioral Research Branch in the Division of Cancer Control and Population Sciences at the National Cancer Institute (NCI) from 1998-2006. Before joining NCI, he was Director of Adult Psychology at the University of Maryland Department of Psychiatry, and Coordinator of Psychosocial Services at the Greenebaum Cancer Center at the University of Maryland. He was on the faculty as Instructor and Assistant Professor, Johns Hopkins University School of Medicine from 1985 -1994, with a full-time appointment with the Johns Hopkins Oncology Center. He was Co-Founder and Co-Director of the Johns Hopkins Breast Surveillance Service, a research focused clinical program of the Johns Hopkins Oncology Center. He has received funding from the NCI and ACS, served on several NCI and ACS grant review boards, and served on institutional review boards at both Johns Hopkins and the University of Maryland Cancer Centers. He was also a recipient of an NCI training grant. He was founder and first Chair of the Society of Behavioral Medicine Cancer Special Interest Group. He has also served on the Behavioral Oncology Steering Committee of the American Society of Preventive Oncology (ASPO), and currently serves as Chair, Task Force on Behavioral Science for the American Association of Cancer Research (AACR). In addition, he is appointed as the 2007 Dukoff Family Visiting Professor to the Department of Psychiatry and Behavioral Sciences at Memorial Sloan-Kettering Cancer Center (MSKCC).

Stephen Taplin, MD, MPH; Office of the Associate Director is a Senior Scientist in the Applied Research Program and Acting Branch Chief of the

Applied Cancer Screening Research Branch of the National Cancer Institute's Division of Cancer Control and Population Sciences. He completed his Family Medicine Residency in Rochester New York in 1983 and his Robert Wood Johnson Fellowship in Seattle in 1985, and moved to NCI in 2003.He built his research career around the problems that arose from his day-to-day practice as a primary care physician and the leader of a breast cancer-screening program that served 100,000 women at Group Health in the Northwest. Dr. Taplin has been conducting research funded by the National Cancer Institute for most of his career and moved to the National Cancer Institute as a Senior Scientist in September 2003 after becoming a Senior Investigator at the Center for Health Studies and Professor in the Department of Family Medicine at the University of Washington.

Vetta L. Sanders Thompson (PhD, Duke University, 1988) is an Associate Professor at the George Warren Brown School of Social Work, at Washington University in Saint Louis. Prior to joining the faculty at Washington University in St. Louis, Dr. Thompson was an Associate Professor at the St. Louis University School of Public Health, Department of Community Health, Behavioral Sciences and Health Education (2004-2008) and a member of the psychology faculty at the University of Missouri - St. Louis from 1989 through 2003. Dr. Thompson is a licensed psychologist and health service provider in the state of Missouri with over 15 years experience in research, recruitment, and data collection with ethnic minority populations, particularly African Americans. Dr. Thompson served as the PI for one of the National Cancer Institute funded St. Louis University 4C (Center for Excellence in Cancer Communication Research) studies. She has received funding from NCI, The Society for the Psychological Study of Social Issues, the American Philosophical Society, and several universities; and participated in mental health research funded by the Centers for Disease Control and Substance Abuse and Mental Health Services Administration.

K. "Vish" Viswanath (PhD, University of Minnesota, 1990) is an associate professor in the Department of Society, Human Development, and Health at the Harvard School of Public Health, a faculty member in the Center for Community-Based Research (CCBR) at the Dana-Farber Cancer Institute (DFCI), and Leader of the Health Communication Core of the Dana-Farber/Harvard Cancer Center (DF/HCC). Dr. Viswanath's research interests include mass communication and social change and health communication in both national and international contexts with particular focus on communication inequities and disparities. He is primarily interested in using a macrosocial approach to the study of mass communication and public health.

Before joining Harvard, Dr. Viswanath was the Acting Associate Director of the Behavioral Research Program, Division of Cancer Control

& Populations Sciences, National Cancer Institute. In this role, Dr. Viswanath was responsible for 50 scientific and administrative staff and for extramural scientific developments in behavioral sciences at NCI. He was also a senior scientist in the Health Communication and Informatics Research Branch. He went to the National Cancer Institute from The Ohio State University where he was a tenured faculty member in the School of Journalism and Communication with an adjunct appointment in the School of Public Health. Dr. Viswanath was also a Center Scholar with Ohio State's Center for Health Outcomes, Policy, and Evaluation Studies. Dr. Viswanath is also active in professional organizations. He was the Chair of the Mass Communication Division of the International Communication Association and just completed his tenure as the President of the Midwest Association for Public Opinion Research. He was the Head of the Theory and Methodology Division of the Association for Education in Journalism & Mass Communication. He is also a member of American Society for Preventive Oncology, the American Public Health Association, the American Association for Public Opinion Research and the Society for Behavioral Medicine.

Dr. Viswanath received his doctoral degree in Mass Communication from the University of Minnesota.

Lindsey Volckmann is the Business Development Manager at Keas, Inc., a new start up focused on utilizing advances in technology to keep people as healthy as possible. Prior to her role at Keas, Ms. Volckmann was a fellow at the National Cancer Institute, within the Health Communication and Informatics Research Branch. While at the NCI, she focused her efforts on facilitating a collaborative, cross-sector partnership between publicly funded, behavioral research and privately funded Information Technology (I.T.) companies and effectively engaged leaders from Microsoft, Google, Intel, and GE Healthcare to explore how consumer health and behavioral research can support the design, development and ongoing adaptation of consumer health technologies. Ms. Volckmann has published works concerning health communication and delivery, and the impact of advances in technology in this space.

William Waldron (BS Mathematics, University of Maryland 2004) is a senior programmer/systems analyst at Information Management Services, Inc. He provides statistical programming support to the National Cancer Institute in data analysis and publication support for multiple health surveys, including the National Health Interview Survey, California Health Interview Survey, and the Health Information National Trends Survey. Mr. Waldron also provides system development support for cancer registry data management/operations software for the NCI's Surveillance, Epidemiology, and End Results Program.

Sherrie Flynt-Wallington (PhD, Howard University, 2006) is a postdoctoral fellow with the Harvard School of Public Health and the Dana-Farber Cancer Institute's MassCONECT program. Her research program focuses on three areas of interest, which target those at greatest risk for cancer disparities. The first area focuses on the cancer information needs, information seeking patterns, and barriers to information seeking. The second area examines the study of new media technologies in the dissemination of cancer information. The third area investigates the effects of mass media in the development, implementation, and evaluation of cancer communication interventions. In April 2006, Dr. Flynt Wallington was awarded the Top Young Scholar Paper Award by the Kentucky Conference on Health Communication in Louisville, Kentucky for her dissertation study, "The Internet as an Emerging Patient Education Tool Among African-American Men with Prostate Cancer: An Exploratory Study." Previously, Dr. Flynt Wallington served as an adjunct professor at Howard University in the John H. Johnson School of Communications and the Howard University College of Medicine's Masters in Public Health Program. She also has held teaching and administrative positions at Bowie State University and Winston-Salem State University. She earned her undergraduate and master's degrees from the University of North Carolina at Greensboro. Dr. Flynt Wallington received her doctoral degree in mass communication and media studies, specializing in health communication, from Howard University.

Zhuoqiao Wang (MS Mathematics, University of Cincinnati, 2005) is a senior statistical programmer at Information Management Services, Inc. He provides statistical programming, modeling, and analytic support for multiple large-scale projects at that National Cancer Institute, including the Health Information National Trends Survey, Polyp Prevention Trial, Costa Rica HPV Vaccine Trial and the NCI Surveillance, Epidemiology, and End Results Program.

Gordon Willis (PhD, Northwestern University) is Cognitive Psychologist at the National Cancer Institute, National Institutes of Health, and previously worked at Research Triangle Institute and at the National Center for Health Statistics, CDC, to develop methods for evaluating survey questions. Dr. Willis attended Oberlin College and Northwestern University. He has co-authored the "Questionnaire Appraisal System" for evaluating draft survey questions, has written the book *Cognitive Interviewing: A Tool for Improving Questionnaire Design* (2005; Sage Publications), and co-teaches a course in Questionnaire Design at the University of Maryland. His work involves the development of surveys on cancer risk factors, and focuses on questionnaire pretesting. His current research interests focus on sociocultural issues in self-report surveys, with an emphasis on the development of best practices for survey translation, and on the adaptation of empirical methods, such as cognitive interviewing and behavior coding, to the development of survey questions that exhibit cross-cultural comparability.

Soye Zaid-Muhammad (MA, MS.Ed) is currently certified as a New York State School Psychologist, and is now working for the New York City Department of Education. In addition, he serves as an adjunct lecturer of psychology at the City College of the City University of New York. He has previously served as a research assistant and research fellow on a number of NIMH and NCI-sponsored research protocols at Memorial Sloan-Kettering Cancer Center, where he participated in studies examining psychosocial issues related to HIV and cancer. He is currently finishing a PhD in Psychology at Pace University in the School Clinical-Child Psychology Program. His doctoral research is centered on HIV+ fathers' perceptions and concerns about psychosocial and health factors affecting their children.

AUTHOR INDEX

SUBJECT INDEX